HEALTHY
TO
100

The Ultimate Guide To Bullet Proofing Your Body
Against Disease, Eliminating Pain, Burning Fat and
Living Longer Stronger!

A SPECIAL NOTE

from Dr. Darrell Wolfe

We all search for good health but how would you like to have great health and experience it on a permanent basis for the rest of your life?

Just as the medical system has made health seem complicated and beyond your reach, so has the natural health industry. By the time patients' call for a consultation with me, they have crashed with the medical system and most have bought into the health fads, ineffective therapies and this season's latest nutritional breakthrough.

Our world is based on Band-Aid therapy, the *'you break it and we'll treat you but never train you'* attitude is a rotating door. Until you become the master of your own well-being - physically and emotionally, on a day-to-day basis, you will always be in emergency care. **You will never have great health until you have a personalized road map built specifically for you and your needs.**

This road map is designed to protect and guide you with gentle baby steps throughout your day, each and every day. Until you become the master of your own health and wellbeing, otherwise, trained - not treated, you will always be left disappointed, continually searching for the next quick fix.

Your potential for self-healing is limitless when you have a Supercharge Your Life road map built just for you! Allow me the honor to build you that road map and to support you along your journey.

May you always be blessed,

Dr. Darrell Wolfe

HEALTHY TO 100 CLUB

Doc of Detox has gone global! We have put together a unique, private club to guide your health, healing, emotional well-being, nutrition and detoxification. Unlock the secrets of living *'Healthy To 100'* - learn foundational tips, strategies & techniques in diet, nutrition, detoxification, exercise, anti-aging and longevity. If you wish to live to your full potential each and every day, then look no further, welcome home to your Healthy To 100 Club!

Club Membership: $6.95/month

Full Access to Teleconferences & Webinars
Your Questions Answered Live & On-Air
(with Dr. Wolfe, the Doc of Detox)

Interviews with the Top Leaders in Natural Health

Recipes For Life & Vitality

Special Access Downloads

How-To Videos

Educational Self-Help Audios & Booklets

Weekly Deals & Monthly Draws

When you become an Elite Member for $19.95/month you will also receive:

LIVE! Webinar Trainings on Mastering Your Emotions & Taking Back Your Life

LIVE! Wolfe Deep Tissue Webinar Trainings on Treating Each & Every Muscle and Joint

Monthly Consultation Lottery: One-on-One Consultation with Dr. Wolfe
(Emotional Awakening Transformation Consultation & Super-charge Your Life Nutritional Consultation)

Register Today at: www.docofdetox.com

Written by: Dr. Darrell Wolfe/Lorie Malcolm
Publisher: Wolfe Publishing

Contact Information for Dr. Darrell Wolfe
www.docofdetox.com
dr.wolfe@docofdetox.com

Training Courses
www.itioh.com

Kelowna, B.C. Canada
Copyright © 2015 Dr. Darrell Wolfe Ac.PhD.
All Rights Reserved
Printed and Bound in Canada

DO NOT HESITATE TO CALL - WE'RE OLD SCHOOL
1 250 448 4544
1 855 900 4544

We love to hear from you, all your questions matter

Yours Truly,
Dr. Darrell Wolfe Ac.PhD.

TABLE OF CONTENTS

TABLE OF CONTENTS

TABLE OF CONTENTS

CHAPTER 13: **RELEASE THE THIN WITHIN**   219

CHAPTER 14: **SPOILED ROTTEN**   236

CHAPTER 15: I AM WOMAN 247

CHAPTER 16: JUST A SPOONFUL OF SUGAR 260

CHAPTER 17: FOODS & FREQUENCY 266

CHAPTER 21: THE BREATH OF LIFE   365

CHAPTER 22: EMF: WHAT THE CELL IS GOING ON   373

CHAPTER 23: THE FUTURE OF HEALTH: ENERGY MEDICINE   391

CHAPTER 24: NATURE'S WAY   417

CHAPTER 25: **WHOLE PLANT BASED SUPERFOOD NUTRITION**   433

CHAPTER 26: **LIVE LONG CORE STRONG**   466

CHAPTER 27: **BEAUTIFUL SKIN**   497

TABLE OF CONTENTS

HEALTHY TO 100:

HEALTHY TO 100:

HEALTHY TO 100:

Thank you to the following individuals for their contributions, support and inspiration:

Lorie Malcolm, Don Wolfe, Jera Wolfe, Laura Dyck, Abby Michelle, Joanna Chase, Carmen Johnston, Evelyn Mulders, Ann Lotwin, Cody Ackert, Tim Toula, Michael Losier, Ronald Klassen, Duane Howes, Kaz Crischuk, Scott Carvey, Chris Kormish, Dave and Marlene Higgins

We hereby acknowledge the following people and organizations for their contributions to this book:

Ty Bollinger: Author of the best selling book *'Cancer - Step Outside the Box'*

Marcel Wolfe and Paula Wood: frequencymatters.com

Dr. Howard W Fisher: Author of *'Moringa Oleifera: Magic, Myth, or Miracle'*

Magna Havis of Rose Lab: magnahavis.com

Ross Andersen: safezoneemf.com

Clayton Nolte: naturalactiontechnologies.com

Jeffrey M Smith: Author of *'Seeds of Deception'*

Dr. Oz: Thanks to Dr. Oz for making a World Wide difference

FOREWORD

Dr. Darrell Wolfe is not only my friend, but he's also a special kind of person whose knowledge surpasses that of most common doctors. In this book, Healthy To 100, you will quickly realize that Dr. Wolfe's nickname is well- deserved, as the "Doc of Detox" takes you on a galactic ride to health, while sharing essential health truths and shattering loathsome lies. *"What lies?"* you may ask.

The fact of the matter is that the majority of what you've been taught about health and medicine is a monumental myth based upon a folklore influenced by the voracious appetite of big business - specifically pharmaceutical giants ("Big Pharma"), multinational food companies ("Big Agra"), and the modern medical institutions ("Medical Industrial Complex").

Big Pharma wants to sell you a "pill for every ill" while "Big Agra" wants to sell you their "franken-foods." All the while the Medical Industrial Complex is more than thrilled to have repeat customers created by their buddies who work in both of the above businesses.

Money, money, money... Lies, lies, lies.

The truth is that the bottom line is the bottom line.

In order to make more money, Big Pharma, Big Agra, and the Medical Industrial Complex have devised a seductive mythology that has been pounded into the consciousness of consumers everywhere. This "mind control mythology" includes some real whoppers such as, "GMO foods are healthy and needed to feed the world" and "cholesterol causes heart attacks."

If we hope to take control of our health, we must learn the truth, dispel the lies, and rid ourselves of the burden of "false thinking." We must embrace the truth that our bodies want to be healthy and are genetically programmed to be healthy. We must realize that the simple avoidance of toxic chemicals in foods, medicines and even household products is, all by itself, a powerful strategy for radically improved health and longevity. We must realize that detoxification is essential if we want optimal health.

This book is a powerful tool. If you are interested in jettisoning the lies, which are so rampant and learning the truth about health, nutrition, and longevity, then you should follow Dr. Wolfe's advice to the letter. Be prepared, profound changes may occur.

This book is truly a gateway to personal freedom. Read it, follow it and free your mind. From there, your possibilities are endless, who knows, you might just stay 'Healthy To 100'.

God bless,

Ty Bollinger
Best-selling Author and Researcher and Host of
'Quest for the Cures'
www.CancerTruth.net
www.TheTruthAboutCancer.com

This book is dedicated to my children for they help me to remember.

Devon, Jera, Genevieve, Sage, Rayleigh, Taylor, James & Jesse

If you need to remember, our younger children have not forgotten.

LOVE IS & LOVE HEALS
Love is the foundation of
E V E R Y T H I N G

**Beside every great man,
there's an even greater woman**

*My partner & co-author,
Lorie Malcolm*

THANK YOU

Feel free to share this inspirational knowledge with family, friends and loved ones. Together, we make the difference by empowering others, showing them that we can Master not just our bodies but our lives and live 'Healthy To 100'.

"The secret of getting ahead is getting started."

- Mark Twain

IT'S ONLY THE BEGINNING

Healthy To 100 belongs to everyone and we're here to share ours with your Whole Family. My name is Dr. Darrell Wolfe. I'm known as the 'Doc of Detox'. I have been compelled to write this story for some time now. Until the year of 1999 I headed up one of the most successful and well-known clinics on the World Wide Web regarding health and longevity. I am now the founder and director of the *'International Training Institute of Health'* and *'Doc of Detox'*. I consult, teach and lecture internationally on longevity, chronic illness, anti-aging, detoxification and deep tissue restoration. Health has been made to look and feel complicated not just by our health care system and supplement industry but also by the outdated information that most have been taught and continue to use as a foundation for their well-being. When we live in a system, we absorb that system and we think only in that system. It's time to reevaluate your **B**elief **S**ystems or settle into the idea that pain and disease are normal but in no way should they be considered Natural. In my former practice we carried hundreds of products and many rigorous, deep cleansing programs. Is more, better? I think not. After 35 years my foundational philosophy on health and nutrition has significantly changed due to a new reality. I feel that I have gone full circle, experiencing an amazing paradigm shift. For me I have now narrowed it down to the Four Pillars of Health. This being Structured High Frequency Water, Gentle Daily Cleansing each and every day, Whole Plant Based Superfood Nutrition and last but not least revitalization of the largest organ of the body, that being your skin. Once you truly understand the cause that undermines your health, your longevity, your weight and the rest of your life, you will be set free of the fear and pain that can keep you feeling helpless and even hopeless. This I promise. This book is about truthful answers, guiding you to have the greatest partnership with your body. This partnership is the most important relationship you will ever have. When two come together there are no limits. You will be The Cure that you wish to see.

This book is all about **U** and how you can overcome even the greatest health challenges. Get ready to break out of the unconscious construct that creates limitations for you without you even knowing it. You may have tried all kinds of personal health programs and/or self-improvement techniques but unless you have a strong foundation from which to come, everything else you do will not give you the desired or permanent results for which you search. What is the real core reason why you don't seem to be in the driver's seat when it comes to your health? What is the real core reason why you seem to struggle no matter how hard you try? Why do some people's lives seem to flow effortlessly when it comes to their health, while others struggle with the same type of recurring health problems? Right now you may be in pain or may know someone in pain or with a debilitating disease. Do you believe that there have been others in this condition or worse, that have completely healed themselves? I can assure you, there have been thousands and hundreds of thousands to come. When you change the rules, you not only change the game... **U** change your life and those around you.

Understanding the rules is the key because it puts you in a powerful position from which you can take and shape your health. For many people, their lives are unconscious living. Not being aware of it, they don't understand why their health is a struggle despite their efforts to do everything right. Once you have a strong foundation from which to proceed you will no longer be doubtful or uncertain or fearful about your health. You will see things for what they truly are and not the way others would have you see. Let's pull back the curtains and make sure that your **B**eliefs **S**ystems are not outdated, that they're truly yours and here to serve only your greater good.

NEW WORLD – NEW RULES

"You will never win the game if you don't understand the rules.
New Game, New Rules, New Life... Get cracking!"

- Dr. Darrell Wolfe, Doc of Detox

People have been using cleansing herbal teas and dietary remedies since the beginning of recorded history. We're talking thousands of years of proven and effective therapies that work in harmony with the human body, without dangerous side effects.

Hippocrates, the Father of Medicine stated, *"Let food be thy medicine and medicine be thy food."*

The reality today is that the M. D. 'Emperors' who created this new reality are only interested in money and the power to control the fate of our health. *Why do I say this?* Well, in order to fully comprehend and understand the current rules and guidelines that our medical system follows in the U.S. and Canada today, we must turn the clock back 100 years to the beginning of the 20th century in order to get a clear picture of the plot to end natural health and self-healing.

The year is 1900 and the American Medical Association, known as the **AMA**, is weak, unorganized and has very little money and very little respect from the majority of the population. Herbalists, Homeopathic Doctors and Chiropractors were the therapists of choice at this time and flourished, while medical doctors were struggling just to make a living.

For the AMA to survive, what was known to be the 'Council on Medical Education' was established in 1904. They stated that their mission was to "upgrade medical education." This, in itself, was a noble goal - if it were true. However, the Council on Medical Education had actually devised a plan, otherwise known as the **'Evil Plot'**, to rank all the medical schools throughout the country. Their guidelines were dubious, to say the least. For instance, just having the word 'homeopathic' in the name of a medical school reduced its ranking because the AMA asserted that these schools taught 'an exclusive dogma'. Otherwise, all viable competition became the target; otherwise, they were now on the hit list.

However, by 1910, the AMA was out of money and didn't have the funds to complete their makeover or should I say takeover. **Around this time The Rockefellers had joined forces with The Carnegie Foundation to create an 'education fund'.** N.P. Colwell, who was the secretary of the Council on Medical Education, approached them.

His request to them was to finish the takeover of the health industry that they had started. Rockefeller and Carnegie both agreed to finish what the AMA could not. **Simon Flexner, who was on the Board of Directors for the Rockefeller Institute, proposed that his brother Abraham Flexner, who knew nothing about medicine, be hired for the project.**

Despite his lack of medical knowledge, the plan was to 'restructure' the AMA, otherwise the American Medical Association, to 'certify' medical schools based solely upon Flexner's recommendations.

Eventually, Flexner submitted his report to The Carnegie Foundation entitled **'Medical Education in the United States and Canada,'** which is also known as the *'Flexner Report'*. Not surprisingly, the basis of the report was that it was far too easy to start a medical school and that most medical schools were not teaching *'sound medicine'*. Let me translate this for you: **These natural health colleges were not pushing enough chemical drugs manufactured by, guess who?** *The companies owned by Carnegie and Rockefeller.*

So to make a long story short, the AMA, who were "evaluating" the various medical colleges, made it their job to target and shut down the larger, respected homeopathic colleges. In 1910, the Flexner Report recommended, *"strengthening medical courses in pharmacology, otherwise drugs, and in addition to this, they establish drug research departments at all schools that they deemed to be qualified."*

Carnegie and Rockefeller began to immediately shower hundreds of millions of dollars on those medical schools that were teaching drug intensive medicine. Predictably, those schools that had the financing churned out the better doctors or should I say, 'the more recognized doctors'.

In return for the financing, the schools were required to continue teaching course material that was exclusively drug oriented, with no emphasis put on natural medicine. I love when a plan comes together. As we all know when it comes to free money, there are always strings attached.

In this case, the Rockefellers and Carnegies were more than happy to place one of "their guys" on the board of directors at each and every medical school that accepted their funding. The end result was that all accredited medical schools became heavily oriented toward drugs and drug research. It was no longer normal to be Natural. *Health now had become patented and synthetic.*

THE BEST DOCTORS GIVE THE LEAST MEDICINES.

- BENJAMIN FRANKLIN

By 1923, the 22 homeopathic 'medical' schools that flourished in the 1900s dwindled to just 2.

By 1925, over 10,000 herbalists were out of business.

By 1940, over 1,500 chiropractors would be prosecuted for practicing "quackery."

By 1950, all schools teaching homeopathy were closed.

In the end, if a physician did not graduate from a 'Flexner-approved' medical school and receive an M.D. degree, then he or she could not find a job.

This is why today M.D.s are so heavily biased toward synthetic drug therapy and know little about nutrition, if anything. They don't even study what makes a healthy body; they study disease. Modern doctors are taught virtually nothing about nutrition, gentle daily cleansing, wellness or disease prevention. Expecting a medical doctor to guide you on health issues is sort of like expecting your local butcher to perform surgery on you. It's simply not an area in which they have been trained.

Since the Flexner Report was released, **have we seen any progress?** 100 years ago if a medical doctor saw a case of cancer he would call on his colleagues because it was felt that they might never see this again, since cancer was so rare. Diabetes was practically unheard of, atherosclerosis (hardening of the arteries) was nonexistent, and the term "heart attack" hadn't even been coined yet.

"Whenever a doctor cannot do good, he must be kept from doing harm."

- Hippocrates, the Father of Medicine

The only thing that remains of Hippocrates is the hypocrite.

Today, cancer is an epidemic.

According to the WHO in a 2010 study, 41% of the people alive today will face a diagnosis of the "Big C" (and that number was pre-Fukushima). **Heart disease is rampant, and diabetes is at epidemic proportions. Infant mortality is up; birth defects are up. Even closer to home, over 66% of North American adults are overweight.**

What did our great-grandfathers and great-grandmothers eat? Fresh vegetables, fresh fruits, bread from fresh grains, meat, butter, and cheese from grass-fed cows and eggs from free-range chickens. None of it was processed with drugs, chemicals or additives.

Amish children are remarkably immune to allergies, says an expert. The Amish, it seems place themselves at risk everyday of their lives, they refuse to vaccinate their children, exposing themselves to disease and they drink raw cow's milk exposing them to salmonella, they even, and this is really disturbing, favor natural food, yet they are far more healthy. What's up with that?

Until the majority of the population is more interested in being than having, we will remain primitive and feed off each other's pain and suffering for power and money. Love is the only answer; ignorance brings chaos. When the innocent are unable to make logical decisions they become prey to the predator.

Our government and medical system is a direct reflection of the self-worth of the majority of the population.

We get what we get because we do not demand better for ourselves, from ourselves. Until we truly become self-centered and look within and doing loving acts for ourselves, we will never claim our universal right, this being the true joy of living.

Why is it that 80% of oncologists, when asked, would not give the standard medical treatments for cancer to their family or themselves, which they give to their patients? Let logic prevail, a 2.3% survival rate after 5 years is not successful, last time I checked, 2.3% was considered a failure, that's why!

Why do those who we've entrusted with our health care, not teach Whole Plant Based Diets and Gentle Daily Cleansing? This information would create individual self-empowerment and an economic crash for those who have been feeding off of us physically, emotionally and let us not forget, financially for almost 100 years.

What is all this health mystery? First, let's be perfectly honest. Medical doctors treat symptoms. Our fear and confusion comes because doctors talk about our symptoms using Greek terminology, which makes us feel helpless and vulnerable, causing a communication breakdown and dis-ease within us. If we cannot even understand what the condition (symptom) even means, then how can we even begin to heal ourselves?

Some examples are:

Polymyalgia: poly means **many**, **my** means **muscle**, **algia** means **pain**, which means you have pain in many muscles. This is not a disease. *When we become backed up with toxins, the body stores these toxins in the muscles to protect our vital organs.*

Fibromyalgia: <u>**fibro**</u> means <u>**fiber**</u>, <u>**my**</u> means <u>**muscle**</u>, <u>**algia**</u> means <u>**pain**</u>. This means you have fiber muscle pain. This is not a disease. *This is pain that moves throughout the body due to inflammation created by a toxic lifestyle.*

Arthritis: <u>**arthro**</u> means <u>**joint**</u>, <u>**itis**</u> means <u>**inflammation**</u>. This means you have inflammation in your joint(s). This is not a disease. *This is inflammation due to acidosis, which is also not a disease but a symptom of an incorrect lifestyle.*

Colitis: <u>**col**</u> means <u>**colon**</u>, <u>**itis**</u> means <u>**inflammation**</u>. This means that you have inflammation of the colon. This is not a disease. *This is a plumbing problem where the body's sewage system has become a cesspool.*

I don't think you will die from this, although it sounds like you could.

I think you get the point. There are hundreds of other symptoms that have been given hard to understand names that can leave you feeling helpless, hopeless and living in fear, *but isn't that the point?* For every new toxic symptom that we experience our medical system will create a brand new disease with another breakthrough drug to suppress the symptoms. **A Pill For Every Ill, Dumbed down and drugged up!**

BREAK THE CHAIN

When treating symptoms is the focal point of your health care you will be lost and forever in pain. *Have you ever noticed when we make pain the enemy and run from it, we're always in it?* **Symptoms are your body's communication system, guiding you to the truth.** Shutting down symptoms by using drugs is breaking communication with your body. It's a partnership, as in a marriage you may end up with a divorce, where as with your body, you're sure to get a disease or end up dying, prematurely.

People will wake up to their own innate healing ability when they can no longer stand this maze of pain, fear and confusion created by the status quo.

We are what we think, say and do. If you live your life and measure the state of your health by the average normal person today, then you have signed up for a life sentence that only you can break free from. Release yourself from the invisible bonds of fear and illusion.

We must filter the information that does not serve or support our health vision.

We must protect ourselves from the "system." Place your focus on the most important system, this being your digestive system.

We will never do better until we know better. Refuse to be spoon-fed! **Educate before they medicate.**

Start keeping a Health Evidence Journal. Become self-centered, you are the only true navigator of your body, and only the body heals. We must learn how to protect ourselves, from ourselves and from those that wish to make money from our lack of wisdom. Please do not forget that you were created by your Creator to create. Take back your power and create that which is your universal right, great health. **Be The Cure that U search for!**

Nature alone can cure disease; doctors cannot heal. They can only direct the sufferer back to the pathways of health. Nature alone can create and healing is recreation.

- Dr. William S. Sadler

BACK TO OUR FUTURE

To understand the cause of our new reality we must go back in time. Until WW2 agriculture in North America increased gradually. After WW2 there were rapid changes in farming methods due to an increased demand for food. The truth be known, drug and chemical corporations were left with tons of nitrates and phosphates from weapon manufacturing. Being savvy marketers this concoction of *N (*nitrogen) *P* (phosphorus) *K* (potassium) became a very cheap fertilizer sold to farmers to boost their crops. From 1940 to 1944 there was a 50% increase in the use of chemical fertilizers resulting in larger crop returns. With the use of DDT and other synthetic pesticides, farmers were able to have continuous cropping on large acreage. Productivity from 1950 to 1975 increased more than any other time in history. This period marked the beginning of the end of nutrient rich food due to the depletion of essential minerals and microorganisms (good bacteria) in the soil. During this period crop output increased by more than half but along with this came a 400% increase in the use of pesticides and chemical fertilizers.

The new reality is that because farmers were forced to use chemicals to stay competitive, our food no longer supports human life as Nature intended. Yes, these crops that we eat look vibrant on the store shelves but fall short for human consumption; all show - no grow, they lack the foundational essential minerals and micronutrients. Our bodies need

59 nutrients on a daily basis including 13 **vitamins** and 22 **minerals** without compromise. *NPK fertilizers* contain no more then 8 of these essential minerals (oops). It doesn't end here, once out of the ground the food is processed, removing more vital nutrients by removing grain husks, blanching, boiling, baking, steaming, bleaching, freezing and microwaving.

It then has to travel thousands of miles to your table in most cases. Don't waste your money; eat local, organic and fresh.

Due to mineral depleted soil, US farmers in particular are now starting to rely on genetically modified (GM) versions of plants to overcome problems of decreasing growth and yield. This is a direct violation against Nature. If there were a third world war this would be it. You must now take a stand and guard against these impostors who tell us they have our best interest at heart.

As a consequence, from trying to outsmart Nature, primitive cultures are now better nourished than we are. You will only be as strong as the soil your food is grown in. We are a direct extension of Earth. If we do not take steps to search out high frequency, Whole Plant Based, nutrient rich, Superfoods, you risk not only your health but also your life.

Whole Plant Based Foods are the cornerstone to life on this planet. Nobel winner Dr. Linus Pauling stated that for every disease, sickness and ailment there is a mineral deficiency attached to it. Without minerals your cells cannot function properly.

Today only 2% of US farms produce 70% of the vegetables, 50% of the fruit and nuts, and 35% of the poultry products grown and raised. As more and more family farms become extinct we are seeing lower quality foods and an increase in disease. The last great battle to keep integrity within our foods was when Willie Nelson was fighting to save *'the family farm'* from the corporate world. *Why is it that there is always an integrity issue when a monopoly is created?* **The bottom line is, the productivity has definitely increased but with many detrimental environmental effects such as rapid erosion of fertile top soils and contamination of our water supply from the chemicals used.** An average of 10 times as much soil erodes from American agricultural fields as is replaced by natural soil processes. For Inch of agricultural topsoil to form it takes up to 300 years, so *'lettuce'* root in and take charge of our own lives, while we still have them.

SOWING THE SEEDS OF DEPLETION

Step One - Use chemical fertilizers to increase productivity (profits). Dr. Drucker of Drucker Labs stated that nutritional crops require 70 trace minerals but currently regular farming methods only use 3-5 of these. Using only three to five minerals makes for a very low vibrational soil supplement, non life-sustaining!

Step Two - Allow minerals and microorganisms to be depleted from the soil and not replaced = low vibrational soil.

1992 Earth Summit Report - Average Percentage of Mineral Depletion From Soil During The Past 100 Years; -*North America 85% -South America 76% -Asia 76% -Africa 74% -Europe 72% -Australia 55%*

Step Three - Crops are now in a weakened state due to lack of minerals so pesticides, herbicides and fungicides must be used to prevent total loss (low vibrational crops). Corporations create the problem and then come to the rescue. Fill your pockets twice and **fill *the humans* with toxins**. *Are you aware that plants can make vitamins, amino acids and fatty acids only if they are grown in soils abundant in minerals?*

Step Four - Feed the Humans and the Animals with vegetables, fruits and grains that are deficient in minerals, chemically laced and genetically modified. **Low vibrational foods create a lower immune system in humans and animals causing pain, sickness and disease.**

Step Five - The Female Humans and the animals are now suffering from hormonal imbalance and consequently require hormone therapy replacement. All are becoming sick and can no longer fight off viruses, bacteria and fungus because of the lack of minerals and the abundance of toxic sprays anointing all of their food. Those who have helped create the problem are the ones coming to the *rescue* with **antibiotics** and **pharmaceuticals** to help combat our infections creating even more pain, inflammation and cellular mutation within us. Fill your pockets three times and ***fill the humans with drugs***. Lower vibration in food weakens the immune system of humans and animals. In turn, they become weaker and they themselves become prey to infectious invaders. You will not experience the negative effects of infectious invaders unless you vibrate at their level. The Swamp always comes before the Mosquito.

My Grandparents

They grew up in a simpler time. At least their environment including the air, water and food were pure. Even the ambient electromagnetic fields were at least familiar to all living things. What was naturally the norm and pure we must now pay a premium for or it is no longer available for many of us.

So Where Did We Go Wrong?

By blindly trusting and following the authorities and experts of the day, we have unknowingly put our family's health, financial worth and their lives at risk.

"A foolish faith in authority is the worst enemy of the truth."

- Albert Einstein

NON-GMO SHOPPING TIPS

How to avoid foods made with genetically modified organisms (GMOs)

What is a GMO?

Genetically modified organisms (GMOs) are made by forcing genes from one species, such as bacteria, viruses, animals, or humans, into the DNA of a food crop or animal to introduce a new trait.

Why Should I Avoid GMOs?

The American Academy of Environmental Medicine reported that, "Several animal studies indicate serious health risks associated with GM food," including infertility, immune problems, accelerated aging, faulty insulin regulation, and changes in major organs and the gastrointestinal system.

Many physicians advise ALL patients to choose healthier non-GMO foods.

Buy Non-GMO Brands

Use your consumer power and invest your food dollars in non-GMO products. A decade ago, a consumer driven tipping point kept GMOs out of the food supply in the European Union in spite of government approvals. If sufficient numbers of US shoppers avoid GM ingredients, then food companies here won't use them. The critical number for a US tipping point could be as few as 5%, which is around 15 million health conscious shoppers choosing non-GMO brands.

Visit ResponsibleTechnology.org to:
- Learn about GMO health risks and safe eating alternatives
- Sign up with the Tipping Point Network to join forces with other non-GMO activists
- Explore their Resources section and Facebook page to share information with others
- Sign up for their free electronic newsletter
- Find out if there is an event or speaker training workshop near you

Frankenstein Foods

Invisible GM Ingredients

Processed foods often have hidden GM sources (unless they are organic or declared non-GMO). The following ingredients may be made from GMOs.

- Ascorbic acid (vitamin C)
- Aspartame (also called Amino-Sweet®, NutraSweet®, Equal Spoonful®, Canderel®, BeneVia®, E951)
- Baking powder
- Canola oil (rapeseed oil)
- Caramel color
- Cellulose
- Citric acid
- Cobalamin (vitamin B12)
- Colorose
- Condensed milk
- Confectioners sugar
- Corn flour
- Corn masa
- Corn meal
- Corn oil
- Corn sugar
- Corn syrup
- Cornstarch
- Cottonseed oil
- Cyclodextrin
- Cysteine
- Dextrin
- Dextrose
- Diacetyl
- Diglyceride
- Erythritol
- EqualFood starch
- Fructose (any form)
- Glucose
- Glutamate
- Glutamic acid
- Glycerides
- Glycerin
- Glycerol
- Glycerol monooleate
- Glycine
- Hemicellulose
- High fructose corn syrup (HFCS)
- Hydrogenated starch
- Hydrolyzed vegetable protein
- Inositol
- Inverse syrup
- Inversol
- Invert sugar
- Isoflavones
- Lactic acid

- Lecithin
- Leucine
- Lysine
- Malitol
- Malt syrup
- Malt extract
- Maltodextrin
- Maltose
- Mannitol
- Methylcellulose
- Milk powder
- Milo starch
- Modified food starch
- Modified starch
- Mono and diglycerides
- Monosodium glutamate (MSG)
- Nutrasweet
- Oleic acid
- Phenylalanine
- Phytic acid
- Protein isolate
- Shoyu
- Sorbitol
- Soy flour
- Soy isolates
- Soy lecithin
- Soy milk
- Soy oil
- Soy protein
- Soy protein isolate
- Soy sauce
- Starch
- Stearic acid
- Sugar (unless cane sugar)
- Tamari
- Tempeh
- Teriyaki marinades
- Textured vegetable protein
- Threonine
- Tocopherols (vitamin E)
- Tofu
- Trehalose
- Triglycerides
- Vegetable fat
- Vegetable oil
- Vitamin B13
- Vitamin E
- Whey
- Whey powder
- Xanthan gum

Tips to Avoids GMOs

Although most Americans say they would avoid brands if labeled GMO, unfortunately labels are not required. Here are 4 tips to help you shop non-GMO.

Tip #1: Buy Organic

Certified organic products cannot internationally include any GMO ingredients. Buy products labeled "100% organic,"

"organic," or "made with organic ingredients." You can be doubly sure if the product also has a Non- GMO Project Verified Seal.

Tip #2: Look for Non-GMO Project Seals

Products that carry the Non-GMO Project Seal are independently verified to be in compliance with North America's only third party standard for GMO avoidance, including testing of at-risk ingredients.

The Non-GMO Project is a nonprofit organization committed to providing consumers with clearly labeled and independently verified non-GMO choices. NonGMOProject.org

Tip #3: Avoid at-risk Ingredients

If it's not labeled organic or verified non-GMO: Avoid products made with ingredients that might be derived from GMOs (see list). The eight GM food crops are corn, soybeans, canola, cottonseed, sugar beets, Hawaiian papaya (most), papaya from China, and a small amount of zucchini and yellow squash.

Sugar: If non-organic products made in North America list "sugar" as an ingredient (and NOT pure cane sugar), then it is almost certainly a combination of sugar from both sugar cane and GM sugar beets.

Dairy: Products may be from cows injected with GM bovine growth hormone. Look for labels stating No rBGH, rBST, or artificial hormones, or check brand listings at: NonGMOShoppingGuide.com

Tip #4: Download the Guide

Visit NonGMOShoppingGuide.com to download the growing list of non-GMO products available and check out the iPhone application, ShopNoGMO free at the iTunes store.

The Institute for Responsible Technology is a world leader in educating the public about genetically modified foods and crops. Founded in 2003 by GMO expert Jeffrey M. Smith, IRT has worked in more than 30 countries designed to achieve the tipping point of consumer rejection of GM foods in the US.

Help Us Reclaim a Non-GMO Food Supply!

Online: ResponsibleTechnology.org

Buy Non-GMO Brands

Spend your food dollars on healthier non-GMO brands!

Visit: NonGMOShoppingGuide.com or download the iPhone app: ShopNoGMO for a list of non-GMO brands.

Educate or Mutate.
Hop to it your body's counting on it.

FOLLOW JACK

OR BECOME A LEADER...

Great health is a right, so it's important to not to give it away. If you have given it away, claim your universal right and take it back. When we do not have the proper tools to make wise decisions for our families and ourselves, we allow others to orchestrate our fate. That ends here with this book. If we do not program our minds with **The Whole Truth About Health**, then we put our families and ourselves in great jeopardy. Our loved ones are counting on us, so don't leave it in the hands of strangers; bring health home under your control.

As my kids used to say, "STRANGER DANGER." When it comes to the medical system and our government embracing and endorsing **Whole Plant Based Foods for a Whole Life**, I have one thing to say, I believe this will not happen in my lifetime because the majority follows Jack. My ultimate desire is that *'Healthy To 100'* will help us remember what we already know and who we really are. Let us rise to our greatness and claim our independence. As you read this please think of others for whom this information may serve to help them remember. ***Are you ready to be the Master of your health and well-being?***

THE LIARS CLUB

Knowledge is great but wisdom is everything. Almost all corporations who grow and process our food have hardly any or no integrity. They starve us nutritionally and poison us slowly, which eventually drives us to the drug companies who have no integrity. In turn, both of these sectors lobby our government, which in turn puts laws in place to strengthen their foothold on our well-being. '***$erve and protect***' went out the door with *'Follow the $'*. If you wish for a health care system to function like one, then the information needs to be based on health, duh! The average drug has seventy known harmful side effects. Whatever happened to *do no harm*?

Whatever happened to the truth, The Whole Truth and nothing but the truth? There is a natural plant for every condition with only one side effect and that being the power to assist your body in its natural healing process. It's amazing how mankind truly believes he can outsmart millions of years of evolution when it comes to Nature, nutrition and the human body. Man can enhance Nature but when Jack tries to '**man**-*ipulate*' her, he is playing a very dangerous and deadly game with your life... **Nutritional Strategy** or **Medical Tragedy**?

IT'S ALL ABOUT U

The only way health will ever become simple and long lasting is when you start making **U** responsible for your health on a daily basis. There will no longer be a need for anyone to save you; you write your own story, you always have. Be the *cure* you wish to see, there is power in keeping things simple. Keeping your health was never meant to be complicated or just out of reach (the shell game). If it's out of reach it's because you made it that way, you put it in someone else's hands because they said they knew better. Our way of thinking must change, we need to look within ourselves and allow Nature to guide us.

Don't look to humanity to fix your body; they never created it. Return to Nature, **the source** of all t rue healing. Nothing is **gentler**, more **life- giving** or more forgiving than **Nature**. It is only Natural to get well and stay healthy when you embrace **her** on a daily basis. We all must awaken the potential that lies within us from a **foundation of whole living;** it's only Natural. Drink Life In, Take Life On, Rebuild, Gently Cleanse Daily and Restore Balance. Your body and your health have always been your responsibility, no one else's. If there's going to be a hero to your story, it must be **U!**

GOOD♪ GOOD♪ GOOD♪ GOOD VIBRATIONS

YOU ARE WHAT YOU EAT, YOU ARE WHAT YOU THINK

Frequency is Everything and Everything is Frequency. Frequency and Vibration are one in the same. Vibrational frequencies can range from high to low. Just as in life, we have light and darkness, health and sickness. They are opposites of each other. Vibrational frequencies can also be negative or positive meaning they either create life force or they drain it. Have you ever walked into a room of people and felt a high vibration that made you surge with energy and happiness? Have you ever walked into a room of people and felt a low vibration that made you feel uneasy and weak, as if something or someone has drained the Life Force from you? If vibrational frequencies are everything wouldn't it stand to reason if you intake low vibrational substances, whether it be water, air or food, over time you would then vibrate at that frequency. Higher frequency food when eaten will eliminate lower frequency substances in the body such as infectious invaders, toxic chemicals, heavy metals and disease. Another effect is increased energy and a higher immune system. When lower frequency food is ingested your cells will take on this lower vibration. The result of low vibrational food is the depletion of minerals, micronutrients, metabolism and vital energy. This opens the door for infectious invaders and acidosis. Low vibration will also affect your emotions causing you to become lethargic and depressed. The emotional body will usually follow the physical body and vice versa. Your body is a living, breathing antenna, so make conscious choices.

BUILD A STRONG FOUNDATION

What if you could have the health and body you always dreamed of and would never feel the need to take another pain **killer**? This is not a tall order to fill. **First we must build a strong foundation** that supports and protects the body on a daily basis. This being the choices we make throughout our day, every day. Then, and only then, is when we should start to fill up our cupboard with more bottles. I will show you why deep cleanses are not ideal in today's environment and that Gentle Daily Cleansing, along with what you take into your body everyday outweighs any medical or single nutrient breakthrough. For years I have been known as the *'Doc of Detox'*. If I could show you the major cause of how we unknowingly become sick, in pain and overweight and how you can truly become the Master of your Body, how would this make you feel? How would this make you change the way you look at life? How would this affect the rest of your life? Never again searching for the next weight loss miracle or miracle cure or painkiller. Near the end of our life when we look back it won't be about the money or the big house. It will be about the difference we have made with our loved ones and with everyone. I know that I can't stop the war on cancer or end starvation, but what I do know is that I can make a difference one person at a time. Small, simple, life changing steps create big change. Thank you for giving me this opportunity.

THE SCOOP ON POOP

"Whether down on the farm or down in your belly if you don't clean it out it's gonna get smelly."

- Dr. Darrell Wolfe, Doc of Detox

THINGS THAT KILL YOU

History shows that methods of internal cleansing date as far back as the caveman days. Although they might not have understood the importance of cleansing, they did respond to instinct. In turn, when they felt bloated or backed up they knew enough to relieve themselves of this toxic load. We all know that when hunting in the prehistoric days if one were plugged up with toxic waste, it would slow you down physically and mentally enough to potentially allow you to be eaten by a dinosaur. That's even in the Cave Man Handbook under the heading '*Things That Kill You*'. As far as man knows it, cave men would use a hollow ram's horn as a funnel; placing the smaller end in the rectum - at least I hope that's how the story goes. Then by pouring water down this homemade device, they would give themselves an enema. Soon after the flush they dropped a few pounds and were off and running again.

Also used by vegetarians was a slender hollow gourd, resembling a squash, through which they poured water to cleanse the colon. Even a bird has the common sense (instinct) to fill its beak when constipated and blow the water through into its back end to relieve the waste caught in its rectum, to lighten the load, so to speak. Fly like an eagle or gobble with the turkeys. Throughout the centuries, colon cleansing is continually mentioned due to its vital importance for health and longevity. Lighten The Load, Flush The Pounds.

EX-LAX GENERATION

My parents were part of the Ex-lax generation, known for helping to usher in the pharmaceutical age (unconscious living), ultimately ridding us of the natural methods used to cleanse and nourish our bodies. These natural methods consisted of herbal remedies that have been with us for thousands of years. *One example 'Moringa Oleifera, The Tree of Life' The most potent and complete Whole Plant Phytonutrient Superfood on the planet has been suppressed for generations.* We turned our backs on Nature, embracing instead the pharmaceutical industry, their ever expanding number of synthetic quick fixes and their false promises of salvation in a pill. Instead of eliminating pain and illness through Whole Plant Based Superfood Nutrition and Gentle Daily Cleansing we use drugs to suppress and cheat (deplete) the body as we do the soil.

Who says advertising doesn't pay. I remember my grandparents had an enema bag under their bed, this was commonplace back then, for their generation. Oh, by the way, try to find one now; and I do not mean a throw away. *Permanent is now temporary. Pain and suffering is now measured in $$$$$.* Soon enough we began giving our money away for temporary relief, along with surrendering our own health into the hands of those who pretended to know better. *"I just wanted to trust them!"* (oops!) If you do not Master your health and life, someone else will always gladly do it for you at a cost and for their benefit only. The more you hand over your power, the more you will be powerless. In addition, you may not like the results because they will never love and care for you as you would for yourself.

A MAN'S HEALTH CAN BE JUDGED BY
WHICH HE TAKES TWO AT A TIME

pills or *stairs*

Everyone has a personal agenda; there is nothing wrong with this, but a word of caution, make sure it matches yours. Drugs are now the #1 accidental killer in the USA, with the vast majority of deaths caused by prescription medications. According to the Centre for Disease Control there is an average of 61 pharmaceutical drug deaths per day in the USA.

Each year 2.2 million people end up in the hospital with adverse drug reactions, 25 million unnecessary antibiotic prescriptions are handed out, 7.5 million unnecessary medical and surgical procedures occur and there are 8.9 million unnecessary hospitalizations. Stats are taken from '*Death by Medicine*' by Dr. Carolyn Dean, MD, ND

As in Nature, the slow and weak of the herd fall prey to the predator. The same goes in the case of infectious invaders and humans with compromised immune systems. Pharmaceutical corporations prey on the weak and unknowing. See what happens when you follow the herd; everyone remembers when it's too late.'

NO ONE SHOULD BE LEFT BEHIND

Let's fast forward to when I was sixteen years old and lived with my grandmother in North Bay, Ontario, where she owned Nipissing Manor. This used to be the home of the Dionne Quintuplets. My grandmother turned it into a nursing home. For myself, this is where the light bulb went on regarding this whole bowel-cleansing fixation. I could never understand the logic on this one. As you know most people in a nursing home are up there in age. I got to know many of the elderly because

I basically lived there. For the life of me, the biggest complaint people had was their bowels and their weight. At the time I had no idea they went hand in hand. We will get back to this later.

At the age of sixteen I started to realize what was really going on. Just like the caveman, these elderly people were jammed up jelly tight. Their main complaints were constipation, intermittent diarrhea, bloating, stomach cramps, low back pain, poor circulation, abdominal pressure, varicose veins, heartburn, heart problems, a foul smelling odor and usually some type of disorder or disease in the pelvic groin region. Go figure. You don't need to be a rocket scientist to know that they were full of poop and rotting from the inside out and from the bottom up. When I was younger I also lived on a farm, so I know how a manure pile can decompose creating a breeding ground for worms, parasites, bad bacteria and nauseous gases. I asked my grandma if she knew that the elderly people in her care were suffering because they were full of poop. Her reply was, yes, and that her staff did the best that they could, under the circumstances. She said that they were not allowed to use herbal medicine or do enemas.

This is when I realized that the medical health practice was really the chemical practice.

The approved protocol was pharmaceutical laxatives and painkillers. This provided some relief, but made the situation even worse by further dehydrating and weakening their already deteriorated state, causing even more toxic build-up, thus lowering their cellular vibration and immune system *(evil plot)*. Drug them up and shut them down - mission accomplished. Remember, history has shown us that all major epidemics and infectious diseases were caused by poor sanitation and sewer back- ups. Poor internal sanitation combined with pharmaceuticals, especially antibiotics, has been shown to reduce resistance to the conditions they were trying to combat in the first place (viruses, bad bacteria and fungus). In other words, this is a rob Peter to pay Paul situation. Yes, these pharmaceuticals would eliminate some of these infectious invaders. Along with this they also deplete your good intestinal bacteria and steal a piece of your **immune system**, only to have these infectious invaders return stronger and more deadly than they were in the first place. Every time you use antibiotics the less effective they will become. Pharmaceuticals are just like street drugs in the sense that the more you use them the more your body needs them and the stronger they need to be. Just like the cockroach that has been around forever, viruses, bacteria, fungus and worms can and will mutate for their survival. You cannot go to war with these infectious invaders and expect to win. You must focus on restoring and balancing your inner terrain. These infectious invaders will survive and thrive in any toxic, low vibrational, nutrient deprived host. Just like a manure pile, you can spray it with pesticides, herbicides and fungicides today, but if you do not remove the manure pile to raise the vibrational frequency of the terrain, the infectious invaders will all be back tomorrow. The only way to send these invaders packing is to **reclaim your inner terrain.**

To put this bluntly, these invaders only become a problem when the host's frequency is vibrating at the same low level as the invaders. When a host is full of toxic waste like the manure pile, they invite the same guests. When a host is deficient in micronutrients and essential minerals their vibrational frequency is lowered, meaning their immune system is weakened. This gives the invaders the freedom to walk in the front door to breed, eat your food and go to the washroom in your body. All of these invaders prey on the weak, the sick, the dying and the walking dead (**zombie nation**). Give me a chronically sick person and my bet is they have unwanted internal guests. Reclaim your inner terrain and take back your home, your health and your life. Restore your body with the most phytonutrient dense plant on the planet, containing every nutrient needed to bring up your vibration to match the frequency of **life**. Whole Plant Based Nutrition, along with Gentle Daily Cleansing will serve these invaders an eviction notice and send them packing for good, the one-two punch for a knockout. Tune in and turn on your life frequency. You're a **living radio**. If you don't like heavy metal turn it to soft rock. **It's all about GOOD VIBRATIONS.**

BRING HEALTH HOME

Okay, let's fast forward to when I am nineteen and I find out that my grandfather has colon cancer and he's coming to stay with us. With cancer you have the full buffet. You would experience chronic acidosis, micronutrient and mineral starvation and as far as infectious invaders go, they have all come to this party. I will try to keep this short. My grandfather has been with us for approximately two weeks and of course his bowels aren't moving. I'm now starting to think to myself that most of the pain and problems I see affecting people are definitely related to a dysfunctional bowel. *What's the big deal? Why doesn't anyone see or smell this obvious answer?* Let's get back to my grandpa; he's off to the hospital. Seven days pass and he hasn't had a bowel movement of any sort. My grandpa is now totally impacted with fecal waste; tighter than a cork in a wine bottle. His biggest complaint right now is not the cancer but the abdominal pain that he is experiencing.

The drugs they have been giving him did not relieve his suffering, but they certainly dulled his brain (**zombie nation**). Mom and I bring Grandpa home and remove the impaction in his colon, getting his bowels moving regularly again (take action; you will always feel better). We used enemas to break up the logjam and an herbal cleansing tea remedy to keep the waste moving. We have now eliminated the pain and the toxic burden placed on his blood stream, organs, and the rest of his body tissues. Even my mother knew better and was aware back then that just cleaning out my grandfather was only half the story. She realized that even though she thought he ate well, he needed additional nutritional support. My grandfather was now out of severe pain and eating again, able to enjoy his life much more because he regained control of his health, dignity and the Mother of all Organs; his colon. Don't waste your life with needless pain and suffering. Invest in your most precious asset... **U**.

MY QUEST

After the experience of living at my grandmother's nursing home and with my grandfather's cancer, I now realized the path that I must take. So bags packed, off I went to the Australian Naturopathic College. This was the beginning of My Health Quest. I knew that I wanted to make a difference. That difference was Natural Health. Even back then, it was the weirdest feeling. I could sense the fear, not just from the person that was sick but from their families as well. I came to realize what this sensation was. It was the smell of being crippled, unable to help themselves or their loved ones because they had given all their power over to the health care system. You're either in control or out of control; there are **no** half measures. Medical doctors were, and are, put on pedestals as if they are the great healers, when in fact; there are only three great healers, **U**, your body and Nature.

So, what became my quest? Not to remain emotionally crippled when it came to my health or the health of those that I love. I had an *'ah-ha'* moment and realized the great betrayal. Health was being deliberately stolen, a piece at a time so those affected would not notice or realize that the quality of their life was being sold at a price. This angered me. Not only for the needless pain and suffering of those who I love, but also for those who wanted to become medical doctors who were unable to truly represent health. I am no longer angry, for this serves no purpose. Just as there is dark, there is light; just as there is sadness there is happiness. This is Planet Earth after all. Where others are front men for *'pharma'*, I support Nature to empower people and wish my end result to be health and happiness for all who I touch. **Remember, everyone has an agenda. You just want to make sure that theirs matches yours.**

CORPORATION CANCER

100 years ago the rate of cancer was 1 in 80 in United States. Now it's 1 in 2 with men and 1 in 3 with women. These are toxic times. A wise man once told me if something stinks follow the

trail and it will always end up at money. I didn't understand what he meant at the time but I do now, and yes, he was right on the money. **The war on cancer** can illustrate one prime example of this analogy. We cannot expect to go to war with anything and find **peace**. When we push something or someone we must always expect to be pushed back. Cancer will never be able to be beaten until all decisions are based from **love** and the **good of all**. As a result, this would allow humanity to empower itself, utilizing a healthy means on both a physical and an emotional level. One cannot beat anything back to balance. **Love heals everything**. We cannot attack the body; instead we need to Love and Respect it, as it should be with planet **earth** as well. According to the EPA's Toxic Release Inventory, 320 billion pounds of toxic chemicals are released into our air annually - and 100 million pounds are carcinogens. Another disturbing point is that only 2,000 of these 80,000 chemicals have been tested for **carcinogenicity**. When we come from the Head we come from the Masculine. As I previously stated one cannot **beat** Cancer with this energy. Instead, one must come from the Feminine, which flows through the Heart. This is where true healing begins and ends. Cancer is a war money machine that will eat one up and spit one out, due to the fact that it's fueled by fear and has no conscience; in turn, many people view it as a death sentence.

This in itself can be more debilitating than the disease. You get and become what you mainly focus on. Oops! Don't focus on corporation cancer. Take back your power - raise your frequency and focus all your energy on Corporation **U**. You become what you eat and focus on, you are your thoughts, you are the Cure!

WHAT'S YOUR ANSWER FOR CANCER?

Embrace the healing power of Nature NOW or Cut, Poison, Burn LATER

According to the World Health Organization, over 41% of the people who are living today will face a cancer diagnosis before they die. Only you can change the rules to this statistic by becoming proactive. Conventional medicine defines cancer as a colony of malignant cells or a tumor. If you have a tumor, then the conventional oncologist will try to cut it out via surgery. After they cut you, then they typically recommend chemotherapy to try to kill any remaining cancer cells with toxic poison. They will finish you off with radiation, to burn whatever cancer cells remain. This is why I, and many others, refer to 'the Big 3' protocol as 'Cut, Poison, and Burn'. The most thorough research study that has ever been done on chemotherapy was at the Northern Sydney Cancer Center in Sydney Australia. They looked at 22 different lines of cancer and the effectiveness of chemotherapy at 5 year survival, which is how we measure if it's successful or not. *What percentage of people live 5 years?* They found that chemotherapy is 2.1% effective at a 5-year survival rate in Australia and 2.3% in the USA - bottom line, it doesn't work.

Natural medicine sees cancer as a multidimensional, systemic total body disease. The cancer tumor is merely a symptom and the purpose of the natural cancer treatment is to correct the root causes of cancer in the whole body. The fact is we develop cancer cells throughout our bodies throughout our lives. Our bodies are normally able to find them, identify them and destroy them before they are able to grow uncontrollably. It is a normal occurrence, which is constantly taking place in a healthy body.

It is only when the healthy body becomes unable to mount its normal defenses and the cancer cells are allowed to reproduce at an uncontrollable rate that cancer becomes life threatening. This is a failure or breakdown of our normal immune system.

The immune systems break down, so it's vital to figure out what's the root cause of the failure and address the cause, rather than just treating a symptom (tumor). Any treatment that does not address underlying causes for the breakdown of the immune system will be palliative at best, and life threatening at worst. That's why the *'Big 3'* treatments are mostly unsuccessful. It's important to remember the basic physiology of all cancer cells. Whether it be breast, prostate, renal or lung, there are many facets that will remain constant.

All cancer cells produce energy the same way: They ferment glucose (sugar). The cancer cell gobbles up the sugar, then, just like a person, it eventually has to poop. So, the cancer cell *'poops'* out some lactic acid and *'flushes it'* into the blood stream. Much like sewer pipes in your house, the arteries then carry the lactic acid (*'poop'*) to the body's amazing poop treatment plant called the *'Liver'*, which takes the lactic acid (*'poop'*) and converts it back into sugar. The cancer cell gobbles up the sugar, then, just like a person, it eventually has to poop. Wait, didn't I just say that? OK, you get the idea, right? It's an endless cycle.

This process is called *'anaerobic respiration'* and occurs in all known cancer cells. Knowing this fact, the wisdom of removing simple carbohydrates and sugars from the diet becomes obvious. The ignorant use of glucose IVs in cancer patients also becomes painfully obvious. The object is to make it difficult for cancer cells to reproduce, so why fuel them with a primary requirement? Cancer cells are unable to efficiently use protein or complex carbohydrates for food. The healthy cells of our body and immune system are able to use these as fuel and for repair. We need to feed our bodies protein and complex carbohydrates and eliminate the rest. It's also important to remember that a large number of cancer cell types have receptor sites for opiates. In other words, opiates used to fight pain will increase the cancer cell's growth rate. Now, concerning the **tumor**, which is only a symptom of the disease and not the cause - the quick shrinkage of tumors that is sometimes seen in chemotherapy or radiation therapy is not a sign of recovery from cancer. It is a complete shutting down of the normal immune response.

Under optimal conditions, tumors will enlarge as they become engorged with CD-cells and macrophages. These cells identify the cancer cells, kill them and then devour their remains. This is an inflammatory response and results in the tumor growing slightly as it becomes engorged with these cells. If the tumor shrinks quickly from chemotherapy or radiation therapy, the ideal healthy response does not have a chance to occur. Never confuse rapid tumor shrinkage with beating the cancer. It is just the opposite. How do you stay healthy and avoid cancer? When you Fuel your Life with Whole Plant Based Foods and Superfood Nutrition you embrace the true healing power of Nature. Either Master your body or others will gladly do it for you; Cut, Poison, Burn. Be the game changer with the densest **Phytonutrient** on Earth; Moringa Oleifera, the body's most powerful healer on the planet. Cleanse daily, fuel your body with Structured dynamic water, the nutrition it needs and it will do the rest. It's only Natural.

Ty Bollinger is the Best Selling author of *'Cancer: Step Outside the Box',* World-renowned Health Researcher and the Host of

'Quest for the Cures', the first ever, complete investigative report *(60 minutes style)* mini-series on natural cancer treatments and the cancer epidemic.

www.cancertruth.net

www.thetruthaboutcancer.com

The Quest For The Cures

In May of 2014, The Truth About Cancer broadcast **"The Quest for The Cures"** which was the first ever investigative report *(60 minutes style)* documentary mini-series on natural cancer treatments. Then, in October of 2014, *"The Quest for the Cures... Continues"* was broadcast.

In these unique documentary mini-series ("docu-series") episodes, the viewer follows Ty Bollinger, who lost both his mother and father to cancer (as well as 5 other family members), as he travels the USA and sits down with the foremost doctors, researchers, experts and survivors to find out their proven methods to preventing and treating cancer.

MASTER YOUR BODY OR PAY $ PAY $ PAY

So here I present the weapon used against us. Spoil people rotten with incorrect information on how to look after their bodies and minds, this is carried out by convincing the masses that having a special degree in health is needed before they could even propose the notion of being Masters of their own well-being. As a result, the public is sold food and remedies based on profit and half truths. Then there is the current Health Care System dilemma, which would be a book in itself.

If it's the truth you seek, here is a book to read: '*The Truth About The Drug Companies*' by Marcia Angell MD. Due to all the factors mentioned above, we are now becoming a nation of people in mental and physical pain. When one is Spoiled Rotten mentally, bad choices are made. When one is Spoiled Rotten physically, pain and suffering become the norm. In turn '*dis-ease*' becomes apparent while pain becomes a normal way of life, but this is not a *Natural Way* to live. They say there is comfort in numbers; in this case I think not, especially when it pertains to needless suffering. This must end. We are one. In turn, when one suffers we all suffer. It is vital that we unite to create the change we all wish to see. I invite you to continue to read on and dwell on the propositions made in this next section. So pull up a toilet, for our journey starts here.

THE CANCER ANSWER

"Cancer is a corporation. It has no feelings because it isn't human. The truth will set you free."

- Dr. Darrell Wolfe, Doc of Detox

CANCER IS A FUNGUS CANCER IS A FREQUENCY

By the time you finish this chapter, you will understand that you are the only answer to cancer, which means you will hold the cure for the fear that has been downloaded into your very cells. With this new information you will move forward with courage and have faith in knowing that only you can master your health and well being. Knowledge is power, heal yourself and rise to your full potential.

In this polluted, low frequency world we live in, it is not difficult see why our bodies accumulate chemicals and other toxins, known as *'carcinogens'*. Carcinogens can cause free-radical damage to our DNA and trigger mutations in the cells, which turns cancer on.

Research has shown that cancer cells develop in every human being, but because of the body's built-in natural defense system, which consists of an immune surveillance system, a repair mechanism and other regulatory mechanisms; cancer cells in a healthy body are identified and destroyed before they become tumors. As long as this natural defense system is functioning properly, the body is able to protect itself from cancer. In all cancer patients, the body's natural defense system is functioning poorly or not at all. In turn, when a cancer cell is present, it is not recognized or destroyed, allowing the cancer to go unchecked. This is why we must be trained on how to manage our body's natural defense system with correct detoxification methods and Whole Plant Based Nutrition.

Your intestines are called the second brain because they are home to 85% of your immune system. Your large intestine is the mother of all organs because it makes up the majority of your precious immune system.

Cancer is the consequence of a weak and toxic large intestine, which kicks off what we call the domino effect. The domino effect of the average, so- called healthy lifestyle eventually weakens, exhausts and undermines the rest of the organs and eventually the whole body, lowering your immune system's healing frequency all the way down to the cellular level.

Infection caused by Candida is what I believe to be a main contributor to the development of cancer. Cancer itself is a fungus. A tumor is your body's attempt at protecting you from the devastating effects of fungus *(Candida Albicans)*.

The good news is that the healthy bacteria in your gut typically keep your Candida levels in check. However, a few factors can cause the Candida population to grow out of control and even explode.

How do you get Candida overgrowth?

- Eating a diet high in refined carbohydrates and sugar
- Consuming alcohol
- Taking oral contraceptives *(birth control)*
- Living a high-stress lifestyle
- Taking a round of antibiotics that killed too many of those friendly bacteria

What are common symptoms of Candida?

- Skin and nail fungal infections, such as athlete's foot or toenail fungus

- Feeling tired and worn down, or suffering from chronic fatigue or fibromyalgia
- Digestive issues such as bloating, constipation, or diarrhea
- Autoimmune diseases such as Hashimoto's thyroiditis, Rheumatoid arthritis, Ulcerative colitis, Lupus, Psoriasis, Scleroderma or Multiple sclerosis
- Difficulty concentrating, poor memory, lack of focus, ADD, ADHD and brain fog
- Skin issues like eczema, psoriasis, acne, hives and rashes
- Irritability, mood swings, anxiety or depression
- Vaginal infections, urinary tract infections, rectal itching or vaginal itching
- Severe seasonal allergies, itchy ears or sinus infections
- Strong sugar and refined carbohydrate cravings

Have you ever smelled an aroma of fish or pepperoni coming from yourself or another person? This is fungus. When there is a fowl odor being emitted from the body you have just become *'Spoiled Rotten'*.

When food begins to spoil, fungus shows up. When tissue cells become compromised, fungus shows up. When a banana is ripe to eat it is absent of brown spots.

When brown spots on the banana start to appear, fungus is on its way. When the brown spots start to turn black the banana is becoming moldy and decomposing. When the skin is healthy it is free of blemishes. When brown spots, sun spots, aging spots, whatever you or the medical system wish to call them appear on the skin, they are fungus and are signs of worse things to come. Just as the banana can go moldy - so can you. This is why when brown spots on the skin change color, turn black or change form, doctors want to remove them because fungus spreads and cancer is sure to follow. Again, this is another case of remove the symptom but not the cause. Fungus gets its foothold first in the large intestine, which is the core of your immune system. The atomic bomb for fungus is the writing of 250 million antibiotic prescriptions every year by our medical system *(immune system wipe-out)*. Your skin is the mirror to the mother of all organs, that being your large intestine. This is why I advocate gentle daily cleansing each and every day with a herbal tea I formulated years ago.

At night when you sleep your body enters into the rest, repair, restore phase. With your body and mind in shut down mode, all excess energy is funneled to the major part of your immune system, that being the friendly otherwise good bacteria in your large intestine. As long as you have not eaten before bed, your good bacteria are on guard and in attack mode ready to devour vast quantities of parasitic microbes such as bad bacteria, fungus and yeasts within your intestines. If you do eat before bedtime and your choice was refined carbohydrates or sugar then you have just been out smarted by the fungus that live within your large intestine. With food in your digestive tract, the vital energy that was needed to devour parasitic invaders has now been diverted to digest the food you just ate. Of all the parasitic invaders your friendly bacteria's favorite food is the yeast or fungus known as Candida Albicans. These fungus are like vampires and will drain you of your life force if your defenses are down. Ask any cancer patient.

As night comes closer most people are tired and exhausted, which affects the immune system, causing it to weaken. The fungus will use this opportunity of weakness to multiply causing you to crave sugar, refined carbohydrates, chocolate, wine, beer and hard liquor. The one glass of wine that you have everyday to unwind is unwinding your immune system as well as tying your body into knots *(internal scar tissue formation)*, and you thought you were in charge. When you feed your cravings, you are actually feeding the fungus within you, the addicts that control you.

It has been shown that people with higher blood sugar levels have a higher risk of developing cancer *(fungus factory)* and have a lesser chance of surviving this disease *(low oxygen, low nutrient environment)*.

Those living unconsciously fall for the false unhealthy cravings caused by the fungus that now reside mainly within the large intestine. Fungus needs these addictive, low frequency foods so that they can thrive and populate. If these parasites can successfully trick you to eat unhealthy addictive foods prior to bedtime, actually anytime, the energy needed for your friendly bacteria to rest, repair, restore and devour fungus will now be redirected to digest the food you just snacked on. You have just weakened the major part of your immune system, that being the large intestine, and strengthened the foothold of these life sucking worms, bad bacteria and fungus. Your good bacteria is your body's major line of defense. You have approximately 85 trillion cells in your body but 10 times more good or bad bacteria depending on the life you live. We are literally walking globs of bacteria. Weather they become good or bad bacteria, solely depends on the choices you make daily.

Talking about choices, look what happens when you let someone else master your health and well being. Like the devastating effects of an atomic bomb, you have just allowed your doctor to prescribe antibiotics (mutate). Your good bacteria will now transform into bad bacteria, which will set off a chain reaction creating hundreds of thousands of microscopic fungus producing factories called Candida Albicans. They will now proceed to undermine the major part of your immune system by rooting pinholes through the walls of the large intestine into your blood stream. The domino effect has now begun and will continue unless you take personal action and master your own health and well being; get trained or stay in treatment.

Candida Albicans is a parasitic fungus that roots itself into and through the walls of your large intestine creating pin like holes. These pin-like holes allow toxic waste, fungus, bad bacteria and worms to enter freely into the blood stream from the large intestine. Once in the blood stream these parasitic invaders now have easy access to the rest of your body.

This yeast, like Candida, is anaerobic, which means they generate their energy and can thrive in the absence of oxygen. Once in the blood stream these anaerobes search out and attach themselves to compromised unhealthy low frequency tissue cells. These low vibrational areas in your body are known as your weak links.

We all have weak links in our body. Just like a weak link in the chain of a bicycle your body's weak links are found in the tissues, bones and vital organs. You know what and where your weak links are. They stick out and scream at you when you're run down, eat unhealthy or when you're emotionally out of balance. When your body's frequency is lowered by physical or unprocessed emotional toxins, these toxins will settle into areas of the body that give off a matching frequency, this being low, otherwise, unhealthy.

These weak links, otherwise compromised areas of the body, will eventually become parasite ridden with worms, bad bacteria and fungus. The weak links within your body are mainly compromised, unhealthy low frequency tissues. These compromised tissues will act as an alarm by creating inflammation, pain and stiffness, continually warning you that your defenses are weak and your immune system is down. If these compromised low frequency tissues are not reinforced and returned to their natural state of health then they will become home base to millions of microscopic, fungal producing factories that will pave the way for a parasitic invasion. This parasitic invasion will begin at your weak links and spread outward consuming the rest of your body one cell at a time. To eliminate disease, heavy metals, bad bacteria and worms you must first remove the magnet that attracts disease and disease causing elements, that magnet would be fungus.

Unless you are trained to master your own body, you will eventually live a life of pain and suffering, end up in the hospital, a nursing home or hospice, prematurely die, become a victim of cancer or some other fatal disease. As the frequency continues to lower in these compromised areas of your body, disease and decomposition will be the result. This compromised or diseased tissue creates a frequency that becomes a homing device, which attracts vampire like microbes such as bad bacteria, viruses, worms and fungus. Compromised and diseased tissue is the perfect breeding ground for micro-organisms such as fungus, bad bacteria, viruses and worms to feed on because these parasites have a frequency that matches compromised or diseased tissue. People with diseases have a low vibrational frequency.

When most people think about parasitic predators, these being bad bacteria, fungus and worms, they think of a manure pile or a decomposing corpse. *Well, how about the chronically sick and diseased?* If these parasitic invaders are not eliminated by raising the vibrational frequency, not just with in these compromised tissues, but within the whole being, then elimination of these predators such as fungus, bad bacteria and worms will be temporary at best.

When your inner terrain vibrates a frequency of life, energy and positivity then these parasites can no longer exist within you. Frequency dictates matter; darkness is only created by the absence of light. These predators will continue to return and invade tissue that matches their frequency; living in it, feeding off it and yes, defecating *(pooping)* in it. If this continues the only possible outcome for these compromised cells is death or mutation, whether it is a vital organ or muscle tissue.

Low frequency tissue is the prey in nature and the parasite is the predator that feeds on those who are chronically depressed, chronically sick, diseased or dying. One of the main objectives of any parasite is to decompose what is already perceived to be decomposing, search and destroy. Draining whatever life force is left in the tissue cells and changing *(mutating)* it to be more like them, anaerobic. Compromised unhealthy tissue are the weak links in your body that live in an environment of decreased oxygen and nutrition. This unhealthy environment leads to the suffocation and starvation of healthy tissue cells.

Fungus is opportunistic; when it finds a weak link it will then set up home and attach itself onto the outer membrane of the tissue cell, preventing crucial receptor sites from working properly. Otherwise blocking the needed nutrients and oxygen from these already compromised tissue cells.

To survive, these compromised tissue cells must either mutate to match the frequency of the fungus, become anaerobic, make sugar its number one food source or die of suffocation and starvation. The main objective of any and all living organisms is survival. For their survival your cells will choose mutation before death whenever possible.

To mutate they must switch their energy production from an oxygen-based system to one that does not use or need oxygen. This new system does not use oxygen to generate their energy from food molecules because they have now mutated into cancer cells.

A cancer cells main fuel source is sugar. What a coincidence, the same fungus that caused these tissue cells to mutate into cancer cells is feeding its sugary-like waste *(poop)* to the cancer cells as a food source.

Otto Warburg won a Nobel Prize in 1931 for telling the world that cancer cells do not need oxygen and that oxygen is now their enemy!

"All normal cells have an absolute requirement for oxygen, but cancer cells can live without oxygen - a rule without exception. Deprive a cell 35% of its oxygen for 48 hours and i t may become cancerous."

- Otto Warburg

Dr. Warburg has made it clear that the root cause of cancer is oxygen deficiency, which creates an acidic state in the human body. Dr Warburg also discovered that cancer cells are anaerobic *(do not breathe oxygen)* and cannot survive in the presence of high levels of oxygen, as found in an alkaline state.

The mitochondrion is commonly known as the *"power house"* of the cell. Recent research from Harvard Medical School has identified that mutations to oncogenes *(by toxins)* in the mitochondria can lead to a process called the *'Warburg Effect'*. Here, a cell is able to grow uncontrollably by utilizing glucose *(sugar)* better and adapting to low oxygen environments whereby avoiding the apoptosis *(cellular death)* pathway.

This is a consequence of improper mitochondrial respiration and must be treated – otherwise cancer is harder to treat and more likely to return. Natural cancer treatments aimed at increasing mitochondrial metabolism are essential.

We understand that the true cause of Cancer is the depletion of your immune system, from your large intestine all the way down and into your cells. To understand this better we must look at the Domino Effect of Cancer, which starts with the first symptom being constipation of the large intestine and the last being constipation at the cellular level ending with the life threatening symptom we call *'Cancer'*.

It's the inner terrain within your body that allows cancer to grow or never show. What we think, eat, drink and do on a daily basis each and every day determines the vibrational health of our inner terrain, because frequency is everything. Function dictates form. We must create and maintain a healthy internal environment to prevent or cure cancer. Biologists studying living cells found that cells can do only what they are allowed to do by the environment that surrounds them. This suggests that if the body's internal environment, otherwise internal terrain changes, it influence's the cells behavior!

Mina Bissell and other scientists have proven that cancer is not only caused by cancer cells, it is caused by an interaction between cancer cells and the surrounding cellular micro-environment, which they live in. Micro- environment and the content that surround those cells is actually telling the cancer cell and the cancer gene what to do. If tissue architecture and context are the message, then tumor cells with abnormal genes should be capable of becoming normal if tissue architecture is restored.

Mina Bissell's conclusions: Growth and malignant behavior are regulated at the level of tissue organization, and tissue organization is dependent on extra cellular matrix and micro-environment. Extra cellular matrix and micro-environment are totally dependent on, as I stated earlier, what you think, eat, drink and do on a daily basis. Everybody produces cancer cells but not every person gets cancer.

Mina Bissell: Experiments that point to a new understanding of cancer can be seen on TED TALKS.

It all comes down to form (tissue integrity) and function. Form and function is dependent on the Architect otherwise whoever is in charge of the body. For most, decisions on health are decided by the media, Pharma, food conglomerates and the Medical System. Neither has majored much less minored on what constitutes a healthy body. The Medical System majors in disease and drugs and the media majors in getting you to buy anything that can generate a profit.

At any given time in your 70 trillion cells, the extra cellular matrix, which is outside the cell, is in continual back and forth communication with the nucleus, which is inside the cell. This is how balance is kept and restored. As I stated earlier, how you live your life physically, emotionally and mentally on a daily basis, that is, the decisions you make and how you process your thoughts will be the deciding factors on whether you turn cancer on or off.

Let us not forget as Einstein stated, *"Everything is frequency."*

Just like a light switch every person has the power to turn cancer on or off. You are the Master controller of whether you will ever have cancer. *Do you really believe the 'Medical Model' that a single cancer gene in just one of the body's trillion cells is enough to turn cancer on?* This medical model will have you living in fear each and every day wondering when your number will be called. But wait a minute, isn't that the way the majority already live each and everyday? Crippled, captive, cursed and controlled. All your thoughts and the food you eat carry a frequency, choose wisely.

As Louie Pasteur stated on his deathbed, *"The bug is nothing, the inner terrain is everything."*

An acidic inner terrain is the only true disease and acidity is cancers greatest ally. An acidic body is the strongest link to ill health and cancer. The increasing acidity, that most lifestyles create today, cripples the cytotoxic T-cells found in a healthy body. The purpose of these T-cells is to attack and destroy cancer cells. In all cancer patients, the body's natural defense system is functioning poorly or not at all. In turn, when a cancer cell is present, it is not recognized or destroyed, allowing the cancer to go unchecked.

Cancer cells produce large amounts of lactic acid. This lactic acid production creates the perfect environment for fungus to multiply and for tumors to grow. For the tumor to thrive it must create and maintain an acidic environment because cancer cells are anaerobic (*a no oxygen environment*). These once healthy cells are now anaerobic, live primarily on sugar and are lactic acid factories. These cancer cells will continue to produce lactic acid because like any other microorganism, survival is first and foremost. Lactic acid is produced to keep the environment in and around cancer cells acidic so they remain strong, propagate, otherwise multiply and conquer. The cancer cell starts out as a life saving survival mechanism created by the body to put cell death on hold. But due to our health care system being built on a foundation of deception, this life saving mechanism called cancer will become a death sentence for millions of innocent loving human beings.

Due to this ongoing acidic condition your body's defense system goes on high alert encapsulating cancer cells and the invading fungal colonies by creating and sending fibrin, otherwise known as internal scar tissue, to the area of concern. This fibrin production is used to wall off and stop the parasitic invasion, inflammation and mutation from spreading to healthy tissue cells. If this perceived threat continues, the area of concern will form layer upon layer of fibrotic scar tissue, with the result being the formation of tumors.

A tumor is similar to the rings of a tree. With every passing year a new ring is formed. With a tumor, the longer this inflammation and parasitic invasion continues, more layers of hardened scar tissue are formed for your protection.

The bigger the tumor, the more fibrotic scar tissue it has, and the more toxic by nature it tends to be. A tumor is mainly made up of dense layers of fibrotic scar tissue, which by the way, is the same fibrotic scar tissue that you would find in any injured tissue throughout the body. Just a few examples of this are arthritis, sciatica and fibromyalgia. This internal fibrotic scar tissue builds up over the years as a protective life-saving mechanism due to an incorrect lifestyle. This fibrotic scar tissue that your body creates helps to wall off the continual attack of fungus, bad bacteria, viruses and worms that prey on compromised, low integrity, low vibrational tissue.

Left unattended the fungi will continue to spread into the surrounding tissue and eventually throughout the body, also known as 'metastasis'. Candida, when left to it's own device, can invade and infiltrate any and all of your tissues and vital organs, due to its highly adaptive qualities. It is able to mutate and adapt itself to whatever environment it is invading more effectively than any other parasitic invader. This is why there are so many different types of tumors.

Over time, your body tissues and its vital organs will become overrun and overwhelmed with this fungal invasion. This will leave you in a weakened state due to the destruction of the immune system, that being mainly the large intestine, where this fungal invasion first took root. The body becomes unable to protect itself from this improperly managed, ineffectively treated fungal invasion, which allows the fungi to spread throughout the body like a raging fire out of control. At this point your body is completely overwhelmed and fighting for its very survival.

To remove the fungus you must raise not just the frequency of the compromised tissues but the whole body itself. To do this you must rid the body of the manure pile that creates the environment for the fungus to grow. To rid yourself of the manure pile you must focus on where the majority of your immune system resides. This would entail gentle daily cleansing of the large intestine each and every day on a daily basis.

The medical system, food conglomerates, pharmaceutical corporations, government and the media, are continually programing the masses to live a toxic lifestyle. This is known as herd mentality. This herd mentality serves one purpose, that being a profit center for pharmaceutical corporations. Create the crisis and then run to the rescue. Our health will continue to be sold off by the pound along with our bodies until we break from the herd and get trained to master our own health and well being. But let me make this perfectly clear, even the Natural Health Industry and the Supplement Industry have learned from their big brother, Big Pharma. It can be very confusing to know what to cleanse, where to cleanse and how to cleanse. This is why I now focus on training instead of treating, information before products.

The most important thing to understand is that you can cleanse the heavy metals, bad bacteria and worms from your body but like a revolving door these cleanses will never end because fungus is the magnet that attracts heavy metals and all other parasites and like super glue, the fungus pulls and sticks everything together. Heavy metals, bad bacteria and worms will continue to return until your attention is on gentle daily cleansing of the large intestine and the elimination of fungus so that bad bacteria, heavy metals and worms cannot and will not return. Fungus will eventually be your downfall if not made a priority.

I would like to leave you with something to think about. ***Does the lack of drugs, chemotherapy, radiation and surgery cause cancer?***

With our current health care system the average person doesn't stand a chance. One out of every two people will experience cancer within their lifetime and I pray they live in a family that supports natural health. Between the medical system, media, family and friends, it is easy to see how we have all been continually downloaded, dysfunctional programs 24/7 distorting the truth, creating a life filled with fear, pain and suffering for most.

Being the director of the International Training Institute of Health, I am dedicated to training you, not treating you, so that you may train your family and friends to become the masters of their own health and well being so they may live a life filled with the joy and happiness they deserve. I am dedicated to training you, not treating you, so that you may train your family and friends to become the masters of their own health and well being to live a life filled with the joy and happiness they deserve. www.itioh.com

THE MOTHER OF ALL ORGANS

"Health and Disease are born inside The Mother of all Organs. A compromised Immune System begins and ends here. Show this Organ respect or all Cell will break loose and U will live in pain."

- Dr. Darrell Wolfe, Doc of Detox

THE MOTHER OF LIFE

Most people believe that their body is mainly composed of cells. **90% of the cells in your body actually belong to bacteria.** Scientists realize that unbalanced microbial (bacterial) communities in the digestive tract, mainly the colon, are the root cause of the pain and disease we suffer today. Almost all dysfunctions of the brain can be connected to the digestive tract as the cause. Hippocrates, the Father of Medicine, stated that 'All diseases begin in the intestines.' The more science learns, the more we realize just how correct Hippocrates was. Your intestines play the most significant role when it comes to diseases such as: Allergic Disorders, Asthma, Hay Fever, Heart Disease, Cancer and yes, Obesity. Good bacteria are absent in those who suffer from Inflammatory Diseases, such as Colitis and Crohn's Disease. **Other conditions greatly influenced by a toxic, unbalanced colon are as follows:** Type 1 and 2 Diabetes, Multiple Sclerosis, Lupus, Kidney Problems, Chronic Fatigue Syndrome, Urinary Conditions, Fibromyalgia, Rheumatoid Arthritis, Ulcerative Colitis, Osteoarthritis, chronic skin conditions, degenerative conditions and other inflammatory bowel diseases. As I stated earlier this is no coincidence; almost all diseases get their foothold in the digestive tract, mainly in the **colon**. This includes both physical and mental conditions. Don't think for a minute that pharmaceutical companies are not aware that you are giving up a piece of your immune system every time you take antibiotics to attack a virus, bad bacteria or infection to find only that your intestines are now overrun by fungus (evil plot). The first rule, that any practitioner with any common sense knows, is that antibiotics should only be used in life-threatening situations because continual use of antibiotics causes life-threatening situations.

"All diseases begin in the intestines."

- Hippocrates

A compromised immune system is the major cause of most disease. As mentioned before, you cannot go to war or attack your body and come out in one piece. The fungus (Candida) you created will leave you vulnerable and open to more and bigger problems than you started with. By taking antibiotics you have given a piece of your immune system away within days, which will now take years to replace or may never be replaced. Oh, and by the way, those bad bacteria that you thought you killed, have now mutated, are becoming immune to the antibiotics and are now seeking revenge. You cannot make your body a war zone and win. The only way to regain your health and keep it is to create an environment in which the invaders cannot exist. Bacteria outnumber our cells by 10 to 1. Your health rests on you keeping a proper balance of 85% good bacteria and no more than 15% bad bacteria.

As long as these bacteria are in proper balance, they will keep you in balance physically, mentally and emotionally. For most it is the exact reverse, or worse, 85% bad bacteria to 15% good bacteria, oops! We have 100 trillion microbes living on our skin, up our nose and on any body surface you can think of. Your digestive tract makes up *'80-85% of your immune system.'* The greatest percentage of your immune system resides in the mother of all organs, the large intestine (colon). These good microbes (bacteria) help break down fibers, harvest calories, and protect us from micro-invasion, when kept in balance. Your gut functions as **your body's second brain**. It produces even more serotonin than your brain does. Serotonin has a beneficial effect on balancing your mood. 1 out of 4 Americans will eat a high fat, high carbohydrate fast food meal each and every day. Because 25% of the population participates in this type of eating, it is widely accepted. These eating habits have a negative impact on the body and because most of the population participates, it is regarded as normal; I call it unconscious living. When your bacteria go from friendly to unfriendly they will become downright pathogenic, leaking noxious by- products (endotoxin), which will cause all 'cell' to break loose; this is the beginning of your demise. When this happens the domino effect begins and these trillions of bacteria will turn on you and make your life a living hell.

Acidosis, inflammation, internal scar tissue, degeneration, cell mutation and disease will be the result. **Dead Meat Bacteria = Endotoxemia** (endotoxin in the blood): After a meal of animal products people suffer from Endotoxemia. Their blood stream becomes awash with bacterial toxins, known as endotoxins that are present in animal products. These dead meat bacterial toxins are not destroyed by stomach acid, pancreatic enzymes, cooking or even boiling for hours. Animal fat triggers immediate inflammation within the body due to being loaded with endobacteria, even if fully cooked. Saturated animal fat then boosts the absorption of these endotoxins into our blood stream causing arterial paralysis (high blood pressure). Another cause of Endotoxemia is a greasy, refined carbohydrate meal. This will cause inflammation due to the release of endotoxin from the outer walls of the bad bacteria that now live in your colon. Endotoxin, if not eliminated daily from your colon through Gentle Daily Cleansing can and will be absorbed into the blood stream causing inflammation to the weakest parts of the body or throughout the whole body; this inflammation is created by the body to warn you of a perceived threat or injury.

If left unattended, the body initiates a secondary support system that starts continual fibrin production to the area of concern in order to wall off the inflammation overload, until you incorporate a Whole Plant Based Lifestyle and gently cleanse on a daily basis. This continual inflammation and fibrin production, if not halted, will drain you of your vital energy, essential nutrients and will create massive internal scar tissue which will gradually immobilize, deteriorate, mutate and distort the tissues, organs and bones in the area of concern. Every disease whether it's a muscle or organ has internal scar tissue involvement where inflammation is present. Hello '***invisible bonds***'.

Many will suffer massive internal scar tissue formation as if there has been a physical injury to the area, all due to mismanagement and misinformation *(evil plot)*. For the body to run at peek performance there cannot be energy wastage. To be at war with one's self for more than short periods, will cripple critically needed defense systems of the body by exhausting the body of its energy. When you continually try to kill the pain using drugs, over time you are slowly and unknowingly killing yourself *(oops)*.

Inflammation comes in many forms. The redness and pain experienced in an affected area of the body is a built-in safety mechanism to help ward off further invasion of microbes. In the case of flu, you will experience fever, aches and pains throughout the body. This represents a body-wide '*seek and destroy*' mission aimed at *'invading virus'*. These symptoms are all essential for our survival. They warn of a perceived threat or injury. Even though these symptoms of inflammation are a protective device for survival they will cause injury if allowed to persist or are suppressed through drugs. Vital energy will be drained from the body leaving you exhausted and unprotected in both cases.

How was your energy level during this time of needless suffering? Low, because your immune system was low (energy leakage). If inflammation is eliminated through drugs or just not attended to, you will become more acidic, create more internal scar tissue, creating crippling invisible bonds and never regain the energy needed to heal unless the cause is dealt with; this being the balance of bacteria in your large intestine. Once you cleanse and heal your colon by replenishing and restoring your body on a daily basis your digestive system will start functioning properly again and disease symptoms will disappear.

When not under threat, the body uses energy for cellular repair, maintenance and yes, sex. Life is great once again. When a threat arises hormone related activity decreases to a minimum. Non-essential tasks will be shut down and other body systems and functions will be rationed. The majority of your energy will go to fight the threat. Forget tomorrow, the priority is to preserve the self today. Right about now you should be having a **gut feeling** where the answer lies. The challenge for most people occurs when they have never had a nutritional strategy to optimize colon integrity.

Health and disease are born in The Mother Of All Organs so Drink Life In and Take Life On with Whole Plant Based Superfoods. Lighten Your Load with Gentle Daily Cleansing and say goodbye to 'Endo'. **Be The Cure That You've Been Searching For!**

THE CURE IS RIGHT UNDER YOUR NOSE THAT WOULD BE U

NOT SUCH A . . . FUN - GUY

Any organism whether from a piece of fruit or a human being can become moldy or infected with fungus if its life force is depleted. When fruit is over-ripe it will get brown spots as it is decomposing. When people become overly toxic or ingest antibiotics and other drugs, street or pharmaceutical, they run the risk of altering and destroying their immune system thus opening the gateway to a fungus frenzy known as Candida.

We then add fuel to the fire when we ingest sugar, refined carbohydrates and greasy foods, thus empowering these parasitic invaders into full attack mode. Your uncontrollable cravings for these foods are instigated only for the survival and propagation of the **FUN - GUY.**

STEPS LEADING TO METABOLIC SYNDROME

1. A diet mainly composed of refined carbohydrates, sugars and fatty, greasy foods.
2. Microbes (bacteria) become unbalanced in the colon due to antibiotic use or foods high in fat and sugar causing the growth of a family of bad bacteria, which produce and release a toxic substance called endotoxin from their outer layer.
3. If the endotoxin is allowed to accumulate and stagnate within the colon it will be absorbed into the bloodstream, which will trigger the immune system to react. When this

happens your body will conserve energy to gear up for a fight and maybe even a full out battle with these endotoxins. You will know when the battle has begun. All 'cell' will break loose and your life will become a living Hell-th.

At least three quarters of the population suffer from this debilitating predator known as Candida and most are not aware of its existence. This parasitic organism can be responsible for your negative health symptoms from the top of your head to the tip of your toes. Your favorite addictions become the fuel to create the perfect breeding ground for these invisible but not so silent killers. Eventually the invaders will enter your bloodstream and create havoc anywhere and everywhere throughout your body.

Here is a list of common Candida symptoms composed by Dr. Mark Hyman, recognized Candida authority, and best-selling author of, 'The Blood Sugar Solution'.

General Symptoms include

- Chronic Fatigue
- Loss of Energy
- General Malaise
- Decreased Libido
- Sensitivity to foods, chemicals, or other allergens
- Eczema
- Psoriasis
- Irritable Bowel Syndrome

Gastrointestinal Symptoms Include

- Thrush
- Bloating & Gas

- Intestinal Cramps
- Rectal Itching
- Altered bowel function such as Diarrhea or Constipation
- Yeast Infections
- Frequent Bladder Infections
- Irritable Bladder

Hormonal Complaints

- Menstrual irregularities like pain or excessive bleeding
- Premenstrual syndrome
- Thyroid Dysfunction

Nervous System Complaints

- Depression
- Irritability
- Inability to concentrate

Immune System Complaints

- Allergies
- Chemical Sensitivities
- Low Immune Function

And If Your Past History Includes

- Chronic yeast infections
- Chronic antibiotic use for infections or acne
- Oral birth control pill usage
- Oral steroid hormone usage

A 2012 study by Dr. Robert Lustig of the University Of California, San Francisco revealed that sugar is just as addictive to the human brain as cocaine, setting off the same dopamine triggers and forcing us to crave more and more of it.

The food conglomerates are always one step ahead of us so we won't see the word *'sugar'* on a food label.

Some other names for sugar are:

- Agave nectar
- Brown rice syrup
- High-fructose corn syrup
- Dextrose
- Evaporated cane juice
- Glucose
- Lactose
- Malt syrup
- Molasses
- Sucrose

Over the last thirty years, more and more of these re fined sugars, artificial sweeteners, preservatives, and other unnatural elements have infiltrated our food supply, creating a life-threatening breeding ground for these invading fungi. The answer is under your nose and has rooted into your intestines and is preparing to invade your bloodstream.

Now you know why more people are getting sick more than ever before, why more people are suffering from obesity and why cancer is predicted to soar by 50% by the year 2020. Food conglomerates will do what ever it takes to protect their shareholders' profit margin.

Back when I was in my teens there was a song that I used to sing. It went like this "Oh Candida, we can make it together."

In no way does this song have any relationship to the Candida (fungus) that sets up shop in your body. This Candida will take you for everything you've got - if you don't keep your digestive tract healthy.

Candida is a naturally occurring organism that lives in your digestive tract. As long as you have a balance of 85% good bacteria to 15% bad bacteria your digestive tract and immune system will function normally. Where the problem lies is that the majority of our population has the percentage reversed. Over the last fifty years the food chain has been dismantled along with our health. The food chain is broken and so is our health care system, and will remain this way if it's left up to those who broke it in the first place.

When you feed the Candida: sugar, refined carbohydrates, pastas, pizza, sodas, fried foods, breads, crackers, chips, etc, you are adding fuel to the fire. The more you eat these foods the longer and more intense your cravings become and the stronger the Candida becomes. They now rule not just your body but your moods as well; welcome to the emotional roller coaster.

I have consulted hundreds of people where their relationships became harmonious when they reclaimed their inner terrain, that being their digestive tract, mainly the large intestine.

Your digestive tract, which makes up the majority of your immune system, contains 60% of the cells in your body.

Gentle Daily Cleansing along with ample Dynamic Structured Water and a Whole Plant Based nutritional lifestyle hold the keys to reclaim not just your inner terrain but life itself.

Read: *'Scoop on Poop'*, *'The Domino Effect'* and *'Eat Whole - Love Life'* for a deeper understanding to who holds the keys. **Get Trained Not Treated - Be The Cure!**

GOT CANDIDA?

Here is an at home Candida Test, one you can do in the morning. We do not know the source of this Candida Test but it has been around a long time and is thought to be quite reliable in the evaluation of Candida symptoms:

DID YOU KNOW - Up to 85% of North Americans May Have Candida?

When you awake in the morning, before you put anything into your mouth, work up some saliva and spit into a clear glass of water. Within 1-30 minutes, look in the glass. If there are strings coming down from your saliva, or if the water turned cloudy, or if your saliva sank to the bottom, YOU MAY HAVE A CANDIDA CONCERN! Healthy saliva will simply float on the top!

(You may want to put out a glass of water in the bathroom or on a nightstand the night before you wish to do the Candida Saliva Test, just to remind yourself not to brush your teeth prior to spitting in the glass.)

THE ROYAL FLUSH

The Royal Society of Medicine did a major study and found that **a dysfunctional large intestine *(colon)* is the contributor to 85% of disease and illness from which we suffer.** I believe and will prove conclusively that if this organ is not cleansed and nourished on a daily basis, it generates the fuel *(absorbed toxic waste)* that creates most of the illness and pain we suffer on an emotional and physical level. Until your colon *(large intestine)* gets the attention and co-operation it deserves, you will not be able to prevent or reverse illness effectively.

Remember, no one is happy when they're feeling crappy and yes, I am referring to the literal sense. For a society so medically advanced and in search of health *(drug based)* breakthroughs, *why is it still so complicated for many to see, feel and smell the obvious?* When it comes to how people feel and look, what was once abnormal has now become commonplace. To illustrate this point, the next time you go to a public place make a conscious effort to look around and maybe even look down. You decide if I am correct. The majority of men and women appear to be 3 to 6 months pregnant. This is not just excess weight, this is also extreme putrefaction *(rotting)* in the large intestine - unconscious living in full bloom. I often have patients in my office constantly telling me how sick and tired they feel. In response, **I propose this question:** *Are you sick and tired of being sick and tired?"* If so, let's change it! In this book, you have the tools to **Master Your Health and Well-being.** Fear of the unknown will become the illusion as opposed to being the reality. Unconscious living is a silent but deadly force and **The Whole Truth About Health**, is the antidote.

A HEAVY LOAD

Statistics show that the average person is overweight, with 1 in 4 carrying as much as an extra 25 pounds of not just weight, but toxic waste within the large intestine. This notion is all too evident once one is able to read the signs. Everywhere I go I see people complaining of the way they look and feel; many of them sporting the middle age bulge, also known as the spare tire, beer belly, potbelly, etc. What we are really dealing with is the large intestine, which, by the way, is a muscle; how's yours hanging? If by chance, yours is hanging, it now lacks muscle tone and has fallen down and outward, or down and inward within the abdominal cavity. Your abdomen is the core to your immune system. If your core lacks tone externally then it lacks tone internally. Limp and in a state of coma.

This problem is caused by a buildup of stagnant waste material along with poor dietary habits, which leads to nutritional starvation and Endotoxemia *(toxic blood)*. Did you know that in our culture, the average adult has 8 to 12 pounds of stagnant fecal waste putrefying *(rotting)* within their body, even if they don't have a protruding abdomen? In this instance, their intestines are falling down and inwards. In today's society people are always eating yet always hungry. Plenty of food but we're always hungry because the food chain is broken. You can eat until you put yourself into a food coma but unless your body gets dense phytonutrients that support life, the brain will not turn off the hunger trigger. Everything is frequency. Unless you raise the frequency of your cells with Structured Water and Structured Air, **Whole Plant Based Superfood Nutrition**, you will never turn the hunger switch off. We will discuss this in further detail later.

Without realizing it, the average person is in fact, toxic *(acidic)*; this condition is becoming both widespread and accepted as the norm because there is **comfort in numbers**. We are rotting from the inside out and from the bottom up. The large intestine is the Mother of All Organs. If it is not managed properly, it will ultimately become a prime breeding ground for disease.

Being the first organ developed in the fetus, it is also the most important organ in the body. Nature understands that without a proper waste disposal sewage system life would cease to exist before it even had a chance to get started. Raise your frequency and lighten the load by flushing the pounds. **Take Life In & Release The Thin Within.**

BACKED UP AND FEELING DOWN

Just picture the catastrophes and epidemics we would face if our cities' sewer systems were not maintained. They would back up into our streets and homes, causing widespread infections and disease. The body is no different. *Where do you think the average, so-called, healthy person stands in this situation?* They have turned their body's sewage system into a living **cesspool**, creating a breeding ground of bacteria, viruses, fungus, worms and toxic gas. There are a couple of sayings that come to mind...

"Cars rust, people rot." The second is: *"An ounce of prevention is worth a pound of cure."* Small steps daily make big changes. I'm sure we can all agree that prevention is the preferred course of action. Gently cleanse and nourish your cells daily with Whole Plant Based Superfood Nutrition. **Go green, get clean or become a Mean Machine.**

THE HIGHWAY TO HELL-TH YOU CHOOSE

The Digestive Process starts at the mouth and travels down the esophagus to the stomach and into the small intestine, which is approximately 22 feet long. It then continues on to the large intestine, which is 5 to 7 feet long. In total, we are looking at 30 feet of highway. That's quite a long distance for food to travel, even when combined properly. Every component has to be digested in its proper order and time sequence for this process to be successful, not unlike any other assembly line. The digestion process is a work of art regarding its simplicity and effectiveness. Improper eating throws this whole delicate process off course, causing pain and discomfort throughout the body. Most people are only conscious of the first 4-inches of the process; only aware of the taste and texture from the lips to the beginning of their throat.

In essence, they get 4-inches of pleasure followed by 30 feet of pain, discomfort and gas. Unfortunately when it comes to food selection, important health concerns such as nutritional value, quality, the degree of toxic chemicals, and digestive ability all take a back seat to the following factors: taste, texture, appearance and smell, which in turn creates one heck of a smell at the other end. Most people only adhere to these four standards while choosing foods to eat. Distorted taste buds cause a distorted shape to the body inside and out.

Often the foods we consume simply end up sitting too long and rotting in the digestive tract, simultaneously releasing poisons and noxious gas into the body. When food enters the body dead and toxic, meaning no nutritional life force, it vibrates at the level of stagnation, putrefaction, inflammation and pain.

Negative symptoms one may experience from this situation are the following: heartburn, headache, nausea, bloating, cramps, gas, low back pain and fatigue. If we eat for energy we should feel energized as a result. Life breeds Life.

Ask yourself this, are you tired or energized by your food?

Are you absorbing nutrients or toxins?

Are you addicted to processed chemical laden foods?

Without food guidelines and logic, we are satisfying only the savvy marketers and our distorted taste buds *(evil plot)*. In the meantime our digestive tract becomes severely burdened and clogged up.

EMPTY FOODS WILL NEVER FILL YOU!

What happens in between the front and back door of your body is a primary factor in deciding whether one will experience vital health or pain and *'dis-ease'* throughout life. We must learn to become our own watchdog, conscious of which foods are detrimental and which foods are supportive to our bodies. The first rule of thumb is the following: The more man touches food, the less you should want it.

The more he advertises it, the more you should run from it. Let me propose a question. *Why do children have so much energy?* Yes, they are young, but most importantly, they are not toxic. They haven't experienced thirty, forty or even fifty years of absorbing toxic waste that migrates from the stagnant fecal debris that is lining the walls of the large intestine into their blood stream. As a result, the poisons emitted haven't had a chance to pollute their blood, lymph system, organs and tissue cells. In addition, they haven't experienced the invasion of fungus, bad bacteria, viruses and parasites, which are the inevitable outcome of a backed up sewer system *(colon)*. **U honestly do hold the keys.**

As I stated earlier, the large intestine is the last 4 to 7 feet of the digestive tract, beginning at the Ileocecal valve, 2-inches left of the right hip and ending at the rectum. The large intestine *(colon)* is a muscle. Therefore, if it lacks tone, every other muscle and cell in the body will consequently also lack tone.

The core is everything. Without the existence of muscular tone within the colon muscle, the leakage of toxic waste slowly begins to filter through its walls into the bloodstream and the cells of the rest of the body tissues. When this occurs your immune system will be more than put to the test. This is the beginning of what's called '*The Domino Effect*' which we will digest later. Emotional stress can also aggravate this, affecting digestion, which in turn slows down the elimination process.

Most symptoms of emotional stress will be experienced negatively within the abdomen. In today's environment, even if you make healthy food choices, bowel management should still remain a top priority. Overall well-being is dependent on the efficiency of the digestive process and the large intestine *(colon)*. If not managed properly on a daily basis this will be the beginning of much unwanted discomfort because these are toxic times on our planet. Your digestive tract in essence, is the Highway to **HELL-TH... U CHOOSE.**

HOT & STINKY
TROUBLE DOWN BELOW

MEET THE BOWEL BROTHERS

Do you suffer from persistent bad breath? If you do, it is not because of what you ate yesterday. It is the result of what you have eaten days, weeks, months and even years before. Hot gases rise up from your large intestine and out through your mouth. This unpleasant taste and smell is the cause of plaque formation due to the years of toxic waste buildup within the colon. For those of you who suffer gum disease just know the root cause is by the back door, your large intestine. Something your dentist forgot to tell you, oops *(evil plot)*. Where there's smoke there's usually fire - hot and stinky.

Mints, toothpaste and mouthwash provide only a temporary fix which masks the symptoms, never resolving the root cause. *Why do people use underarm deodorant and perfumes?* One of the main reasons is to camouflage odor. The real cure is to remove the waste from the large intestine thus removing the toxic load from your lymph system and sweat glands. So get to the root cause and quit being such a stinker! *Why is it that young children do not smell? Why does the strength of body odor increase as we age?* The answer is the following: The more waste we have and the older it is, the worse it smells. As a result, we're a stinking mess. In an attempt to mask unpleasant odors emitting from the body, we have turned to a billion-dollar business for guidance: The toiletry industry. It is important to note that almost all bathroom toiletries and perfumes are toxic and harmful to the body. Another example of the *(evil plot)*, they make worse what they are meant to hide. Even some of the so-called *'natural'* products are questionable. Underarm deodorants such as antiperspirants *(aluminum)* shut down the sweat glands, quite possibly contributing to the cases of lymph ailments and breast cancer increasingly apparent in our society. Therefore, it's best not to tell your body to shut up and shut down, but instead, to clean it out so you can be the sweetie that you truly are. Do not get consumed by savvy marketers, remember what they want and who they are; **REMEMBER WHO U ARE.**

WHEN YOU SMELL TROUBLE

Why do some people avoid going to the washroom when away from home? Is it because of the odor that they may leave behind? *(Oops! No, I mean poops!)* Imagine walking into your own house, confronted by a foul odor and not knowing from where it was originating. Would you try to find the source or just simply spray deodorizers through the house to mask the odor! Most of us would try to find the source. Why is it that when we smell the odor of putrefaction originating from within our own body we hide it as if it's something dirty, pretending it doesn't exist. Is this from embarrassment, or have we been brainwashed to believe it is normal? Maybe that's why we sometimes joke when a friend leaves a horrible smell in the bathroom. Unfortunately, it's because we don't know any better. It's no laughing matter; they are rotting from the inside out. It's a downhill slide when we accept putrid smells coming from the body as normal, for it certainly is not Natural. These smells are signs of worse things to come. This is called unconscious living. **See, Zombies do exist!**

TO THE TIPS OF YOUR TOES... THEY LIE YOU STINK

Most products advertised in the media are designed to mask the symptoms of health problems. Body deodorizers, breath and body fragrances, pills for headaches, lotions for dry skin, topical creams for yeast infections, arthritic pain relievers, weight loss programs, allergy relievers, gastrointestinal remedies and many, many more cure-alls are marketed. Yet none of them address the origin of the problem. This is because if the manufacturer did truly cure the problem, their product would no longer be in demand. Marketing teams are generously paid to convince you that, *'instant and temporary relief'* is what you really want and need. It's a quick fix that ensures the product will be purchased time after time, while never getting to the root cause of the actual problem, only leaving you to suffer. As a result, society is left continually paying, reaching into their wallets to fund fixes that are only temporary at best. Insanity is doing the same thing day in and day out but never reaching the desired outcome. Gentle Daily Cleansing, Structured Water and Whole Plant Based Nutrition not only clean and restore your digestive tract but also take the toxic load off your bloodstream, liver, kidneys, lymph system and skin. Why pay them to mask the problem only to become toxic and sick when you can embrace Nature and restore balance and become the Master of Your Health. Invest wisely in your future; you're worth it. **Don't be a stinker, become a thinker.** Love and respect your body from the inside out and the bottom up and you will become as sweet as a rose.

THE WORMS CRAWL IN THE WORMS CRAWL OUT

Willy The Worm,
Will he or wont he come out?!

Most people in our society suffer from pain in the abdominal area, specifically in the large intestine. Stagnation of fecal waste causes trapped gas, infection and inflammation that lead to pain. The large intestine has pockets called haustras from the beginning to the end. These pockets contract in a manner similar to the movement of a snake, pushing the waste along for elimination.

As previously stated, the Ileocecal valve is located at the beginning of the large intestine. Its role is to regulate the passage of foodstuffs, allowing them to pass through on a gradual basis. When pain is experienced in this area, gas is usually the culprit. Gas can hold the Ileocecal valve open, causing waste and parasites to back up into the small intestine. This one-way door will malfunction when fecal debris stagnates in this area. Worms can enter the small intestine from the large intestine, migrating to other parts of the body, creating even more complications. It is important to remember that worms and parasites always accompany every stagnant manure pile, whether down on the farm or down in your belly.

As stated earlier, the average adult has approximately twelve pounds of old stagnant fecal debris and excess mucus hardened along the walls of the large intestine. The most important step towards reclaiming and keeping the health you deserve or reversing sickness is to learn the true art of Gentle Daily Cleansing and Whole Plant Nutritional restoration. Your body is your temple, or better still, the vehicle that you use to drive your energy body around in. Let me propose a question regarding your motor vehicle: *Do you get regular tune-ups and maintenance on your car?* Of course you do, because you want it to last and stay safe. *How about one more example for those who use a vacuum?* When the vacuum bag is full, would you switch it out for an empty one, or leave the full one in and burn out the motor and stink up the house?

Even if you change your diet and start eating properly, you will never experience the vibrant health you could have unless you do two important steps on a continual basis. Flush old toxic waste out of your body daily and restore the vital nutrients that have been depleted from even our fresh and raw foods during the last 50 years. This ultimately allows for the restoration of body tissues and your immune system. Without future buildup of toxic waste, along with an ample supply of dynamically Structured Water and essential vital nutrients, you not only get rid of disease and parasites, but also those who have their hands in your pockets with false promises and cures. It's your choice, a Whole Plant Based Nutritional Lifestyle or pharmaceutical drugs. Toxic fecal waste is the home and breeding ground of parasites, viruses, bad bacteria and fungus. We must break their foothold and hand these low vibrational invaders a well deserved eviction notice!

PARASITE PARTY TEST

Take The Parasite Self Test

1. Do you experience unexplained muscle aches and pains?

 YES_____ NO_____ (YES=1 NO=0)

2. Do you experience normal bowel movements with bouts of intermittent diarrhea or constipation?

 YES_____ NO_____ (YES=1 NO=0)

3. Do you have unexplained weight loss and/or fever?

 YES_____ NO_____ (YES=1 NO=0)

4. Do you have a distended belly?

 YES_____ NO_____ (YES=1 NO=0)

5. Do you grind your teeth while you sleep?

 YES_____ NO_____ (YES=1 NO=0)

6. Do you experience have dark circles under your eyes and/or acne?

 YES_____ NO_____ (YES=1 NO=0)

7. Do you have insomnia or disturbed sleep?

 YES_____ NO_____ (YES=1 NO=0)

8. Have you traveled outside of North America?

 YES_____ NO_____ (YES=1 NO=0)

9. Do you regularly eat unpeeled raw fruits and/or vegetables?

 YES_____ NO_____ (YES=1 NO=0)

10. Do you have pets that sleep in bed with you or do you eat after contact with your pets?

 YES_____ NO_____ (YES=1 NO=0)

Total Score
A score of 3 or higher indicates you may be suffering from Parasites.

SAD SITUATION

Studies have shown that a Whole Plant Based diet not only prevents but also can reverse conditions that a SAD diet creates. Because of the so-called Standard American Diet, aptly called 'SAD', digested food becomes so sticky due to lack of fiber, nutrients and Structured Water, it does not move along at the proper rate. This creates advanced putrefaction (toxic waste) by the time it reaches the large intestine due to the lack of vital life force. The large intestine is a living, breathing organ made up of billions of cells which are too often bathing in this SAD, stagnant, toxic waste. This toxic debris becomes absorbed into the bloodstream, polluting the rest of the body's organs and tissue cells. Sooner or later, the colon can no longer handle this toxic load and all Hell-th breaks loose. Your kids are not lazy or bad. They're just spoiled rotten from the low vibrational water and foods that you bring home. Keep your home a **Freaky Frank** free zone. Either we train ourselves and our family or we end up in treatment.

DOWN & OUT RAISE A LITTLE HELL-TH

A toxic condition over time causes the colon muscle to degenerate. In turn, it begins to lose its tone, becoming spastic but flaccid due to constant infection, which leads to the inflammation and energy drainage of its tissue cells. When your abdominal muscles become soft and begin to lack tone both internally and externally, your lower back muscles will tighten and go into spasm. This is due to its futile efforts to compensate for the lack of tone in the abdominal area. The back muscles must pick up the slack for the intestines and abdominal muscles, which are in a state of coma. In this case the colon is falling down and out causing decreased circulation in the pelvic region. This is where your belt is no longer visible and you can't tell if your shoes are tied.

This will severely reduce circulation to this part of the body affecting the ovaries, uterus, bladder, prostate, and testicles and cause a detour when it comes to your sex drive. Plus everything below such as the hips, legs and feet will experience swelling *(water retention)*, pain, achy joints, gout, poor healing and varicose veins. If the abdominal area is not toned and cleansed, other conditions may arise such as Crohn's Disease, Colitis, Mucoidal Ulcerative Colitis, Diverticulosis, Fistula, Fissures, Hemorrhoids, Ulcers, Hiatus Hernia, Inguinal Hernia, Fibroids and Cancers. How can something so obvious and so debilitating be commonplace? People's intestines are falling outward and downward everywhere I look; it's an epidemic. Is there anybody out there? We need your help. We have become a **zombie nation**. Fight back, people. Eat your veggies, gently cleanse daily, **Take Life In** with Whole Plant Based Superfood Nutrition and become a **Whole Nation**.

HEART ATTACK OR FART ATTACK

Another condition known as the hot air balloon effect is characterized by a super tight stomach protruding outwards. This occurs because of the large amount of trapped gas being produced by the toxic fecal waste, causing a ballooning effect in the large intestine. It can be compared to being six months pregnant. Just think about all the additional pressure that is exerted on the lungs and heart. Remember, hot air rises. This is no different from the manure pile down on the farm. I can remember when I used to go fishing at the pond. We would take a shovel and dig into the manure pile to look for worms. When we dug the shovel into the manure it would release hot, toxic, noxious gas with an ammonia smell that would irritate our eyes. These chemicals are silent but deadly whether outside or inside the body. Many are rushed to the hospital with symptoms of a heart attack when it's just a gas attack. Cry *'Wolf'* too many times and it just might happen.

Lighten up before you tighten up. For those of you around retirement age you may want to say a little prayer regarding your prostate, uterus or ovaries if you are not doing four things. A Whole Plant Based Superfood Diet, Gentle Daily Cleansing, drinking plenty of Dynamically Structured Water and have two healthy, well-formed bowel movements daily. Don't live normal... Live Natural, Live Whole, Be The Cure.

BACK PAIN OR JUST BACKED UP

Do you ever go to the chiropractor because your hips and spine are hurting or out of place? Why not deal with the major cause of the problem first? Then, if needed, see a chiropractor. You need to clean and tone your digestive tract! Weak and toxic abdominal muscles will create many problems for the hips and spine. Remember, a strong core holds everything in place. If it falls apart so will you. About two inches past the Ileocecal valve is the beginning of your large intestine. Here you will find the appendix. This is an endocrine organ that acts as protector, creating infection fighters *(good bacteria)* for the large intestine. Many children and even adults suffer from appendicitis, an inflammation of the appendix. You won't have inflammation unless you have an infection. Usually you won't have infection unless you have putrefaction (rotting waste). One will not have putrefaction if the art of Gentle Daily Cleansing is understood. **It's Tea Time**. Now your digested foodstuffs are sitting in the cecum, at the beginning of the large intestine. Hopefully your haustras *(normal bowel pockets)* are not encrusted with fecal waste or hardened mucus and your colon has the necessary muscle tone to start the last seven feet of the journey to the rectum, where its content is hopefully eliminated. I say, *hopefully* because if your colon can't get rid of it, it becomes stored and has the potential to be leaked through the intestinal wall, back into your bloodstream, similar to seepage from any other waste dump. As you can see by the diagram below, your large intestine sits in front of your spine and on top of your hips. When you back up, you will have back problems. How many times have you gone to the washroom and felt that elimination was incomplete. *If you add this up over the years, where do you think you stand?* **Maybe at the top of a pile**.

THE WALLPAPER EFFECT

What happens when the large intestine lacks proper tone? If the waste cannot be eliminated effectively, it must be stored. The body removes the water from the stagnant waste and compacts it. Layer upon layer of dehydrated fecal waste builds up along the walls of the large intestine, creating a *wallpaper effect*. This toxic waste will gradually leak into the bloodstream causing toxins to build up. This is known as **Toxemia**, which means dirty blood, which leads to acidosis. Imagine a garbage truck working all day. *Where does the garbage go?* Each truck has a compactor; your body is very similar. If it cannot eliminate the fecal waste, it dehydrates it and stores the waste in the lining of the haustras *(normal bowel pockets)* of your large intestine until its Master takes control. Oh, what a toxic silent bomb. Talk about a breeding ground for *bugs*. I guess you can see that we may have a chronic constipation problem on the rise and an intestine ready to fall down and out. I once had a patient who came to the clinic for colon irrigation. While cleansing his large intestine, a red berry was seen leaving his colon, which he said he had not eaten in years. This occurs because if the body cannot eliminate it, the berry will be dehydrated and stored in a cocoon of mucus until you take charge and cleanse, nourish and restore. **Berry Good!**

Layer upon Layer of old fecal waste is like Layer upon Layer of old wallpaper.
THEY BOTH TAKE WORK TO REMOVE

CAPSULES OF CONTAMINATION

When a block is created in the large intestine it will become either herniated or ruptured resulting in a breakdown in the muscular wall. When the wall becomes impacted with fecal waste diverticulae are formed. These are abnormal out-pouchings. This is a lifestyle disease. Diverticular disease was almost unheard of in the 1900s. When these out-pouchings become inflamed due to the infection stored within them, it turns into a condition known as diverticulitis. The majority of the population over the age of forty has diverticulae. They just don't know it because they haven't experienced pain nor had an X-ray to show it. This condition is a symptom of chronic constipation. The waste within the diverticulae is called faecoliths, they can be one-half to three inches in length. These can be brown and spongy or black and brittle, they look like herb capsules. When the large intestine wall heals, these *capsules* are forced out into the intestines and eliminated from the body. Get to the cause and restore this vital organ with Gentle Daily Cleansing, Structured Water that hydrates and heals and Whole Plant Based Superfood Nutrition. This may sound too simple but I assure you, when you remove the blocks you will Naturally Heal. This is Nature's Way, the only way. Put on your boots and return to your roots.

BUN ON THE RUN

The main cause of diarrhea is constipation. It is caused by a block of encrusted fecal waste within the large intestine. Constipation doesn't mean that you do not have a bowel movement. Constipation occurs when you are not experiencing complete evacuation. *Do you strain to go to the washroom? Have you ever had the feeling that you wished a little more would come out? That you need to wipe more than twice, or wished there was a TV in the bathroom?* Stop, Look and Listen. These are all signs that your body is telling you that you need to cleanse the colon or it will do it for you in the form of diarrhea.

Diarrhea is a safety mechanism to save your butt when it's in a constipation rut. Constipation is the perfect breeding ground for parasites, bad bacteria, viruses, fungus and digestive tract diseases from A to Z. Diarrhea becomes the solution to remove your personal manure pile pollution along with these infectious invaders. These deadly invaders give off noxious gas, toxic waste and chemicals, causing infection throughout the large intestine, leading to inflammation. This eventually results in bowel disorders such as Colitis, Mucoidal Colitis, Diverticulitis,

Hemorrhoids, Hiatus Hernia, Inguinal Hernia, Malabsorption Syndrome, Candidiasis and a severe toxic spillover into the bloodstream. As you can see, constipation has a detrimental domino effect on the body that can lead to life-threatening conditions. You can either go to the washroom gently or you will be forced to lighten this toxic load. Get the job done or it's bun on the run. **U** choose.

IGNORANCE IS NOT BLISS

Most people do not want to talk about their poop. They stick their heads in the sand hoping you, or it will go away, because they have been taught that this is an embarrassing topic. There is big money in keeping you embarrassed and from properly understanding how to look after your body's waste management system. Unfortunately, a toxic colon (large intestine) is the breeding ground for disaster. Don't think for one minute that drug companies aren't aware of this scientific fact. The major cause of disease is acidosis, acidity in the blood and tissues. The major cause of acidosis is putrefaction (rotting) of fecal waste being absorbed into the bloodstream from the large intestine. Toxic overload equals increased acidity, which equals fat cell production, pain, inflammation, infection, internal scar tissue formation, cellular mutation, which in turn equals pharmaceutical profits. It can be a crappy life when you choose to live on autopilot (**zombie**). Let me again propose a question, do you believe that you could have any of the following: systemic Candida (fungus in the blood), leaky gut, chronic fatigue, headaches, sore throat, skin disorders, heart disease, gout, arthritis, sinus problems and even cancer without your blood becoming toxic and the t issues throughout your body becoming acidic? The list of illnesses is endless. With mismanagement, the colon becomes like a screen door in a submarine; allowing toxins, viruses, bad bacteria, fungus and parasites into the bloodstream, which accelerates the condition we know as acidosis. Some call this **leaky gut syndrome**. The proper term being malabsorption syndrome. I call it preventable and absolutely unnecessary.

TAKE LIFE IN

What do you think the chances are of your body breaking down prematurely or chronic illness emerging if your blood was pure and oxygen and nutrient rich? The reality is that I don't know of anyone who doesn't suffer from toxemia or acidosis on some level in these toxic times. This condition is epidemic and only becoming worse because of processed fast foods, **environmental toxins and pharmaceutical drugs**. To counteract this environmental imbalance each of us must travel greener pastures if a healthy life is our desire. Pure dynamically Structured Water, a fresh and raw alkaline diet, proper gentle daily cleaning and **Whole Plant Based Superfood Nutrition** on a daily basis. The result being an alkaline lifestyle, balanced pH and a pain-free, *dis-ease* free, energetic body. The grass is always greener on our side of the fence. **Take Life In** and raise your vibrational frequency so you can **Take Life On**.

HEAL THE GUT CURE YOUR BODY

"Candida, the drill bit immortal predator that will not just eat you, but out-live you." Gently Cleanse Daily!

- Dr. Darrell Wolfe, Doc of Detox

CANDIDA ALBICANS: DRILL BIT PREDATORS

Gut bacteria, which number more than 100 trillion cells, have more of an impact on our health than medical experts previously realized. But not all gut bacteria are created equal. Among other things, 'good' gut bacteria improve digestion, strengthen the immune system, and manufacture the vitamins your body needs. On the other hand, 'bad' gut bacteria can cause digestive disorders, mental problems, skin conditions, autoimmune disease, internal scar tissue formation and all kinds of other challenges and that's just the tip of the iceberg.

When you think of the potential consequences of unhealthy gut bacteria, digestive problems are probably the first thing that comes to mind. Many doctors will begin by prescribing drugs like antacids to help people struggling with these issues and then move to even stronger drugs, such as antibiotic and steroids, but those medications only address surface level symptoms. They don't get to the root cause of the problem, which are unhealthy gut bacteria and an out of fungal control problem.

A healthy gut isn't made by trying to rid your body of gut bacteria altogether, as the medical system attempts to do by using antibiotics. Doctors will even use antibiotics on viral infections, which is useless. The food industry uses antibiotics indiscriminately on factory-farmed animals and fish. Antibiotics will wipe out the bad bacteria, but will also wipe out the good bacteria; this will weaken your immune system, which is essential for your vital health. Research also suggests that good bacteria destroyed by antibiotics will not replace themselves, to re-establish your good bacteria; the only permanent way is to take personal action on a daily basis. A healthy gut is made by balancing the bacteria—limiting the bad guys through lifestyle and encouraging the good guys to grow strong through gentle baby steps daily - you're only as strong as your good bacteria. The gut is the gateway to health; if your gut is healthy then so are you - end of story.

The bacteria in your gut will either be your body's strongest alliance for getting or keeping you vibrantly healthy or it will become your worst enemy. Most people don't realize it but what and how you eat, drink, think and do on a daily basis is the main contributor in causing a mutation to your gut bacteria, which represents the majority of your immune system. Your immune system is a complex network of specialized cells and organs that work hard to differentiate between what is beneficial and what is harmful to the human body. Groundbreaking studies are being released every day, revealing the connection between gut bacteria and practically every aspect of human life, for example, the skin and the gut. There's been a lot of confusion about skin conditions over the years. Much of it comes from the common misguided idea that the symptoms of a condition must appear in the same spot as the condition itself. For many skin conditions, the problem isn't with the skin itself, it's with an unhealthy gut. Your large intestine and your skin are one in the same, meaning your skin mirrors the state of your large intestine's health.

Yeast overgrowth, often referred to as Candida, is the most common condition I see in my clinic at the Doc of Detox. These days, almost everyone I consult has become prey to this drill bit predator known as, Candida. A Candida yeast infection is the baby brother of the full- blown Candida fungal infection.

In the 'so- called average, normal' person, Candida yeast infections exhibit problems in the gastrointestinal tract, mouth, genital area and on and in the skin. It is important to treat this yeast infection quickly and effectively because without taking personal action it will become a full-blown Candida fungal infection. Taking a treatment for a yeast infection will not kill or eliminate the fungus, it will reduce the symptoms temporarily but it will not get to the root cause. Candida fungus is the silent killer that robs you of your life force, controls how you feel, and even how you think. The only place that you will find a cure is within yourself when you make a permanent healthy lifestyle change. This is why at the Doc of Detox; our first goal with our patients is to create a daily road map for success tailored to suite each and every person taking into consideration age, condition and how they process their emotions. First, we must know where we are going, second is how to get there and third is to be trained so that we become the master of the body that we have been given.

How do we know when something is wrong with our gut bacteria in the first place?

If you suffer from symptoms such as regular headaches, irritability, brain fog, low energy, recurring fungal infections, skin problems, scar tissue formation, ongoing pain and inflammation, mood swings, depression, digestive disorders, bloating, fatigue, if you have a pepperoni- like odor, have a fish-like odor coming from your vagina or if you have white deposits on the back of your tongue and if you have cravings for sugar, or carb-rich foods like pasta, or bread - then it's very likely that you have systemic Candida, which at the very least creates an unhealthy internal environment. Systemic Candida means these drill bit predators have created microscopic holes through the mother of all organs, your large intestine. When these drill bit predators, known as Candida fungus drill pin-like holes through your intestines, this creates inflammation, which sets up a reaction called scar tissue formation. The scar t issue is formed to prevent pain, inflammation and fungus from spreading.

As we know scar tissue cuts off circulation, which in turn can cause the intestine to lose muscle tone and become flaccid. If this condition continues, just like weeds in a garden, the scar tissue will also continue to spread out of control. As the scar tissue spreads and takes over the intestine it will become what we call, 'lead pipe disease.' Lead pipe disease is when the intestine lacks tone but is stiff with scar tissue. You know the saying, 'Grandpa is getting weaker, and he is becoming stiff as a board!' Once the Candida drills its holes into the intestines it gains access to the river of life, your arterial system, its game on or should I say, game over for the uninformed and mistreated.

How do you know if your gut bacteria are out of balance? Here are the common signs and symptoms of Candida overgrowth:

- Skin and nail fungal infections such as athlete's foot, ringworm and toe/ toenail fungus.
- Feeling tired and worn down or suffering from chronic fatigue, fibromyalgia, chronic pain and muscle weakness.
- Digestive Issues: Gas, bloating, heartburn/acid reflux, constipation, diarrhea and IBS/IBD.
- Ear, nose and throat infections: Oral thrush, sore throat, ear ache, sinus infection/sinusitis.

- Autoimmune Diseases: Hashimoto's Thyroiditis, Rheumatoid Arthritis, Ulcerative Colitis, Lupus, Psoriasis, Scleroderma and Multiple Sclerosis.
- Migraines, headaches and dizziness.
- Mental Disorders: Autism, difficulty concentrating, poor memory, lack of focus, ADD/ADHD, OCD, brain fog, irritability, mood swings, anxiety and depression.
- Skin Issues: Eczema, Psoriasis, Rosacea, Acne, Hives, Rashes and Itching.
- Vaginal infections, urinary tract infections, rectal itching, or vaginal itching.
- Low sex drive.
- Severe seasonal allergies or itchy ears.
- Strong sugar, alcohol and refined carbohydrate cravings.
- Vitamin and Mineral Deficiencies.

You might be wondering, *"What on earth is Candida?"* Candida is a fungus, which is a form of yeast; a very small amount naturally lives in the mouth and intestines. Candida's job is to aid in digestion and nutrient absorption, but when it is overproduced it breaks down the walls of the intestine by drilling microscopic pin- like holes through it, thus gaining free access to the bloodstream, releasing toxic byproducts into the body, causing what is known as the leaky gut or malabsorption syndrome. Over the short term, this isn't such a big deal since our immune system is designed to handle short breaches in security. But over the long-term the immune system becomes overwhelmed, allowing toxins to flood into the bloodstream. This can lead to countless different health problems ranging from emotional disorders, digestive issues to autoimmune diseases. Due to the domino effect created by leaky gut, autoimmune diseases can be difficult to manage because the body is literally attacking itself. When it comes to the medical system and the average health care practitioner, it is difficult for them to find the true cause of the condition due to how they were educated. When a practitioner is educated into weakness, they do the same for their patients. More and more research is linking autoimmune diseases to an unhealthy gut.

9 Major Signs of Leaky Gut

1. Digestive issues such as gas, bloating, diarrhea or irritable bowel syndrome (IBS).
2. Seasonal allergies or asthma.
3. Hormonal imbalances such as PMS or PCOS.
4. Diagnosis of an autoimmune disease such as rheumatoid arthritis , Hashimoto's thyroiditis, lupus, psoriasis, or celiac disease.
5. Diagnosis of chronic fatigue or fibromyalgia.
6. Mood and mind issues such as depression, anxiety, ADD or ADHD.
7. Skin issues such as acne, rosacea, or eczema.
8. Diagnosis of Candida overgrowth.
9. Food allergies or food intolerances.

The primary purpose of the immune system is to produce antibodies against germs and large particles. Unfortunately, when a person starts to enter into autoimmunity, the immune system can sometimes mistakenly identify its own cells as foreign. The immune system fails to recognize its own cells and produces antibodies against its own tissues, also known as auto-antibodies. It's like your body declared war on itself, your healthy cells on one side and your immune system on the other – you have actually become allergic to yourself. Chronic inflammation and tissue degeneration, pain, and loss of function are all signs of autoimmunity. A large part of the population suffers from autoimmunity. One out of five people with autoimmunity will move onto an autoimmune disease, this is because our health care, medical and natural, is based on treating patients instead of training them on how to take care of themselves on a day-to-day basis. Approximately 90 percent of the North American population is struggling with chronic low-grade inflammation that eventually leads to more serious problems like autoimmune disease, accelerated aging, obesity, diabetes, and other serious problems. Most conventional medicine approaches are aimed at masking symptoms, not addressing the true cause.

Regardless of the particular disease, the underlying cause is an overactive immune system attacking the body. What distinguishes one autoimmune disease from another is simply the body part that is under attack. This is caused by leaky gut, which causes a domino effect on the rest of the body.

In fact, there are over 100 different diseases that can be experienced from Candida overgrowth, but in actuality, these diseases are just symptoms from a leaky gut but more specifically a dysfunctional large intestine. The symptom name depends on where the fungus is located. The initial stages of a Candida infection will very often start within the mouth, urinary tract and gut then work its way inwards.

As more studies are done on Candida infections, it is being realized that this yeast is a serious contributor to many illnesses that now includes:

- Alcoholism

- Asthma
- Addison's Disease
- Chronic fatigue syndrome
- IBS
- PMS
- Depression
- Anxiety Disorders
- Psoriasis
- Arthritis

A healthy gut is full of good bacteria that feed on yeast keeping the levels low, which stops the yeast from becoming a problem. The yeast becomes problematic when it grows beyond normal levels and spreads throughout the gastrointestinal tract. The healthy or 'good' bacteria in your gut typically keep your Candida levels in check. However, the Candida population can get out of hand if a round of antibiotics kills too many of those friendly bacteria, causing leaky gut syndrome. The main causes of leaky gut are bad bacteria, Candida fungus, parasites and diets high in refined carbohydrates, gluten, sugar and dairy, consuming alcohol and medications such as oral contraceptives, acetaminophen, ibuprofen, antibiotics, steroids and acid-reducing drugs. Environmental toxins like mercury, pesticides and BPA from plastics also cause fungus to create pin-like holes in your intestines. Some other clear-cut signs of leaky gut syndrome are premature aging and the inability to cope with stress.

Unless you are trained to master your body, *you will never escape the maze of unconscious living!*

Here at the Doc of Detox, we discovered a long time ago that there are two sides to creating permanent healing, one being the physical and the other being emotional, which is overlooked by the medical system and most natural health care practitioners. There have been countless studies done by prestigious medical hospitals and universities around the globe. Their conclusion has been unanimous, that all physical pain and ailments have a minimum of 85% emotional attachment. This is why we recommend all of our patients go through our Awakening Transformation Consultation, so that they learn the simple and effective strategies in removing dysfunctional belief systems, which block their healing. Stress can wear you down, make you anxious, increases your blood pressure as it wreaks havoc on your gut! Stress is inevitable, no matter how hard we try to avoid it. Stress isn't the issue — it's learning how to harness your subconscious and overriding dysfunctional belief systems so that you can release your full potential and become the master of your emotions and your own healing. Unmanaged stress raises cortisol levels, which can stop the gut from working properly. If you've been stressed for the past few months (or years, or decades) but haven't acted to manage your stress, you're more likely to have an unhealthy gut. When you finally heal your leaky gut, you will be restoring the largest part of your immune system.

The intestines have a natural permeability that allows small molecules through its lining to absorb vital nutrients. In fact, regulating intestinal permeability is one of the main functions of the cells that line the intestinal wall. Gluten can cause the gut cells to release zonulin in sensitive people. Zonulin is a protein that in time can break these cells apart in the intestinal lining. Other factors such as infections, toxins, stress and age can cause this protective lining to the intestinal wall to break apart.

Once this protective cell lining comes apart, the domino effect is triggered, and you now have a leaky gut. When your gut becomes like a screen door in a submarine, toxins, unfriendly microbes, undigested food particles, and more can escape from your intestines and travel throughout your body via your bloodstream, settling in the weakest links wreaking havoc on your health. Your immune system will then target these "foreign invaders" as pathogens and attack them. The immune response to these invaders can appear in the form of pain, inflammation and rampant scar tissue formation if not addressed in a timely fashion.

Once this infection gets access to the bloodstream from the large intestine it will set up residence in the weakest links - that being the lungs, sinuses, skin, brain, liver, heart and so on. Fungus has a protective coating that prevents the body's immune system from being able to eliminate it effectively. It is the Candida fungus that undermines the immune system causing a vast range of debilitating symptoms. Take the brain for example, Candida is one of the few things that can actually cross the blood-brain barrier and when the fungus roots itself in the brain and sets up its mycelium-like network, the most common symptoms are depression, anxiety, and foggy thinking. Scientists have discovered that your gut bacteria produce neurotransmitters, which directly affect your mood; this is why they call the large intestine the second brain.

Candida fungus cannot root itself into healthy tissue; it has to match itself up with the same vibration, which is unhealthy, low-vibrational tissue. When Candida fungus roots itself into unhealthy tissue, it is the perfect environment for a fungal colony to take over and eventually will spread throughout the whole body. The fungus then begins to wreak havoc on the body, excreting (poops) over 300 different mycotoxins into the blood stream - everything that eats poops. Normally, before this gets out of hand, your immune system would identify and fight off this intruder without any problem. However, that's not the real problem with Candida, the real problem is the 'armor' that this fungus wears. The Candida fungus is protected from your immune system's attack by its cellular membrane; a powerful armor called a "chitin layer." When your immune system becomes depleted, it will no longer have the strength to punch through the chitin layer. Chitin is made up of the same material that the hard exoskeletons of insects like cockroaches are made of! This is why Candida can be so hard to conquer, making it very difficult for a weakened immune system to attack the fungus and win. It is vitally important that you understand that everything is frequency; the frequency within the tissue will determine the health of the inner terrain. The health of the inner terrain will determine what lives there. When the inner terrain has a high-vibrational frequency flowing through the tissues, you will only see the good bacteria flourishing. When the frequency, otherwise, the immune system lowers within the body, the weakest links will lose their vitality first and become prey to the predator, as in the case of your intestines being attacked by Candida fungus. This is why if you wish to eliminate Candida fungus from your body, you must raise the frequency on an emotional and physical level on a day-to- day basis, for this is the only permanent cure. Just like an opera singer can hit the right note that causes the wine glass to shatter, you too can hit the right frequency to cause the Candida to crumble by creating an inner terrain that vibrates vital health. This is why I am adamant with my patients that it is what they do on a daily basis that will determine whether they live a life of joy and happiness or one of pain and suffering.

There are numerous treatments for Candida and strict diets that promise to rid the body of this fungal invasion. Just as there are plenty of weight loss programs and weight loss diets, if they worked, people wouldn't have to do so many. Cleanses will not permanently rid the body of the fungus, they cause the fungus to go dormant. The fungus can stay dormant in your body for months or even years, and the moment you slip up with your Candida diet or maybe you just have a stressful week because you do not know how to process your emotions and your immune system takes a dive, then the fungus will show it's ugly head and your systemic Candida problem erupts like a volcano once again. I have seen countless people continually fail by implementing Candida diets and Candida cleanses into their lifestyle.

GENTLE DAILY CLEANSING?!

In my 35 years, the only thing that I have seen work for my patients is having a personalized lifestyle plan designed specifically to fit their age, condition and routine. It's what you do daily that matters - simple, gentle and effective baby steps repeated daily or you can call in a bulldozer every few weeks or months to lighten the load temporarily. We are crisis driven; why do we continue to create a health crisis? Because the medical system has programed us to believe that we need them to run to our rescue because we are not intelligent enough to look after our bodies and our bodies have forgotten how to heal us. Have you ever noticed how the word extreme has been introduced into the lives of the majority of the population? Whether it's extreme sports, extreme diets or the extreme deep cleanse, it usually does not turn out the way we wished it had. When you take personal action with gentle, loving daily baby steps, you hold the key to a life of joy. It's what you do daily that will create happiness or madness in your life, for the rest of your life.

Candida Albicans is a fungus that is only able to overrun the body when the immune system is compromised or the body is dying or dead. When we pass on, Candida fungus will still be alive and well, eating you from the inside out, because it's designed to break down the body after death. Candida Albicans is anaerobic, just like cancer – being its baby brother. This means Candida fungus require no oxygen to thrive, which makes it immortal.

There are a ton of would-be "cures" and special diets and protocols one can do to try to deal with the overgrowth of Candida. However, this only deals with the symptoms of the problem, not with the root cause. The simple fact is Candida cannot be "starved" to death by a special cleanse or diet. It is an unhealthy low- vibrational lifestyle that caused it and only a healthy high-vibrational lifestyle with day-to-day easy, and gentle steps will cure it. You'll be shocked at how fast and how many of your aches and pains will disappear when you introduce gentle daily cleansing, a whole plant based diet, core exercise, energy medicine, high-frequency nutritional and structured water into your lifestyle.

I have seen thousands of patients over the years, and most of them have been sold on the idea of continually searching for the ultimate Candida cleanse, and then others have spent tens of thousands of dollars on silver bullet therapies such as chelation, drips and the latest greatest breakthrough. I have yet to see anything work more effectively than teaching and training the patient gentle baby steps daily so that they may live a life filled with joy. This is why the Supercharge Your Life Consultation and Awakening Transformation Consultation exist and are so effective at the Doc of Detox. I've given you a bellyful of reasons to rethink the choices you make. Make the right choice, get trained and release the healer within and live Healthy To 100.

"Knowledge is power."

- Thomas Jefferson

DON'T RUSH TO FLUSH

What your poop tells you could save your life

"Everyone Poops, Lighten the Load and Flush the Pounds!"

- Dr. Darrell Wolfe, Doc of Detox

TOILET TRAINING & HABITS

RULES FOR SUCCESS

- Always answer nature's call or prepare for a toxic
- After each meal go to the washroom. This will help to restore the rhythm. Fake it until you make it. Don't wait for the signal, encourage it!
- A stool or small box in front of the toilet will aid in easier elimination. The lower the toilet, the higher the stool, the easier the movement, the bigger the jewel.
- Slow, deep breathing on toilet; no straining. Raise arms over head. Twisting side to side may also help.
- Abdominal clockwise massage after meals, upon rising, and when on the toilet is also beneficial.

FROM THE INSIDE OUT AND THE BOTTOM UP

STOOL STATUS

The stool can tell many things, including the state of your health, what your diet is like and what kind of stress you are under. It's a *'compoohter'* printout. Many doctors believe that people have regular bowel movements whether it is one a day, once every two days, once every three days, four days, or five days. I had one client, who after telling her doctor that she had a movement every seven days, was told that this was normal for her. I believe that you should have two bowel movements a day at the least. The quality of your bowel movement is Nature's way of telling you the level of health you are currently experiencing. Just as you need to monitor what goes in your mouth, stool investigation will give you valuable information regarding your highway to health: the digestive tract.

Your digestive tract is the assembly line for the food you eat. Your bowel movements can give you a clear daily picture indicating whether the most important process of your health is heading in the right direction. Learning what to look for in your bowel movements can prevent illness and suffering now and in the future. **Signs that your digestive system is not functioning properly are:** bad breath, smelly stool and the need to use deodorant in the bathroom and under your arms as well. What indicates a good bowel movement is that the stool does not smell. If you eat three meals a day, you should have three bowel movements per day. If you eat two meals a day, you should have two bowel movements per day.

The bowel movement should start naturally, without any straining or pushing. A normal bowel movement occurs rather quickly, taking no more than about three minutes. If you feel you have the time to read the newspaper while on the toilet then read the comic section and lighten up.

Having books in the bathroom is a good clue that you have internal hemorrhoids and probably external hemorrhoids are here or on their way. A hiatal hernia is just around the corner for this grunter groaner due to all that straining and pushing.

In a normal bowel movement, the stool should have a diameter, which is approximately half the width of your wrist. It should not be so large that it is hard to pass, causes pain or bleeding of the rectum or hemorrhoids. It should not be long and stringy, pencil-thin or composed of small and hard balls.

The stool should be about the same consistency *(density)* as regular toothpaste squeezed from a tube. It should not be soft and watery. It should not be hard and compacted nor cause the toilet to become plugged up, or break the bowl. The stool should be a medium brown color and should not contain dark material from old feces nor black material which may indicate bleeding in the upper GI tract or stomach. It may be slightly colored from certain kinds of foods you recently ate, such as grapes or beets or very dark green vegetables. It should not be yellow, maroon like burgundy wine nor gray. The stool should not have a foul smell if it is entirely composed of the waste from food which was consumed less than 24 hours ago. If you pass gas it should not have a foul smell. Smelly farts may indicate that old, decaying fecal matter is stuck to the walls of your intestines.

The stool should float in the toilet if everything in it is waste material from food that has been properly digested. Stool that has become too compacted, hard and dense due to constipation will usually sink. The stool should not contain a lot of mucus. There should not be any small or large worms or other parasites visible inside or near the stool.

We want to be able to wipe clean and feel a sense of complete evacuation. Wiping clean should only take a few pieces of toilet paper - not a roll. It's amazing how often people do **not** have a sense of complete evacuation. This is a job worth doing right before you're unable to do it at all, so get moving! **It's Tea Time.**

HOW TO TELL
IF YOU HAVE A GOOD STOOL

♦ Is it soft, firm?

♦ What is the color, is it light or medium brown?

♦ Is it free from foul smell, odors?

♦ Does it float?

♦ Was it necessary to strain?

♦ Does elimination take place 15 - 20 minutes after a meal?

♦ Banana shaped?

♦ Is it 5 to 7 inches long?

When You Take Life In

There Will Be NO WASTE!

COMPOSITION OF THE FECES

1. Remnants of undigested foods (Cellulose, fibers, etc.)
2. Remnants of digestible foods which, for one reason or another, did not get digested.
3. By-products or fermentation and bacterial breakdown of foodstuffs.
4. Mucus and salt secretions from the intestines.
5. Bacteria and parasites.
6. Broken down products of blood tissue salts.

Bacteria both dead and alive, usually constitute a quarter to half of the dried feces. With every dump, you eliminate One Hundred Trillion bacteria so it's about time to let go that which does not serve you or Endotoxemia will be your fate.

DID YOU ELIMINATE ONE HUNDRED TRILLION BACTERIA TODAY?

if you did you're on a roll...

STOOL INVESTIGATION

- **Bright red blood** means that the blood is from the anus. It could be from an internal hemorrhoid or from a fistula or other rectal problem. Visit your doctor.
- **Dark red blood** has come from further up in the digestive system. It could mean ulcers or colitis in the splenic flexure area. Visit your doctor.

- **Blackish-red blood** indicates ulceration and bleeding around the hepatic flexure. Visit your doctor.
- **Blood totally black** in color could be from the stomach. Visit your doctor.
- High protein diets with mostly meat produce a dark colored stool. Spinach and other vegetables containing chlorophyll can stain stools green; dark colored food such as blackberries or cherries will stain the stool a darker color.
- **Yellow or orange stool** indicates insufficient bile and is mixed with intestinal contents, or a sign of jaundice or liver disease. Visit your doctor. Carrot juice can also make stools turn an orange color.
- **A reddish wine colored stool** can be caused from eating beets.
- **Iron medication or anemia** could cause slate gray or blackish stool.
- **Excess protein** can cause a black stool.
- **Very dark, olive blue stool** may indicate a diet too rich in protein and fat - putrefaction within the bowel.
- **Dark, hard, offensive smelling stool** may indicate very severe bleeding high in the intestinal region. It may come from an ulcer in the stomach, duodenum, colitis, or Crohn's Disease. Visit your doctor.
- **Gray or chicken soup-like stool** can indicate liver or gall bladder trouble. Visit your doctor.
- **A hard, black stool** means constipation.
- **Flat and thin stool** indicates an obstruction in the lower part of the bowel or spastic colitis (usually around the splenic flexure of sigmoid area).
- **A stool with many small bead-like bubbles** shows fermentative conditions.

- **Slick, slimy stool** could be caused from **jaundice** or cleansing the intestines.

The stool is made up of different kinds of secretions; the color of it will depends on what food we eat.

The transverse colon contains only waste products and no more nutrient absorption occurs beyond this point. The amount of debris, composition, color and odor of feces depends on whether the frequency of the food and water taken in is low or high, meaning dead or alive.

For that perfect stool have a Whole Plant Based Superfood Lifestyle.

THE SCOOP **ON YOUR POOP**

Log yourself for 30 days!

STOOL STATUS	Day **1**	Day **2**	Day **3**	Day **4**	Day **5**	Day **6**	Day **7**
Are you Constipated?							
Do you have Diarrhea?							
Is Stool of Uneven Formation?							
Is it Hard?							
Is it Soft?							
Is it Firm?							
Is it Cracked?							
Is it Smooth?							
Is it Loose?							
Is it Jagged?							
Stool Length (in.)?							

1 of 2

THE SCOOP **ON YOUR POOP**
Log yourself for 30 days!

STOOL STATUS	Day *1*	Day *2*	Day *3*	Day *4*	Day *5*	Day *6*	Day *7*
Stool Width (in.)?							
Does it Float?							
Does it Sink?							
Does it have Little Bubbles on it?							
Does it have Big Bubbles on it?							
Does it contain blood?							
Does it contain mucus?							
Does it Slide out Easily?							
Do you Have to Strain?							
How many bowel movements do you have?							
Stool Length (in.)?							
Time of day							

2 of 2

POTTY TRAINING 101

EDUCATE OR CONSTIPATE YOUR CHILDREN
(POOH-TEA)

Children have worse bowel problems than any other sector except for seniors. Our children ingest all the toxins that we do, plus all the treats and sweets, which create an imbalance to their delicate digestive tracts. The first step is to stop using our children as an excuse to bring home a truck load of junk. The second step is to do your research on antibiotics and what they can do to these delicate little digestive tracts. Antibiotics should only be considered in life-threatening situations because they can alter your child's inner terrain in a very negative way.

Antibiotics will wipe out your child's good bacteria along with the bad, creating a compromised immune system in their digestive tract for years to come. The third step we must teach our children is that having bowel movements daily is as normal as breathing. They must be taught at an early age what a good bowel movement looks and feels like.

If your desire is to have happy, healthy children then proper bowel management is foundational for vital health and the prevention of disease in our little ones.

The most important questions you will ever ask your children are:

How is your tummy?

Did you have a bowel movement today?

Did it come out easy or did it hurt? What did it look like?

We have been taught that poop and bowel movements are an embarrassing topic. This point of view is crippling our children's health. We need to avoid passing on our old worn out beliefs that cause our children needless pain and suffering. These worn out **B**elief **S**ystems may just turn them into **zombies** in the future when they try to medicate their pain away instead of being free of it. Teach your children to answer Nature's Call, instead of ignoring it. This is Nature's Way, the only way, or pay, pay, pay. I can remember, as you may too, countless times of stomach pain and cramps throughout my childhood that scared the heck out of me. I remember being too scared to tell my parents because I thought I was dying and I didn't want to worry them. All this needless pain and suffering could have been avoided if I had been properly informed that what comes out matters but what stays in matters even more. Dollars to donuts you were in the same situation that I was, when you were a kid.

Talk with your children, don't let your children pile their poop up as we did. Teach them well and lighten their load on both emotional and physical levels. Open up to them so they open up to life. One poop at a time. It's **pooh tea** time. www.docofdetox.com/tea

BABIES STOOL

NEWBORN - The first few stools of a baby are a black ointment-like substance called meconium. After a few days the stool will go from black to a greenish brown to greenish yellow. After a week the stool should be a golden yellow with no offensive odor. Breast fed babies have two to four stools a day. A formula-fed baby will have only one to two stools a day due to this being a low vibrational food. Bowel troubles and gas are already on the way for the little one because this is not Nature's Way. This is *'**man**-ipulation'*. Have you ever noticed that a baby will have a bowel movement within ten to fifteen minutes after it has been fed.

This trigger mechanism begins to break down over the first few years because proper toilet training was not taught to toddlers.

Do not cripple your children before they even get started. Make pooh a celebration event. Do not underestimate the power of Pooh. Don't forget about the *'com**pooh**ter'* printout.

TOILET TRAINING FOR BABIES

During the first two years of life, the emphasis is on feeding; after the second year, elimination comes into focus. Children should be applauded and congratulated when they eliminate. From this we will be promoting a child who is proud, assertive and self-sufficient. Do not rush to flush. Take this time to teach your child what having a good bowel movement feels like, smells like and looks like. This will instill in the child that poohing is something worthwhile. When you do flush, put the lid down so the noise does not scare the child.

Be patient and tolerant, keep any ancient ideas and habits you may have away from your children. Do not constipate their thinking with **B**elief **S**ystems that are neither true nor empowering.

Be The Cure - Make them #1 in the business of #2!

Teach your children well, and they
will stay that way. Remember they
are here to help **U** remember.

POTTY TRAINING CHART

...for the little ones

My Potty Training Chart Name:_____					
Monday					
Tuesday					
Wednesday					
Thursday					
Friday					
Saturday					
Sunday					

Log your child for 30 days

ACIDOSIS

WHAT THE CELL IS GOING ON!

"Learn to Eat Right or Be Eaten Alive. Nobody Likes a Bad Acid Trip."

- Dr. Darrell Wolfe, Doc of Detox

WHAT'S EATING YOU

Acidosis is the primary cause of all the symptoms, ailments and diseases we suffer from today. Acidic bodies will experience a rapid decline of their immune system, which in turn creates a low vibrational internal environment where harmful bacteria, viruses, and other pathogens can thrive and multiply. The **pH balance** and the frequency at which your cells vibrate will dictate what and who will live there. The bloodstream is the most critically buffered system of the entire body, far more sensitive than any other. Arterial and venous blood must maintain a slightly alkaline pH: arterial blood pH = 7.41 and venous blood pH = 7.36. Because the normal pH of arterial blood is 7.41, a person is considered to have acidosis when the pH of blood falls below this value.

When excess acidity (acidosis) must be neutralized, our alkaline reserves (minerals) run the risk of becoming depleted, leaving the body in a weakened condition. Just as your body so is the soil. Calcium is the main mineral drawn from your bones to buffer down an acidic condition in an attempt to protect and keep your body in an alkaline state. This can lead to early onset Osteoporosis.

BONE UP - It's Not A Disease Osteoporosis is not a disease, it is a natural course of life. All elderly people have Osteoporosis to some degree, but to suffer from it is not normal. Medicine has turned it into a disease at the wishes of the drug companies just as they have now made Obesity into a disease *(evil plot)*.

For every new disease there is a new drug, the promise of a new breakthrough and a brighter future. It's wake-up time for the unconscious living. We need to eat right or be eaten alive. Osteoporosis is a very confusing condition for people. Most people think they can eliminate it with milk, eating plenty of dairy products and ingesting calcium supplements. In reality, the instances of osteoporosis are very rare in countries where the people do not consume milk or dairy products. Milk and dairy products are acidic so we are being milked for our money. The largest mammals on the planet do not take in dairy products or calcium supplements; they stay alkaline by eating a fresh and raw Whole Plant Based diet and by drinking plenty of high frequency water, the way nature intended.

Osteoporosis is a symptom of chronic acidosis. The body is literally being eaten away. It is in a state of emergency. The body, in its innate intelligence, will steal calcium from the bone in attempts to delay, as long as possible, a heart attack, stroke or even cancer. As the bone mass becomes depleted, the condition is called Osteoporosis. Just as a raging forest fire eats anything that gets in its way, an acid pH out of control, will rage through your body. Similar to the way we put out the forest fire by drenching it with water, the only way to effectively treat Osteoporosis is through an alkaline lifestyle.

Osteoporosis is reversible. We need to saturate the body with dense, **Phytonutrient Rich Superfoods** and cleanse the body gently on a daily basis to remove the toxic waste build-up. This is our only choice. It is our only true defense. Calcium deposits are likely to form if action is not taken. They can be found in any part of the body from your nose to your toes, wherever acidosis is prevalent *(weakest link)*. Examples of this are: calcium deposits in the breasts, kidney stones in the kidneys and gallstones in the gallbladder.

The wastes produced from most foods we consume are highly acidic. Acidosis is a main contributor to premature aging whether it's a crack in your face or a crack in your bones. Acid waste is excreted from the body by the colon *(large intestine)*, kidneys and sweat glands. If this waste is not excreted in a timely fashion it will circulate in the blood and migrate throughout the body tissues. When your liver gets overburdened and can no longer process this acidity, fat cell production must take place as a storage site for this acid to protect vital organs, bones and blood from further damage. **Embrace an alkaline lifestyle** or embrace a bigger, unhealthy **U.**

When you keep your blood clean, your body will be lean and your mind will be keen!

- Dr. Darrell Wolfe

THE PRESSURE'S ON

Acidic waste, if not eliminated, will gradually accumulate in the capillary blood vessels, resulting in plaque buildup. To neutralize the acidity within the blood, the arterial walls must give up their minerals thus causing microscopic cracks within them. Your body, in all its wisdom, repairs these mineral deficiencies by producing cholesterol to goop up these cracks. Cholesterol has the consistency of candle wax. As long as this blood acidosis continues so will your high cholesterol problem. The medical system and the pharmaceutical companies, in all their wisdom, will try to convince you to go to war with your cholesterol levels instead of creating harmony within your body. Cleansing the toxins out and restoring the vital nutrients that are needed for your vital health and well-being must be done on a daily basis to be permanent. If you do not learn to work in harmony with your body then thickening of the arterial walls and the blood will occur. This can cause blood clots which can lead to a heart attack or stroke. Currently in North America 50 million people have been diagnosed with hypertension. Just like a river, if you dump enough garbage and toxic waste in, the river will not flow at a proper rate and stagnation will occur. In this situation high blood pressure may become a concern due to the extra force needed to move the blood.

People go to doctors concerned about high blood pressure more than any other condition. The cells will be deprived of their normal supply of oxygen and essential nutrients, thus creating cellular dysfunction and mutation. Moreover, with the capillary blood vessels becoming clogged, the function of every organ is in jeopardy. Accumulating acidic waste will begin to deteriorate organ tissue causing internal scar tissue and serious illnesses in the long run. Let's say your body is like a chain on a bicycle and every link an organ. With the chain, the weakest link will break first.

With your body the weakest organ will accumulate the acidity and '*dis-ease*' will overtake it. Common examples: the pancreas with diabetes, the heart with heart disease, the liver with liver disease, the stomach with ulcers, the small intestine with Crohn's Disease, the large intestine with colitis and on and on. If the cause of premature aging and other diseases lie in acidosis, then the answer to longer life must lie in eliminating such acidic wastes and replenishing alkaline reserves with a **Whole Plant Based Superfood** lifestyle. Invest wisely, your body's counting on **U**.

THE HEART OF THE MATTER

"TICK TOCK... I've got a block!"

- Dr. Darrell Wolfe, Doc of Detox

MY ACHY BREAKY HEART

Heart disease is the number one killer in North America. The number one cause of heart disease is Dead Meat Bacteria. **Dead Meat Bacteria = Endotoxemia** *(endotoxin in the blood)*: After a meal of animal products people suffer from Endotoxemia. Their bloodstream becomes awash with bacterial toxins, known as endotoxins that are present in animal products. These dead meat bacterial toxins are not destroyed by stomach acid, pancreatic enzymes, cooking or even boiling for hours. Animal fat triggers immediate inflammation within the body due to being loaded with endobacteria, even if fully cooked. Saturated animal fat then boosts the absorption of these **endotoxins** into our bloodstream causing arterial paralysis *(high blood pressure)*. Another cause of Endotoxemia i s a greasy, refined carbohydrate meal. This will cause inflammation due to the release of endotoxin, from the outer walls of the bad bacteria that now live in your colon. Endotoxin, if not eliminated daily from your colon through Gentle Daily Cleansing, can and will be absorbed into the bloodstream causing inflammation to the weakest parts of the body or throughout the whole body. 785,000 people will have their first heart attack this year. Forty million plus suffer from heart disease in North America today. 70 million have high cholesterol and one hundred million have elevated LDL, but less than half are being treated for it. Almost 75% of heart attack patients fall within recommended targets for LDL cholesterol, demonstrating that the current guidelines may not be low enough to cut heart attack risk in most who could benefit. Medical studies have stated that we need to get our cholesterol down to the 150mg/dl area. In other words the serum total cholesterol must be lowered to that of the average pure vegetarian. Statin drugs do lower heart attacks but increase the incidence of diabetes. *How would you like to decrease your chance of a heart attack and diabetes at the same time?* A Whole Plant Based diet or drugs, it's your choice. Studies have reported possible links between cardiovascular disease and PCBs, dioxins and pesticides. Because these compounds are fat-soluble, they can be stored in the body and accumulate over time. Studies indicate that these toxins can specifically accumulate in the vessel walls and contribute to arterial plaque formation. Common sources of these compounds include: plastics, fish and seafood *(especially farmed fish)*, processed foods, non-organic and **GM** *(Genetically Modified)* produce, tap water and many cosmetic/beauty/hair products.

In Sweden and many other countries most of these substances, including heavy metals such as lead, are now forbidden. Since they are so long-lived they are persistent and ubiquitous in the environment. The older we get, the higher these levels become within our body tissues. Accumulate, degenerate, mutate or cleanse, hydrate, nourish and restore or you may find yourself on the floor.

Have a Heart - Play it smart Go green like me.

LIGHT HEARTED EATING

The first step is to eliminate animal products, refined carbohydrates and sugar whenever and wherever possible. The second step is to avoid exposure to chemicals, as much as possible. The third step is to learn the art of Gentle Daily Cleansing. We must detoxify to flush out the build-up of cholesterol, endotoxin created from bad bacteria and other acidic wastes that have accumulated and stagnated within the large intestine. This prevents any toxic waste or cholesterol from entering or re-entering the bloodstream. We must take on a Whole Plant Based Food Alkaline Lifestyle approach and eat a good and generous variety of organic vegetables and fruits, as much as possible. These foods contain anti-oxidants and enzymes that assist the body in eliminating toxic substances. You know what they say,

"An apple a day keeps the doctor away." Well, an apple a day can also keep statin drugs and even a heart attack away due to the pectin, enzymes and fiber. Take in plenty of foods that contain healthy fats, these being organic olive oil, coconut oil, nuts, seeds, avocado and fish. Incorporate plenty of organic garlic, onions and cilantro into your diet as these compounds are natural 'chelators' *(binders)* of cholesterol, heavy metals and toxins. Along with this the body needs an ample supply of pure Structured Water daily to eliminate toxic build-up and to prevent further damage. Daily exercise is also a very important factor. We should incorporate 20 minutes a day of core exercise. When you tone your core, you tone your heart. Learn to '*Live Light Hearted*' in all areas of your life.

A HEAVY HEART

The large intestine is the major waste disposal system for the body. Just like an artery, waste can build up along the walls and even become blocked without us being aware. It's not how much comes out but what stays in that can be your downfall. This accumulated toxic waste will eventually be absorbed into the body and overburden the liver. In turn the waste will not be eliminated efficiently and will be left to circulate in the bloodstream. All blood goes to the heart so it is just a matter of time before the waste that clogged your large intestine will now clog the vital arteries of the heart.

From here we see mineral depletion, decreased oxygen, infection, inflammation and internal scar tissue formation on and within the heart. The more fresh and raw live foods you eat the more Life you will have surging through your arteries. Lighten the load in your large intestine, bloodstream, liver, kidneys and lymph system. Lighten up - don't tighten up. Open your mind so you may open your heart and get to... **The Heart of the Matter**. Let Love In. Let Life In. Be The Cure **U** Wish To See!

ALKALIZE OR DIE

Dr. Theodore A. Baroody states in his book *'Alkalize or Die'*, *"The countless names of illnesses do not really matter. What does matter is that they all come from the same root cause - too much tissue acid waste in the body!"*

Dr. Otto Warburg states, *"Cancerous tissues are acidic, whereas healthy tissues are alkaline."* He then states, *"All normal cells have an absolute requirement for oxygen, but cancer cells can live without oxygen, a rule without exception."*

Dr. Warburg states, *"Deprive a cell of 35% of its oxygen for 48 hours and it may become cancerous."* He then states, *"Even though cancer cells are eliminated entirely through an operation, they reoccur because the acidic surroundings still remain after the operation."*

To help prevent this, we should stop the domino effect that creates acidosis by having an alkaline lifestyle. To support this reduce stress, exercise, drink plenty of Structured Water, gently cleanse daily and restore all essential nutrients on a daily basis. Nothing is permanent unless done daily. Welcome to Planet Earth.

Almost 99% of the components of food that we consume every day are composed of carbon, nitrogen, hydrogen, and oxygen with only 1% minerals. Our vegetables today only contain very few minerals in small amounts. That is why even a very large quantity of vegetables eaten is unable to meet your nutritional needs in neutralizing these acidic wastes and building the real **U**. Hippocrates, the Father of Medicine stated, "***Let food be thy medicine and medicine be thy food.***"

"Every single person who has cancer has a pH that is too acidic"

As I stated before, the food chain is broken and those in power have no intention of fixing it. Medicine has not been about food for 65 years and the food has and is being adulterated and depleted as you read this, even the fresh and raw is limping to the grocery stores. The United States Senate Bill 284, Dr. Charles Northern states, "*In the absence of minerals, **vitamins have no function**. Lacking vitamins, the system can make use of the minerals, but lacking minerals **vitamins are useless**.*" The Biochemical Institute of the University of Texas examined changes in food composition of nutrients in 43 garden crops from 1950 to 1999.

Their findings were as follows: 6% decrease in Protein, 16% decrease in Calcium, 9% decrease in Potassium, 15% decrease in Iron, 38% decrease in B2, 20% decrease in Vitamin C.

The food grown today no longer has all the vital nutrients nature intended for our body. This is why I have my patients incorporate the planet's most dense Phytonutrient Whole Plant Based Superfood into their diet for whole body healing and protection; so they may thrive and Master Their Health. This is foundational for everyone. Do your research. Trust no one until they have earned it. **Your body depends on U**.

THE DOMINO EFFECT

"Have you ever thought that if one thing hadn't happened, a whole set of things never would have either? Like dominoes in time, a single event repeated enough kicked off an unstoppable series of changes that gained momentum and spun your health out of control, and nothing was ever the same again. Until you Take Life In."

- Dr. Darrell Wolfe, Doc of Detox

WHAT A BLOODY MESS

Once this game starts you will definitely want it to stop. Toxemia, also known as dirty blood is caused by a lack of essential nutrients and a multitude of chemicals in the foods, air and water we ingest everyday. To add fuel to the fire, the absorption of stagnant toxic fecal waste from the large intestine *(colon)* into our bloodstream, is creating an acid spill-over. It follows, that if the large intestine is operating properly, you won't absorb this toxic fecal waste. Unfortunately, this is not the case with the majority of the population, including the people we love. We have been downloaded incorrect information. We have been duped.

The average healthy diet will give you a life of misery because it is mineral and nutrient deficient and loaded with chemicals. **We are what we eat**. It is hard to measure misery when everyone you know is in the same Bloody Mess.

You hold the power of Life and Death in your hands.
We either create or destroy.

You choose.

PH ON

When your bloodstream becomes overburdened by these deadly bowel toxins *(poisons)* and lacks essential nutrients to support Life, acidosis is the result. The liver is called into action to help filter out these toxins from the blood stream. The blood stream is the most critically buffered system of the entire body, far more sensitive than any other. Arterial blood must maintain a slightly alkaline pH: arterial blood pH is 7.35-7.41, the ideal pH of arterial blood is 7.41. A person is considered to have acidosis when the pH of blood is 6.8-7.24. A Blood pH drop below 7 can lead to a coma and even death due to severe acidosis. Under 6.8 pH, *'death'* will come knocking. pH is like a light switch: only **U** hold the power to turn it ON or OFF, so tune in and turn on. **Embrace Nature, Embrace the Real U!**

LIVE R DIE

When we are dealing with a malfunctioning large intestine, the liver must work much harder to keep the sensitive balance in the bloodstream. Your liver already plays a role involving over 500 different functions for the body. In addition, it now must pick up the slack and handle the toxic waste developing from the large intestine.

The liver says to the large intestine *(colon)*, *"I can't believe this! Sewage disposal is your job; are you trying to deplete me of my energy and poison this glorious body?"*

"No of course not," replies the colon, *"I can't do my job. My Master eats glicky, sticky, gooey, processed, fried, chemical-laden food and has been made to believe we can handle this. She watches too much TV, gets her health tips from magazines and her friends who know just as much as she does. My Master keeps talking about* **new and improved** *but I never get to see it, much less feel it. Now I've got twelve pounds of toxic fecal waste stuck to my walls, I've lost my muscle tone and I'm pooped out."*

Please forgive her, she knows not what she does. *"I now understand your plight, my dear colon, and I realize the responsibility must always fall back to our Master. Does your*

Master not know that Gentle Daily Cleansing and Whole Plant Based Nutrition is the key to end all her pain and suffering? The word around the body is, she thinks all this pain and suffering is normal and out of her control."

The colon suddenly bursts out in a chuckle and says, *"I'll show her what out of control is when she has diarrhea and I turn her **brown** eyes **blue**."*

The liver, being a team player, works overtime until it becomes chronically fatigued. In turn, the owner of the body starts experiencing Chronic Fatigue, go figure, as well as aches and pains throughout her whole body. Off to the doctor.

The doctor says, *"You're doing great for an average person of your age."* He adds that the Chronic Fatigue and Fibromyalgia *(pain in the muscles throughout body)* she suffers from, are average and quite ordinary.

He writes a prescription to numb her senses. **Thanks a lot, Doc!** He may consider her an average person, but the occurrences inside her body are anything but normal or ordinary.

"You are EVERYTHING! Choose Wisely on how someone treats you. That's why they call it a treat."

- Dr. Darrell Wolfe 'Doc of Detox'

ACIDOSIS ON THE MOVE

Symptoms are simple, fast moneymakers. Instead of society drugging her to shut her down and to shut her up, why don't they just get their hands out of her pockets and search for the true cause. Causes take dedication; being involved does not mean dedicated. Why don't they just come from their heart and find out why she's truly hurting? Roughly 5 million Americans have Fibromyalgia. This means that 1 in 50 or 2% of the entire American population suffers from Fibromyalgia, the second most common musculoskeletal ailment, after Osteoarthritis. 90% of Fibromyalgia fighters are female. Fibromyalgia is acidosis and internal scar tissue formation of the muscle tissues, **end of story**. You're getting eaten from the inside out. Read: '*Web of Destruction*' and '*Scarred For Life*' for a deeper understanding. Fibromyalgia is a symptom of a poorly managed body. Being compared to the average person is not a good thing. Our medical system changes its definition of normal every few years to suit the majority, due to the decline of the so-called average person's normal health. How convenient *(evil plot)!*

Liver toxicity is becoming more common as a result of our exposure to higher toxicity levels in our daily lives. Liver toxicity develops as a result of being overwhelmed by too many toxins. This will exhaust the liver of its vital energy and essential nutrients resulting in lowered immunity.

Damage can be done to the liver by chemicals, toxic substances such as heavy metals, prescription medications, cigarettes, recreational drugs and alcohol. The liver plays a crucial role in the detoxification of the body by cleaning the blood of toxic chemicals. Harmful toxic substances that enter the bloodstream from the large intestine *(colon)* are broken down and metabolized by the liver into a water soluble form. Made harmless, they now can be flushed out of the body through the bile or the kidneys. Truly, the real problem is, everybody wants a piece of the action. The problem always starts off as something small but turns out to be a nightmare because we turn our backs on Nature and embrace **man**-ipulation. You know what has to be done. **Take control - Be The Cure!**

**NEVER LOVE ANYBODY WHO
TREATS YOU LIKE YOU ARE ORDINARY**

- OSCAR WILDE

NOWHERE TO RUN NOWHERE TO HIDE

Symptoms of liver toxicity may be acute, severe and very noticeable or come on gradually as a chronic problem. It is possible for non-severe liver toxicity to cause chronic conditions such as, fatigue, depression, mental illness, headaches, skin conditions, low libido, fibromyalgia and even cancer. Skin disorders often develop as a result of toxins flooding the bloodstream as they cannot be detoxified by the liver fast enough. Since the blood cannot be cleansed at this rate, excess toxins are then released, as a safety valve, through the skin to protect vital organs and bones thus causing breakouts of red, itchy patches. Age makes no difference to toxemia.

Allergies are another symptom of liver toxicity. A liver that is overwhelmed with toxicity will malfunction and will not be able to effectively break down any new incoming toxins. This will create a hypersensitivity to the external environment, chemicals and foods ingested. Foods that were once digested with ease will now turn on you. If your body cannot process it then it becomes a poison. In other words, you are becoming allergic to life. 60 million people now suffer with seasonal allergies, a large percentage of these being children; this is the worst it has ever been, go figure. Check their bowels, Mom and Dad.

Fatigue, loss of appetite, nausea, abdominal pain and vomiting are also often symptoms of liver toxicity. Palpation of the liver is a method used by physicians to check whether there is tenderness or enlargement of the liver. Do not confuse trapped gas caught in the upper right side of the colon for gall bladder or liver problems.

Rising levels of ammonia in the blood is another symptom of liver malfunction. Ammonia is a by-product of protein being broken down by bacteria in the intestines. This is resolved by proper food combining, better food choices and Gentle Daily Cleansing to eliminate the stagnant putrefaction. Now let's get back to our story. The liver now has to do much more than its share of cleansing because of the toxic blood condition caused by the failing large intestine *(colon)*, which is in a coma. What do you think is one of the major side effects when the liver is overloaded with toxins?

It can no longer burn body fat efficiently and the toxins are now stored in fat cells... Hello, weight gain! Let me say this another way. When the body is overloaded with toxins it transfers its energy away from burning calories and redirects the energy to support detoxification. It's in a state of crisis. This burden of toxic waste caused by a sluggish large intestine that is still in a coma, has exhausted the liver. The liver now has to call on a neighbor for help. The next in line in the domino effect are the kidneys. **Hello kidneys.**

ARE YOU KIDNEY-ING ME?!

The kidneys aren't so happy about taking on this extra burden either. They've already felt the added pressure both physically and chemically. The kidneys sit just behind the large intestine which has become a cesspool leaking toxic waste for many years.

"Great, now I'm going to get calcium deposits, internal scar t issue and crystallization from taking on this acid waste." The kidneys scream out, *"You P me off. Our job is to purify body fluids. We're not meant to take on these heavy bowel toxins. What are these poisons?"*

They're not toxins occurring from normal metabolism. These are chemicals and toxic waste from the large intestine that should never have entered the body's system in the first place.

"I demand a clear answer not a toxic one and don't Kid Me." The liver answers back, *"Nothing is clear anymore, especially the body fluids, I have done my best. Talk to the large intestine, but I doubt he will answer, he's been in a coma for some time now."*

The kidneys then shout back, *"Easy for you to say, you can still function on 25% and rehabilitate much easier than I can. Once I get into trouble, I am in big trouble and it usually just goes from bad to worse. Call me a worrywart but I don't want to end up on life support (dialysis)."*

The kidneys must now carry this acid torch and they're burning mad. They do their best but as the months go by, chronic lower back pain sets in due to the overload of toxic waste causing severe acidosis, mineral depletion and oxygen deprivation. Other warning signs are beginning to show up from the overworked kidneys: Kidney stones *(calcium to buffer acidity)*, sweaty palms *(kidneys in a fever state)*, under-eye baggage, frequent urination and bladder infections. Internal scar tissue and crystallization are now forming in kidney tissues due to severe acidosis, and last but not least, excess weight gain around the kidney region. Most people know these as *Love Handles*.

Fat cells must be created to store toxic acidity or someone may have an unexpected trip to the hospital with kidney failure. The kidneys can no longer take on the brunt of this cesspool *(large intestine)*. They are waking up at night in a cold sweat from dialysis nightmares. From here, the next domino falls into the holding tank known as the bladder. Skitter scatter, she's getting fatter.

A BLADDER MATTER

Let's talk about the bladder. It sits just in front of the sigmoid colon, the last part of the large intestine. The tissues of the bladder have been under attack physically and chemically for quite some time now, soaking in the toxic waste that has entered the body from the large intestine; this being the root cause of most bladder infections. The same situation is true for the prostate, ovaries and uterus that reside in the same neighborhood as the colon *(large intestine)*. It is no coincidence that there is a high incidence of fibroids *(mutated scar tissue)* and cancer in this area, go figure. Increased acidity equals tissue inflammation, which leads to internal scar tissue formation resulting in decreased circulation and increased stagnation. Hello, cellular mutation. This results in fibroid formation for the **zombie nation**. Skitter scatter, back to the bladder.

How many people do you know who find themselves going to the washroom two, three or four times a night? This toxic waste that has come from the colon is now forced into the kidneys and will irritate and in flame any tissue it encounters. Remember, it's an acid trip. This toxic sediment is not only irritating the bladder but also its neighbors: the prostate, ovaries and uterus. This toxic waste is now settling and building up on the bottom of this sac- like organ known as the bladder. The tissue becomes inflamed and irritated due to this toxic waste. The bladder becomes hypersensitive contracting into spasm to protect the inflamed tissue. It can now only hold small amounts of urine. The toxic waste will continue to irritate, inflame and degenerate the bladder tissue, causing internal scar tissue and crystallization to form.

This will continue until the root cause is released from its coma through Gentle Daily Cleansing and Whole Plant Based Nutrition. So Take Life In or check out. Now you understand the mystery of why you have to urinate so often. It is 3 o'clock in the morning and it's the fourth time you feel pressure in the bladder area. So it's out of bed and off to the bathroom again. Relief is only seconds away. Finally you get to the toilet but – what's this? Only a few drops come out. Remember, your bladder is hypersensitive from the inflammation and lack of elasticity due to the internal scar tissue. Many people now have to wear '*Depends*' because of the constant **drip, drip, drip**.

The valve that holds the urine back has been infected and inflamed for so long that the tissue has become weakened and unable to shut down properly due to hardened internal scar tissue, just like the bladder. Maybe you recall, I said that scar tissue spreads like a weed if not dealt with. Just as a steel valve will rust, scar tissue and crystallization will make a tissue valve sticky. How will we ever rest and repair with all this interrupted sleep... **drip, drip, drip.** *How many people wear Depends?* It's a multi-million dollar business. These companies are counting on you never to take control or have control. That's right, there's nothing you can do for yourself, so you better pick up some more big boy diapers. We have a choice. **Depends or Cleanse.**

IT'S YOUR BUDDY

Your body talks to you continually; Stop, look and listen, learn to feel what it is telling you. Unless you answer its call you will have more than a broken heart. Your body talks to you continually whether you're listening or not. A negative emotion or pain is your body's way of telling you that you are not in line with your health or your higher purpose. Ignore this loving communication or try to suppress it with drugs and you will pay more than just financially. Your body will warn you until all hell-th breaks loose. We call this the domino effect. First a sluggish toxic colon, then the blood, liver, kidneys, bladder, prostate, uterus, ovaries and soon the lymph system will become toxic and highly acidic. These occurrences all come into effect because you've never been taught to understand what your body is trying to tell you.

Pain and odor are major signals from your body crying out for your help. You are the Master of this body. You hold the power to create or destroy. Choose wisely. You have a choice to detoxify with Gentle Daily Cleansing, hydrate with Structured Water and nourish your body with Whole Plant Based Nutrition or turn to drugs to suppress and shut down these warning signs. Ignoring or shutting down these symptoms (warning signs) does not make for a good relationship. When couples do not communicate they suffer and create pain in their relationship. If harmony is not reached, divorce may be the outcome. If you have not learned how your body communicates with you or you continue to ignore your body then pain, premature aging, disease and maybe even premature death may be the final chapter. When an issue is not dealt with it only gets worse. It would be wise to have a *'heart-to-heart'* talk with your body. Learn to listen. It's your buddy.

COMMUNICATION BREAKDOWN

So here we go. There is still no proper communication happening between you and your body. The first logical and most basic step has not been taken, *'Potty Training 101'*. The kidneys can no longer take on the extra burden of toxic waste once they have reached their maximum threshold. They become overworked, starting to malfunction and now your bladder is in a tatter. Your skin may be showing signs of the toxic burden; it is known as the third kidney. Signs of this may include premature aging, wrinkles, age spots, dry skin, itchy skin, dry patchy skin, eczema, psoriasis, boils, abscess, acne and even skin cancer. If action is not taken, then the lymph system is next in line to carry the acid burden.

By the time the Domino Effect reaches the lymph system it will be under full attack. The **lymph system** has been backing up on itself since the beginning of the Domino Effect. It has been unable to dump its toxic waste into the colon (large intestine) due to the colon walls being clogged for years. So, how's that for **communication, constipation breakdown?**

WATER LOGGED

The toxic burden of the Domino Effect is now attacking the lymph system - a major part of your immune system. Welcome to the puffball age, when we begin to look and feel bloated! When the body reaches a state of toxic, acidic overload as such, it will retain water, causing the body to gain excess weight *(safety mechanism)*. *Why?* It retains water to dilute the toxins, hoping to put off the inevitable: internal scar tissue, crystallization, cellular degeneration, disease and even organ failure. There will also be a sharp rise in fat cell production to keep the body safe from the increasing acidic condition. No one suffers this long and this much through choice. You suffer because of unconscious living.

What are some of the symptoms that come with a toxic lymph system? Potential symptoms are the following: a sudden increase of weight, hard to keep weight off, swelling of lymph nodes, foul smelling armpits and/or groin region, profuse sweating or never sweating due to lymph system blockage by toxic waste. There can also be water retention, swelling of face, hands, feet, legs, abdomen, dry skin, skin disorders, achy joints, achy muscles, cellulite and a lowered immune system. In addition, toxic waste overflow to breast tissue from the lymph nodes creates swelling, tenderness, pain, cysts, fibroids and may even be linked to breast cancer. The body will always choose fat cell production first to store the toxic waste that it cannot remove. This is to keep the toxic waste as far away from bones and vital organs as possible. Since breasts are composed mainly of fatty tissue they are ready made storage tanks for the unconscious. The majority of the population when they start to retain water, their first impulse is to stop drinking water. This will only add fuel to the fire creating more of a toxic burden. Now is the time to introduce plenty of Structured Water to hydrate and eliminate this toxic burden.

THE WEIGHT ELEVATOR

You know when you have become a human elevator when you eat or drink something and swell up like a balloon. At this point not only your size but also your weight will fluctuate on a continual basis. At this stage in the Domino Effect the only thing still working properly is the elevator. Due to the weakening of the immune system, allergies may begin to appear. Foods or toxins that could be digested and eliminated before can no longer be tolerated due to the excessive burden placed on the liver by a colon in a coma. This morning your belt is on the fourth notch and by tonight it's on the second. Today you can take your rings off, tomorrow you cannot. This morning your shoes fit, but by supper they are too tight. When you're tired these elevator symptoms magnify, becoming even worse. You go on a weight loss program and lose ten pounds in the first ten days but by the following week a couple of pounds are gained back. This happens because you have not opened the door to proper Gentle Daily Cleansing and Whole Plant Based Nutrition. These acidic toxins that are not being eliminated efficiently must now be diluted by retaining water resulting in a false weight gain to protect your tissue cells, bones and vital organs. This is a built-in safety mechanism to shield and reduce the damage until you flush the pounds and restore vital nutrients. If you get tired of this ride push 'L' for **Lighten the Load and get off on Life.**

ORGANS UP IN ARMS

Now all the major eliminating organs are up in arms while one of them still remains in a coma. First, the bloodstream took on this toxic waste from the colon. The burden then traveled to the liver, kidneys, bladder, skin and lymph. The body has more built-in safety mechanisms than one can even imagine. The brain calls a meeting with all the organs showing up except for one: the large intestine; still in a state of a coma.

They all agree that the large intestine has become a breeding ground for toxic chemicals, parasites, viruses, bad bacteria and fungus which are poisoning the rest of the body.

A consensus is reached to temporarily help remove the burden of toxic overload on the other organs caused by the large intestine. Whatever water they can retrieve from the organs or the body's tissues without causing severe dehydration must be sent down to the large intestine. Action needs to be taken in order to flush out some of the encrusted fecal waste, which is causing this acidic problem in the first place. All for one and one for all until the Master Heeds The Call.

EXPLODE, IMPLODE OR LIGHTEN YOUR LOAD

Guess what? Now you have diarrhea. Why diarrhea? Well, almost all cases of diarrhea are caused by chronic constipation. Constipation does not mean you do not go to the washroom. It means that the waste from the colon is not being eliminated completely. There are people who go to the washroom three times a day but still have colon cancer. Also, not everyone will have diarrhea at this point, they are the unlucky ones. They are unlucky because diarrhea is a safety valve and without it you run the risk of heart attack, stroke or other life-threatening conditions. I know diarrhea is an inconvenience but don't we feel much better when the cause of the problem has been temporarily reduced in hopes of buying time until the Master of this body takes charge. Pooped out, but relieved. Even though you feel tired, your body can finally start to rest, restore, and regenerate itself with some of its toxic load eliminated. Your large intestine is now eliminating loose stool. This will continue until the chemical and physical pressure is removed from the other organs. This Domino Effect will keep repeating itself until you have learned the importance of Gentle Daily Cleansing and Whole Plant Based Nutrition. **Answer Nature's call, Lighten the load and flush the pounds. Be The Cure!**

SUPERSIZE ME MEGACOLON

A Toxic Mega Colon is a life-threatening condition. It is also known as toxic dilatation of the large intestine. The dilation is often accompanied by a paralysis *(comatose)* of the muscle movement of the bowel. In more extreme cases, the feces become hard masses inside the colon, called fecalomas **(literally, fecal tumor)**, which may need surgery to remove. A mega colon can either be an acute or chronic condition. Toxic mega colon is usually a complication of inflammatory bowel disease, such as ulcerative colitis, Crohn's Disease and other long-standing infections of the colon. Toxic mega colon can come on very quick in people with severe Inflammatory Bowel Disease. In some cases, it can be triggered from the overuse of certain drugs, including narcotics, drugs used for pain relief and from drugs used for depression, anxiety and nervousness.

Medication can cause abdominal distention *(bloating)*, and sometimes fever, abdominal pain or shock. Other symptoms are rapid heart beat, decreased blood Leukocytosis *(high white blood cell count)* and dehydration. Those who suffer with toxic mega colon often appear quite ill and have a history of several days of diarrhea and abdominal pain. As stated previously, days of continual diarrhea is the body going into rescue mode to lighten the toxic load. Balance would be the main goal for such a process. To restore, one must adhere to a fresh and raw alkaline lifestyle, ample Structured Water, Gentle Daily Cleansing, Whole Plant Based Superfood Nutrition and core exercises to restore balance and tone to the colon. Your body has amazing healing powers when you embrace Nature and support a healthy lifestyle. Take Life In and let go of that which does not serve **U**.

HOLLYWOOD HALL OF PAIN

WORLD FAMOUS GIBB BROTHER

Maurice Gibb, best known for being one-third of the pop band the Bee Gees, died Sunday, January 12, 2003. Gibb was reportedly working on new music with brother Barry *(also of the Bee Gees)* and Michael Jackson before his unexpected death.

Gibb played keyboard, guitar, bass and percussion in the Bee Gees, and sang the high notes in their 3-part harmony. The multi-faceted musician also wrote many of the group's hit songs. The Bee Gees are regarded as musical pioneers, and were inducted into the Rock and Roll Hall of Fame in 1997.

An Unnecessary Untimely Death

The 53-year old Gibb was rushed to Mount Sinai Medical Center on Wednesday after experiencing intense abdominal pain. Doctors discovered the pain was due to a twisted section in his small intestine. Before the operation Gibb reportedly went into cardiac arrest, which weakened his condition. After surgery to remove the damaged section of intestine, Gibb was listed in critical but stable condition. He passed away at 1:00 AM Sunday morning, January 12, 2003. **Lighten the load and cleanse or you may find yourself with a case of Saturday night fever.**

THE ALL AMERICAN COWBOY

John Wayne donated his body to science and was found to have over 40 pounds of dried fecal waste lodged in his intestines. Hey partner, take a load off and sit a spell.

ELVIS HAS LEFT THE BATHROOM

It is said that when the beloved singer/ actor Elvis Presley died, the autopsy revealed that his bloated body had about 80 to 90 pounds of impacted fecal matter in his digestive tract! No amount of laxative would help. It was reported that Elvis died of a heart attack while on the toilet. The straining to pass hard stools can raise blood pressure and even trigger a heart attack or stroke. One might wonder if cleaning out all of that impacted fecal matter might have reduced his suffering and added healthy years to his life. The King died on a porcelain throne.

With all his money and a top medical team at h i s disposal the obvious was overlooked. What a waste! *"When looking for solutions, don't see what everyone sees. See what everyone else chooses not to see." - Dr. Patch Adams*

You can be the victim or the super star and save the day. Better still, save your life.

- Dr. Darrell Wolfe

All the other body parts laughed at the Large Intestine and Insulted The Mother of All Organs, so in a huff, she shut down tight.

Within a few days,
The **Brain** had a terrible headache,
The **Stomach** was bloated,
The **Legs** got wobbly,
The **Eyes** got watery,
And the **Blood** was toxic.
They all decided that the **Large Intestine** should be the boss.

THE MORAL OF THE STORY?

Even though the other organs do all the work.
The Large Intestine almost Rectum - Now who's in charge!

GO DEEP

Scar Tissue & Crystallization are the major cause of your pain and physical limitations

BREAK FREE FROM THE BONDS WHICH BIND YOU

"The Whole Truth never lies on the surface. Pull back all the curtains and go deep to release the real U."

- Dr. Darrell Wolfe, Doc of Detox

CONTRACTION THE CHAIN REACTION

Let me explain why almost all body pain, physical degeneration and chronic recurring injury are not just preventable but unnecessary when you come from a proper foundation on all levels. The secret to the fountain of your youth does not lie just within the physical but also the mental. When the mind over reacts it causes contraction, shutting down our life force. The fuel is fear, doubt and worry, the result is pain, inflammation, energy depletion and a life ruled by chaos, and last but not least, a severe drop in your pH causing you to become acidic thus forming crystallization and internal scar tissue. The heart creates, causing expansion of our life force. The result being a life filled with an abundance of love, laughter, forgiveness, gratitude and a body free of pain, able to rest, repair, restore, and regenerate - The Natural Way because we are now raising our pH to an alkaline state. Every person and every thing has a frequency ranging from high to low, meaning strong to weak. A large percentage of society today is in a contracted state thus vibrating at the low level of fear, doubt and worry. This low vibrational frequency promotes a lowered immune system and sickness because like attracts like. Toxic, processed, fried, microwaved food contracts, lowering the body's frequency and energy. This causes acidity, pain, spasm, crystallization, internal scar tissue *(invisible bonds)*, mutation and disease.

Whole Plant Based Superfood expands, raising the body's frequency to repair, regenerate, restore and revitalize. Dancing, laughter, yoga, swimming, stretching, meditation and praying are expanding forces; whereas weightlifting without stretching is contractual leaving one acidic, stiff and out of balance.

Running without stretching is also contractual leaving one acidic, stiff and out of balance.

Hurting oneself or someone else without forgiveness is contractual and will leave you acidic, stiff, in pain and out of balance. One might say we live in a downright uptight society. If we do not learn to lighten up, there is only one outcome; to tighten up *(invisible bonds)*. On the topic of *'lighten up'*, what do you think the most common mineral deficiency is in the North American population? The clue, I stated most of us live in a contracted low vibrational frequency, so we're basically uptight physically and drained emotionally. *What is the main mineral used up by the body when we are uptight and out of balance?* **The answer is magnesium**. This mineral is used to rest, relax and repair; to keep things open and keep things moving. One example when this mineral becomes deficient is heart problems such as heart attack. If we look at the digestive tract in the way of contraction and expansion, contraction is constipation and two to three well-formed bowel movements a day is expansion. **How's that working for you?**

It would be best to embrace and learn how to effectively raise your vibrational frequency and live an expanded lifestyle. You can lighten up or tighten up on many levels; it's always been your choice. Love is the greatest expander (healer) but even drinking a glass of Structured Water is a start. All negative emotion such as fear, doubt and worry are contractual in nature and will shut down proper circulation, reducing the supply of oxygen and nutrition to the cells. This will cause a lower vibrational frequency, creating an acidic environment throughout the body.

You will know when you have created an acidic environment within your tissues and joints for they will feel stiff, sticky and painful. This is where it all begins, so if you are not aware of how this develops then this dysfunctional program will continue, internal scar tissue will form and you will prematurely age with invisible bonds. You can become crippled physically, at any age, but there is a greater chance of this happening as you get older.

We usually become more toxic and stuck in our ways with age, due to the accumulation of toxic waste and a colon that lacks tone. You have been unconsciously programed with **B**elief **S**ystems that do not serve your greater good *(evil plot)*.

Is it a physical problem or a mental one that rules the physical, **U** choose; *but haven't you already chosen?!* Every negative emotion and thought if held longer then 30 seconds will cause muscles to tighten, breathing to become shallow, or more shallow and, of course, old faithful, the fight or flight response. This is where your adrenals kick in, responding to the illusion of a life threat. *How many times do you trigger this program everyday, consciously or unconsciously?* The result from this; **drained of vital energy**, painful stiff muscles from the acid you have just created with your mind *(mind over matter)*. Continual knee-jerk reactions repeated enough times means your joints won't be able to move because of all the acid, crystallization and internal scar tissue *(invisible bonds)* from your *stinkin' thinkin'*.

Shoulders rounded almost permanently to protect your heart against the big, bad world and head down because that's where you are heading *(low vibrational frequency)*. If you have a distorted view of the world, life, love or yourself, you may just distort your health, heck, even your muscles and bones. Muscle spasms, inflammation, internal scar tissue and premature degeneration are all due to continual physical contraction, whereas with sickness and crippling conditions you must totally dedicate yourself to a low vibrational contracted lifestyle, for these are chronic and more severe in nature.

Reactive or Creative, make a choice but choose wisely. Love and life depend on it. For myself I've lived through a thousand deaths within my mind, it gets tiring, to say the least. I've done the drama queen show but realized that the world was not going to change for me or save me. Enough already! I am ready to take total responsibility for my life and well-being. I realize that true happiness is not found externally and that all answers lie within the changes that I make for myself.

This is where all true change must take place if we wish to be the Master of our life and the body we live in. Oh, but to free up your joints and muscles you must open the mind, open the heart, become pliable, flexible mentally and physically. Flow freely into life and embrace Nature's Whole Plant Based Foods and Structured Water, so your body may do the same. Take Life In to set your body free from these invisible bonds. **Feed your spirit and live to your full potential. Be The Cure!**

WEB OF DESTRUCTION

THE MAJOR CAUSE OF SCAR TISSUE FORMATION

The internal scar tissue that we all find within the body gets its foothold from years of incorrect treatment and guidance on diet and detoxification, which creates an unbalanced digestive tract, mainly that being within the large intestine. Your health rests on practitioners teaching you how to maintain a proper balance of 85% good bacteria to 15% bad bacteria, no greater. As long as these intestinal bacteria are in balance, the friendly bacteria will keep you in proper balance physically, mentally and emotionally. For most people it is the exact opposite or worse, 85% bad bacteria to 15% good bacteria. This reversal with the percentages regarding bacteria is no coincidence when the majority of the population choose to go to Medical Doctors for their day-to-day healthcare without questioning the fact that they haven't received any real training in nutrition or detoxification, they were trained entirely on emergency care and prescribing drugs.

Refined carbohydrates, animal products, GMOs, processed foods, a high sugar diet and almost every other man-made ingested "new and improved product" will turn your friendly protective bacteria into destructive, invasive, inflammatory, fungal producing bacteria. However, nothing even comes close to antibiotics when it comes to the annihilation and mutation of the good bacteria, the creation of fungus and the destruction that this causes to the major part of your immune system, this being your large intestine. Yes, these same antibiotics that most doctors prescribe for sore throats, earaches and acne will force the body into an over-productive, out of control state, forming internal scar tissue and fungus. Like an atomic bomb, your doctor just helped you transform your good bacteria into hundreds of thousands of microscopic fungus producing factories called Candida Albicans that will now undermine the major part of your immune system by rooting pinholes through the walls of the large intestine into your blood stream. *Thanks Doc! Wait a minute isn't Cancer a fungus?* So begins the domino effect to inflammation, pain, internal scar tissue formation, tissue degeneration, bone degeneration and yes, cellular mutation.

250 million courses of antibiotics are taken every year. When bacteria go from friendly to unfriendly they will become downright pathogenic, leaking highly acidic chemical byproducts called endotoxin from their outer wall. These endotoxins are absorbed into the bloodstream from the large intestine causing the body to go into 'high toxic alert mode', creating a defensive and protective inflammation response known as pain. Your body talks to you on a continual basis but the majority of the population have been programed to ignore these warning signs of pain, inflammation and disease. It all starts with excess acidity in the blood and tissues from the toxic spillover from stagnant waste, fungus and bad bacteria in the large intestine. If the large intestine is not addressed and brought back into balance in a timely fashion with gentle daily cleansing, the domino effect will begin with the first warning sign of inflammation, then pain and continue onto crystallization, internal scar tissue formation and finally a fungal invasion that leads to degeneration and mutation - Hello, Cancer! This is all due to the toxic chemicals being released from these mutated bacteria and fungus created by antibiotics, sugar, refined carbohydrates and the stagnation of putrefactive waste within your large intestine.

If this toxic parasitic breeding ground is not brought back into balance within the large intestine through gentle daily cleansing, the toxic waste created by the bad bacteria and the fungus, can and will, continue to be absorbed into the bloodstream, causing ongoing inflammation and pain with continual scar tissue formation that will overtake the weakest parts of the body, and in time, travel throughout the whole body, if this process goes unchecked. This ongoing inflammation is a symptom created by the body as a built-in safety mechanism to warn and protect you of a perceived threat to your tendons, ligaments, muscles, vital organs, tissues and even life itself. If your body did not experience pain as a warning sign you would be dead already, I know I would be.

If the inflammation is left to run its course, which happens in almost all cases, due to the ineffective therapy and guidance that most patients receive with today's health care system, the body will initiate a secondary support system, which is continual fibrin production *(internal scar tissue)* to wall off the area of inflamed tissue.

The body's built-in protective intelligence does this for three reasons. The first reason is to help prevent the spread of tissue inflammation and mutation to the surrounding healthy tissue. The second reason is to stop the infiltration of bad bacteria, fungus, viruses and parasites from invading the compromised inflamed tissue.

Insanity: doing the same thing over and over again, expecting different results.

- Albert Einstein

The third reason, which is a much more chronic state, is to deaden the area of inflammation and pain with thick fibrotic scar tissue so it does not continually drain the host and the immune system of its life-giving energy.

The body has now deadened the pain but now the patient is stiff as a board. This preventable degeneration process will continue until you have this internal scar tissue broken down and are taught how to become the master your digestive tract to reclaim your inner terrain. This continual fibrin production will create a web of destruction throughout the whole body if not halted. It will drain you of your vital energy and essential nutrients and will create massive internal scar tissue buildup, as if you have been in a severe accident.

This will eventually immobilize, deteriorate and mutate the tissues and organs causing calcium to be pulled from the bones involved. This is one of the final safety mechanisms the body initiates in an attempt to buffer down the acidity in this compromised area in the hopes of preventing chronic diseases such as arthritis and cancer. All calcium deposits found in body tissues and all calcium stones that are found in the gallbladder and kidneys are by-products of a highly acidic body that has never been properly treated or guided. Examples are Bursitis, Tendinitis, Arthritis, Osteoarthritis, Rheumatoid Arthritis, Carpal Tunnel Syndrome, Sciatica, Endometriosis, Breast Cancer and every other sore acidic muscle, joint, organ and disease you can think of because of incorrect information and ineffective therapy.

It does not matter what symptom, condition or disease we discuss they all are created by the domino effect, which gets its start in a compromised large intestine. When patients receive ineffective therapy or incorrect information on how to treat a symptom, that symptom will continue to escalate until it becomes chronic. Then we are taught to call the symptom a disease by the health care system and now the patient becomes initiated into the pharmaceutical system no longer believing they have the ability to look after themselves. An example of this is tendinitis; when not treated properly, will become arthritis and then escalate to rheumatoid arthritis, osteoarthritis or both.

These symptoms are all essential to your survival and will continue until you wake up and take charge. Even though these symptoms of inflammation, pain and internal scar tissue are a built-in, protective safety mechanism for survival, they will cause injury to body tissues and joints if they persist too long because the correct therapy and guidance has not been given.

Vital energy will be drained from the body leaving you exhausted and unprotected, forming internal scar tissue and even tumors that will undermine the quality of life for your whole life. Internal scar tissue lacks elasticity, flexibility and eventually will have the same consistency as beef jerky if the correct treatment does not occur in a timely fashion. This internal scar tissue will block proper circulation to the cells causing nutrient and oxygen depletion backing up toxic waste that can lead to mutation and even cancer.

The majority of the population suffers from massive internal scar tissue formation as if they have had a physical injury to the area. Not only our health care system but also our Natural Health Care System calls it a normal process of aging, go figure. For the body to run at peak performance, there cannot be continual energy wastage. When the body is continually at war with itself, it will weaken the immune system and leave the body open to parasitic invasion such as bad bacteria, fungus and worms creating a life of pain, suffering, prescription drugs and yes, even cancer.

"Pain is our friend, not our enemy. When you make pain your enemy and run from it, you will always be in it."

– Dr. Darrell Wolfe

PHARMA NATION-ZOMBIE CERTIFIED

What if there was a plan to drug the masses of a powerful nation so that they could be controlled and ***man***-ipulated? 50% of Big Pharma's drugs are taken by 5% of the world's population, yours truly the United States of America. It's time we unite and send these drug pushers a message. Make no mistake about it, these drugs are meant to dumb us down and open the gate to a life of pain and suffering; the very thing that they promise to CURE. It's time to say no and kick the drug habit (addiction), get out of the way and allow your body to heal itself. Please get this, drugs do not and will not heal. Drugs suppress you physically and mentally so **you can't truly heal**. Drugs suppress you emotionally so **you can't truly feel**. You're not there for yourself or anyone else, sounds like the definition of a **zombie**.

We need to put these drug pushers on notice - Merck, Pfizer, Novartis, Roche, GlaxoSmithKline, Abbott, Astra-Zeneca, Amgen, Eli Lilly, Bristol- Myers Squibb, and Sanofi (along with the FDA and CDC).

It's a sad day when we know names of the top selling drugs of Big Pharma like - Abilify, Nexium, Humira, Plavix, Crestor, Advair Diskus, Enbrel, and Cymbalta, instead of words like - Whole Plant Based Food, Structured Dynamic Water, Gentle Daily Cleansing and Moringa Oleifera, a plant that has healed millions around our globe for centuries.

Annual sales for the Humira cancer drug: One drug - One year - $9.3 billion. Desperate, uninformed people make pharmaceutical corporations rich.

When you have been taught to Master your life one day at a time you will need no one to come and save you. Desperate people make bad decisions. **Be The Cure U Wish To See!**

ALL TIED UP IN KNOTS

When we give a gift of love we wrap it up with beautiful paper and tie it with a silky bow. When we give the gift of fear, doubt and worry to others or ourselves we wrap it up in a nice, little package of internal scar tissue and crystallization until we are ready and willing to deal with it. How knots is that? This is where emotional problems tie themselves up into the physical body. We all have **B**elief **S**ystems that handicap us emotionally. We typically inherit these beliefs at a very young age to protect ourselves from a perceived threat that could cause us pain physically, mentally or emotionally. Many of these dysfunctional beliefs are stored away deep within our subconscious, long forgotten and difficult to access.

These subconscious invisible bonds cripple our relationships with family, friends and associates but most importantly with ourselves, creating pain and inflammation on an emotional and physical level that can and will create disease if not looked at. A good part of the pain we experience in the body can be attributed to stored toxic emotional waste and trauma. These emotions are buried and stored deep within the body's tissues and joints. They will create pain and inflammation, crystallization and internal scar tissue formation until you are willing and able to reevaluate your **B**elief **S**ystems. Your habits are an extension of your **B**elief **S**ystems. First you make your Habits and then your Habits make **U. Choose wisely or live a knotty life.**

You know the saying, *'lighten up or tighten up'*? As long as we take things personally, which we are all good at, stress and body tension will always plague our lives and body tissues *(realize or crystallize)*. When we learn to practice observing instead of judging, on a daily basis, we will then free ourselves of much unnecessary pain. Give me a person that's in continual emotional pain and I will show you a knotty person riddled with crystallization and internal scar tissue. How do you feel on a physical level when you have been emotionally upset for more than a few minutes? An achy, tired body is usually the answer for many. When we are emotionally upset, two of the main side effects are headache and stomach ache.

This is the beginning of an acidic condition *(acidosis)*, which will lead to pain, inflammation, crystallization and internal scar tissue formation. Continue this program, of not being flexible mentally and you will become as stiff and rigid as your thoughts. We all know that if you want to Master something, you must practice everyday until it becomes second nature.

Many things we do are robotic; some good, some not so good. To Master your life you need to download a new program and practice it daily without fail for months if you wish to release the invisible emotional and physical bonds. The choice is yours; pharmaceutical drugs, alcohol, cigarettes, sugar or reprogram yourself to become **the real U.**

When I perform deep tissue restoration on a patient I can get a sense of how they deal with the emotional side of life by the location, consistency and quantity of the crystallization and internal scar tissue within their body. Following the breaking down of crystallization and hardened internal scar tissue there is also an emotional release some of the time. This emotional release can vary in intensity from the sense of a burden being lifted to a more intense release such as a crying spell. A patient can experience an immediate release or one within that twenty-four hour period.

Many years ago a very experienced deep tissue therapist told me that the emotional release of tears after breaking down scar tissue and crystallization is the crystallized emotions melting and leaving the body in liquid form. For some an emotional release is not needed. For others they're not ready yet to deal with that which binds them, so they keep it suppressed and in lock down mode deep within the body tissues. When we are ready to embrace our **B**elief **S**ystems and only keep those that serve our greater good, along with Gentle Daily Cleansing, hydrating with Dynamic Structured Water and a Whole Plant Based Lifestyle, we will then Master our lives.

WOLFE DEEP TISSUE RESTORATION

Wolfe Deep Tissue Restoration reaches structures far beneath the superficial fascia to reverse chronic muscle, tendon, ligament problems and chronic injuries where other therapies fall short. Our Philosophy at the International Training Institute Of Health - if you cannot guarantee your therapy then you should not don't charge for it!

"He who runs from pain lives in Pain. Go Deep and live pain-free!"

- *Dr. Darrell Wolfe, Doc of Detox*

WOLFE TECHNIQUE & THEORY

Wolfe Deep Tissue Restoration was created 30 years ago by Dr. Darrell Wolfe Ac.PhD., C.C.H., D.M.T. due to the internal scar tissue and crystallization he found in almost all of his patients; this being the underlying cause of physical pain experienced in the body. This unique therapy is taught by the International Training Institute of Health and has been taught and successfully used in the treatment of muscle, tendon, ligament and joint conditions since 1985.

Crystallization and internal scar tissue are the major underlying cause of physical pain experienced in the body. Wolfe Deep Tissue Restoration has shown to be the most effective form of bodywork therapy ever created to reverse the underlying cause of chronic and acute muscular and skeletal problems, injuries, sports injuries, muscle loss *(atrophy)*, pain and internal scar tissue and crystallization in the body. Internal scar tissue and crystallization are the major causes of premature aging, pain and physical limitation. All therapies have their place but unless the underlying cause, that being internal scar tissue, is broken down and eliminated in the process, then the therapy becomes useless or temporary at best.

With every muscle, tendon, ligament and joint problem, if the therapy does not eliminate the internal scar tissue and/or correct guidance is not given by the practitioner to the patient, the body will continue to create fibrin *(internal scar tissue)*, which is a defense mechanism within the body to wall off the inflammation from spreading to the healthier tissue and wall off the bacteria from invading the already inflamed and compromised tissue.

If this inflammation is left to continue or is suppressed by drug therapy the body will go into full production mode of fibrin to deaden the pain and stop the spread of the inflammation in the affected area to end the energy wastage and depletion of the immune system. The end result will be massive internal scar tissue formation leading to a chronic muscular, joint or organ disease, which is actually a symptom of the inflammation allowed to go out of control and unchecked. The area will feel as if a physical injury has taken place, when all this scar tissue is just a symptom created by the body's built- in safety mechanisms due to incorrect therapy and/or incorrect information given to the patient.

Superficial techniques applied at a distance from a lesion cannot be expected to correct the problem. They can help by reducing inflammation, aiding circulation and soothing hyper-toned muscles, but the cause will always remain and will reveal itself time and time again in the future. The true cause of physical disorders is never on or near the surface. For any long- lasting results you must release the deep invisible bonds and empower the patients with true wisdom. Wolfe Deep Tissue Restoration reaches structures far beneath the superficial fascia to reverse chronic muscle, tendon, ligament and joint problems. It is remarkably effective for aligning skeletal structures that lie deep within the body that cannot be reached effectively with other therapies. Even in cases of severe fibromyalgia where the patient is in constant pain, we can still remove the invisible blocks and remove the cause of their pain without any further pain to the patient. It is called 'Wolfe Deep Tissue' but when the technique is done properly, it can even put a patient to sleep. We will break the cycle of pain within the very first treatment. All of our therapies and consultations come with a 100% satisfaction, money-back guarantee. If we can't guarantee our work then we should not charge for it. Deliver lasting results!

The actual manipulation is a controlled, precise, short, concentrated transverse movement with a penetrating action applied directly on individual muscles, tendons or ligament fibers that have lesion (internal scar tissue) involvement. By using a transverse manipulation on the origin and insertion of the deeper tendons and ligaments, we release the whole muscle belly and the involved joints. The origin and insertion is found on either end of muscles where the tendon or ligaments attach onto the bone.

What is a tendon? It is the fibrous cord-like part of the muscle found on either end of the muscle belly that is attached to the bone. With contraction of our muscles, where do you think the most stress would be? In the muscle belly or in the tendons attached to the bone? If I hang from a rope, where is the most stress placed? That's right, at the end of the rope, where it is tied! The tendons get the most stress; they will experience micro tearing and become matted with internal scar tissue and crystallization, which will form knots that will cause the muscle to shorten in length. Why is there spasm in the muscle belly when the damage lies mainly within the origin and insertion, where the tendons attach? This reaction is a built-in, protective safety mechanism for the damage that has occurred in the tendon at or near the origin and insertion point. The muscle belly will stay in spasm and even in pain so that it remains contracted thus limiting range of motion. This reduces the movement of the muscles, which in turn protects the tendon from any further tears until the cause is eliminated, that being hardened internal scar tissue at the joint.

The conclusion is: work deep at the insertion and origin of tendons and ligaments to remove scar tissue and crystallization or become the average, normal person, who experiences premature aging with pain and inflammation continually off and on throughout their whole life, because the true cause was never addressed or eliminated.

"Pain is our friend, not our enemy. When you make pain your enemy and run away from it, you will always be in It."

– Dr. Darrell Wolfe

When you release the internal scar tissue at the insertion and origin of the muscles you automatically release the muscle tension and spasm within the muscle belly, which was only there as a protective safety mechanism against further injury in the insertion and origin of muscles. Wolfe Deep Tissue Restoration is applied by using the base of the phalange, forearm, epicondyle or elbow.

This technique is used to mobilize the muscle, tendon or ligament, separating the adhesions between the individual fibers that are restricting natural movement. Traditional techniques, where they stretch out the muscle in an attempt to widen the distance between the muscle fibers, are temporary at best. During stretching, the muscles lie more closely together. Adhesions within the tissue cannot be broken down by stretching, but only by using a deep transverse manipulation, which broadens the tissue, opening it up and allowing circulation and nerve flow to be restored. This is particularly true of the fibers that attach muscle to bone, where the vicinity of stationary tissue restricts the mobility of adjacent muscle.

Wolfe Deep Tissue Restoration Therapy restores proper blood flow and increases range of motion instantly. In any form of injury, chronic muscular problem, or crippling condition, there will be internal scar tissue *(lesions)* or atrophy *(decreased muscle tone)* developed by the physiological process. Even in the case of arthritis, I personally would not label this as a disease. '*Arth*' stands for joint and '*itis*' stands for inflammation. The inflammation at the joint is increased acidity attacking the tissues within the joint, which causes crystallization and internal scar tissue formation. As the internal scar tissue hardens, mineral depletion of calcium from the bones will occur to buffer down this chronic inflammatory tissue created by acidosis. As long as you receive ineffective therapy there will be continual degeneration to the tissues and joints involved, so the symptom called 'Arthritis' that has received ineffective therapies now has become 'Osteoarthritis'. As you can see, these are not diseases; these are symptoms that only become worse overtime due to improper treatment and incorrect guidance.

As the scar tissue hardens, mineral depletion to the bones of the joint will occur along with degeneration to the tissue involved.

Anyone who runs marathons would be shocked if they could see inside their body. Running creates internal scar tissue in the muscles, tendons, ligaments and also in the heart. Inflammation and pain is the first sign of internal scar tissue formation.

CHAPTER 11 - DEEP TISSUE RESTORATION

There is nothing worse than an injury that won't heal. It does not matter how much ice, heat, Advil, Motrin or anti-inflammatories you take or apply, they may suppress your pain but only to have you unknowingly rip and tear because they have numbed out the warning signs of re-tearing the internal scar tissue that has never been addressed properly with the correct therapy to break it down and remove it in the first place. Sometimes a chronic injury will last for months or even years with no real end in sight.

Repeated visits to the doctor for prescriptions to numb the pain, visits to physical therapists, registered massage therapists, chiropractors and acupuncturists will help reduce the problem but until the crystallization and internal scar tissue is removed and the patient is taught how to prevent it from returning, their search will go on. The major cause of injuries now and always will be the invisible bonds that bind and restrict; internal scar tissue formation that eventually turns into knots will shorten the muscles, ligaments and tendons they are attached to.

This cannot be stretched out, even though most therapies and trainers teach this, for it will only rip and tear again because of the lack of circulation and elasticity due to it being fibrotic internal scar tissue. The same scar tissue that attempts to prevent damage will also constrict future movement, binding tissues and organs, causing unnecessary pain and suffering when the 'healing' has supposedly already completed. A transverse penetrating technique is clearly necessary if such tissues are to be restored to their healthy state. Proper guidance on diet, detoxification and exercise is essential to restore and maintain your health on a permanent basis.

In the majority of the population the internal scar tissue has hardened like cement and a change in diet alone will not be enough for true healing to take place. Tissue that was once elastic, pliable, toned and self-healing now receives hardly any blood flow due to its fibrous, crystalline structure. This tissue now lacks needed oxygen and vital essential nutrients and has the consistency of beef jerky.

From a frozen shoulder to a cancer tumor you will have crystallization and scar tissue formation when incorrect guidance and treatment is given. When you remove the hardened internal scar tissue, crystallization and scar tissue knots, then you will be free of pain and able to perform at your optimum once again, as a healthy active person at any age. This hardened internal scar tissue must be manually broken down and then flushed out of the system with ample quality Structured Water, Gentle Daily Cleansing, a Whole Plant Based Diet along with Superfood Nutrition and Core Exercises.

This is why we believe at the International Training Institute of Health that any physical therapist without proper training in the art of deep tissue restoration and a correct foundation of nutrition, detoxification and **exercise** will never provide what their patients truly need – whole body healing needs a whole body, **whole life approach. Be the Cure you wish to see.**

Make sure your practitioner is well trained in the removal of these invisible bonds **and has the wisdom to teach you how to become the Master of your own health and well being. Release that which binds U.** For more information, go to: www.itioh.com

Wolfe Deep Tissue Restoration & Whole Life Coach Certification

Professional Certification in the Art of Longevity and a Pain Free Disease Free Body

THE MOST ADVANCED TRAININGS IN THE ART OF NATURAL HEALING

This 13-Day in-depth Professional Training Course is designed to give practitioners and those who wish to be practitioners the most advanced, cutting-edge strategies, tools and techniques in the art of Natural Healing in the most empowering, but simplistic way. Dr. Darrell Wolfe is known worldwide for his Whole Life Coaching Methods and his Wolfe Deep Tissue Therapy. His Whole Life Coaching and unique Deep Tissue Therapy leads the way in advanced bodywork therapeutics.

His philosophy has always been, 'If you can't guarantee your work then it should be for free!' Dr. Wolfe takes this one step further, his guarantee is that this 13-Day Intensive Training will give you the tools, strategies and techniques for you to become the therapist that you always knew you could be. Let us train and teach you – we will surpass your expectations and will continue to do so by supporting you with weekly online webinar and teleconference trainings, so that you remain a leader in the field of health. We will teach you how to build and maintain a successful and financially lucrative practice, featuring top industry specialists to help you with marketing, media and business planning strategies.

WHOLE LIFE COACH CERTIFICATION

Whole Life Coach Certification has earned the reputation as being the most effective, life-changing course for practitioners and their patients. We provide our practitioners with the most powerful techniques and strategies along with ongoing support to ensure that your practice is always on the cutting-edge. Teaching the medicine of the past with today's health breakthroughs, along with fundamental tools and strategies, will create the strongest foundation for building a long-lasting, financially successful career in the Natural Health Care Industry.

The successful reputation that we have achieved with our Whole Life Coach Certification Program is based on years of success with our practitioners and our patients; you cannot have one without the other. With this course and our ongoing support, you will have the confidence and the knowledge to create a personalized health plan tailored to suit each individual patient by their age, condition, lifestyle and emotional state. Creating a strong foundation in the regards to Whole Plant Based Superfood Nutrition and Whole Body Detoxification are monumental for a long and vibrantly healthy life. Our nutritional program is not based on fads or the latest, greatest breakthrough or cure but is based on the science of nature. The Whole Life Coach Certification course will create a financially successful business because we teach strategies, techniques, protocols and provide foundational products that have stood the test of time and remain the cutting-edge still to this day. We are a new breed of practitioner, our focus is on training our patients – not treating them.

Too many patients fall through the cracks with the standard protocols that are used by the majority of health practitioners today. If we continue to practice the same old techniques, we will continue to get the same ineffective results. Truly, how many practitioners out there actually halt their patients' degeneration, less turn their condition around? The health manual that is used by the majority of Natural Health practitioners today was written or at the very least manipulated by pharmaceutical corporations, food conglomerates and petrochemical companies and has been spoon-fed to the North American population by the media and the medical system. I would like to say that we learn through logic and wisdom but repetition is still the weapon of choice when educating the average practitioner.

We spend the first half of our lives wasting our health to gain wealth. And the second half of our lives spending our wealth to regain our health. By 2030, 20% of the population will be 65 or older and in retirement. Practitioners that have been trained to empower their patients will naturally be in high demand.

Awakening Transformation Training

Just as there are two sides to every story, there are two sides to health – physical and emotional, you cannot heal one without the other, they must heal together as a team. If you have researched health coaching programs as we have, you will come to realize that with most courses, the emotional part of the training falls drastically short. Our Whole Life Coach Certification Program takes a serious and in-depth look at how emotions and emotional attachment can create dysfunctional belief systems that undermine our health and wellbeing. Every dysfunctional belief system comes with a specific symptom, which becomes labeled as a disease. Our goal is to teach you the tools and strategies so that you can become more aware to help your patients have a greater understanding that their illness is not just physical by nature.

When emotions are not digested, assimilated and eliminated properly, they become stored in the weak or damaged tissue or joints of the human body. We will be looking at the difference between a physical injury and an emotional one, so that you will be able to tell the difference and treat it for what it really is. Dysfunctional Belief Systems programmed into each and every one of us, by not just the medical system but also the natural health care system, keeps everyone in treatment because practitioners are focused on treatment and not training their patients to Master their own health and wellbeing.

With years of research under my belt, consulting thousands, and learning from the best, I have put together what I call Awakening Transformation. How would it make you feel to be able to teach your patients simple but effective techniques to remove the blocks that have prevented them from releasing their limitless potential physically and emotionally? I will teach you how one session will outweigh hundreds of hours and thousands of dollars of therapy by implementing simple, powerful and enjoyable techniques in your patients' daily routine. They say people cannot change – well now they can, with Awakening Transformation Training.

We will teach you how to build a successful and financially lucrative practice, featuring top industry specialists to help you with marketing, media and business planning strategies.

All certified practitioners will be featured on the International Training Institute of Health website. Practitioners will also be invited and encouraged to participate in ongoing, online trainings, webinars and teleconferences to stay abreast of new techniques and nutritional breakthroughs. Do not hesitate to call with any questions, your success is our success. – Dr. Darrell Wolfe, 1 855 900 4544

WOLFE DEEP TISSUE CERTIFICATION

Good Day Dr. Wolfe here! The first thing I would like to do is put the record straight. No, not all deep tissue is deep tissue. To actually be called deep tissue, one must first be using their elbow. Second of all, it is not about how hard you work but how effective the technique is that you use.

If a therapist uses their phalange, fingers or hands, there is no possible way that this can effectively pull muscle fibers apart, remove crystallization, calcium deposits, adhesions from organs, joints, ligaments or tendons. Whether you are talking about the Pfrimmer technique, Rolfing or any of the other countless wannabe deep tissue techniques, nothing else compares to Wolfe Deep Tissue in it's effectiveness, speed and longevity.

Wolfe Deep Tissue Restoration was created by Dr. Darrell Wolfe Ac.PhD. 30 years ago due to the crystallization and internal scar tissue he found in all of his patients. Wolfe Deep Tissue has been shown to be the most effective form of therapy in the elimination of internal scar tissue and crystallization, which is the major cause of premature aging, pain and physical limitation whether it is an acute or chronic situation.

When you remove the hardened internal scar tissue, crystallization and scar tissue knots, then you will be free of pain and able to perform again as a healthy active person at any age. This hardened internal scar tissue must be manually broken down and then flushed out of the system for elasticity, flexibility, strength and complete range of motion to return to normal.

Wolfe Deep Tissue Restoration works by performing a 45 degree angle, cross-fiber technique on body tissues, which restores balance in the muscles on a cellular level. Wolfe Deep Tissue stimulates the lymphatic and circulatory systems, which helps to deliver nutrients while removing toxic waste from the cells.

When we relieve the body of unwanted scar tissue and crystallization, we naturally find balance and alignment. Through Wolfe Deep Tissue, the elasticity of the tissue can be restored and the body realigned so that it can function with ease. Better posture and improved movement can be expected in the first treatment.

Wolfe Deep Tissue helps to release nerves that are being strangled, irritated and inflamed by the scar tissue in your body. Wolfe Deep Tissue also greatly increases the removal of toxins and congestion, that is trapped in the tissues and organs. With the very first treatment, you will see edema (water retention), inflammation and pain are greatly reduced and cellular function is restored along with improved range of motion!

Wolfe Deep Tissue Therapy is most known for its ability to remove topical and internal scar tissue, correct and prevent serious muscle and joint conditions, including MS, ALS (Lou Gehrig's Disease), Muscular Dystrophy, Parkinson's, Cerebral Palsy, Brain Injury and Stroke. **To join our team, go to: www.itioh.com**

SCARRED FOR LIFE

"U will no longer be imprisoned by your invisible bonds when you take charge of your life and Break Free."

- Dr. Darrell Wolfe, Doc of Detox

ACIDIC TISSUES = INVISIBLE BONDS

It is important to remember that **acidosis** is the root cause of the pain, inflammation and **degeneration** of your body tissues and joints. This condition known as acidosis only started to become prevalent after the introduction of chemical fertilizers, sprays, factory farming, processed chemical laden foods and pharmaceutical drugs. Over the years the depletion of vital nutrients from the soil caused a chain of events that left our food chain broken and our body starving of these vital life-giving properties. In addition to this, we bought into the notion that drugs heal so we turned our backs on Nature to suppress the pain instead of seeking balance. Before farming became big business, chronic achy muscles and joints were not an everyday occurrence. This kind of pain was temporary, just a part of the Natural Healing process. You cannot wait for mainstream medicine to embrace this fact; there is just too much money involved for them to change the bottom line.

When your daily habits do not support an alkaline lifestyle such as Gentle Daily Cleansing, Whole Plant Based Nutritional Support and Structured Water then an internal acidic environment will be the result and you can expect pain. When you become acidic your body will always protect your vital organs and bones first and foremost. The body must and will find ways to store the acidity in your tissues until it's cleansing and nutritional needs are met, no compromise. I promise you this, recurring pain; until you turn your back on **man**-ipulation and **Embrace Nature**. Remember who **U** are. You are the key so set yourself free - from pain!

OPTION ONE OR TWO

With an acidic condition there are two main options. The first one is fat cell production to store the acidic waste and the second is to store the acidity in the body tissues such as muscles, tendons and ligaments to protect your bones and vital organs. When your digestive system is not cleansed and toxins stagnate they are absorbed into the bloodstream. Your bloodstream has a very narrow margin on how acidic it can become. The liver must filter the toxic burden. When this extra toxic load overburdens the liver, it will enter into a state of chronic fatigue along with you. If proper action is not taken, pain will persist and the symptom will be called fibromyalgia. As long as you focus on only part of the problem such as: symptoms, single supplements or pharmaceutical drugs, you will never get to the cause or experience for yourself, **The Whole Truth About Health.**

Acidosis is not a disease but a symptom of mismanagement that can be eliminated when you embrace the cause with Nature leading the way; or you can pay physically, emotionally and let us not forget, financially. You have a choice to go deep into your pockets and still live in pain or go deep within and cleanse, nourish and restore your body's tissue. **You are stronger than you think when you remember who U are.**

REALIZE OR CRYSTALLIZE

When acidosis becomes prevalent, elimination has become stagnation, resulting in aching and swelling of muscles and tissues in and around joints. Due to lack of circulation, crystallization of these acidic wastes will form in body tissues such as muscles, tendons and ligaments. These acidic wastes will create a low-grade inflammation that will block oxygen and nutrition at the cellular level causing premature degeneration of tissues and joints. The excessive toxins in our blood become the breeding ground for internal scar tissue and crystallization formation in the weaker points of the body. The weakest link will always crystallize first. This recurring pain is a gentle warning that you are not in balance and that you have not been taught how to properly take care of your body. Those around you have always suffered with pain so you also have accepted pain to be a normal way of life. Your **B**elief **S**ystem might very well be, *'as long as I'm alive, I will be in pain.'* Realize you have always had a choice. Stay mainstream and crystallize or take action and realize. **Go deep within, cleanse, nourish and hydrate. U will release your invisible bonds and heal yourself - Naturally.**

A KNOTTY BODY

Where there is constant inflammation there is pain, degeneration and internal scar tissue formation *(invisible bonds)*. The more severe the toxic buildup, the greater the inflammation which causes a reduction of blood supply and degeneration to your muscles and joints. This in turn, causes your body to produce excessive fibrin (tissue fibers) to be sent to the area in crisis to repair the micro-tearing to wall off the pain and crystallization. Fibrin is what internal scar tissue is made from. The body always overcompensates in cases of inflammation when it comes to fibrin production *(internal scar tissue)*. *What do you think happens if the inflammation is not eliminated and is allowed to continue?*

Believe it or '*knot*', you can have a huge build-up of scar tissue even if you've never had an injury. This internal scar tissue will create a web around your joints, which will prevent the red blood cells from delivering oxygen and from eliminating cellular waste. This is what causes your muscles and joints to cry out in pain. This acidity and crystallization will continue to grow and become trapped until the web of scar tissue is eliminated. Welcome to the beginnings of a knotty body caused by the buildup of scar tissue and crystallization. The more scar tissue and crystallization that forms in your muscles, tendons and ligaments the shorter these structures will become with every knot created. When you take a shoe lace notice what happens to it with every knot you tie. You lose a quarter inch with every knot; the more knots, the shorter it becomes.

I will give you a few life examples. I can't get my arms over my head to get my shirt off. I can't tie my shoes. I waddle like a duck. I can't shoulder check when I drive, my neck is frozen. 'I remember when I used to...' You get the picture. Give me a joint problem and I'll show you a knotty body. Give me a knotty body and I'll show you how to make it young again. The fibers of a ligament, tendon or muscle are like the strings of a guitar in that they run parallel to one another.

When fibers tear or degenerate through inflammation, it's as though the strings were cut. Ideally, the fibers should heal parallel again, like getting new guitar strings, but often this does not happen. Instead, in the body's enthusiasm to heal, the fibers are not only joined end to end but they also stick to those running parallel to them, as if all the guitar strings were glued together. **The Sound Of Muscle Music** has now become a painful party with no relief in sight.

ACTIVE BECOMES INACTIVE

Now you have a situation of matting and clumping of scar tissue which will reduce elasticity of muscles and normal range of joint motion. For the average person who generally lives an acidic lifestyle, this area of the body may very well plague them for a long time, maybe even a lifetime. When this area is stretched through normal use, the strings or the fibers will re-tear due to the decreased range of motion caused by crystallization and scar tissue formation *(invisible bonds)*. The resulting pain and inflammation caused when over-stretching is there to protect against further damage until the cause is removed, this being the internal scar tissue. The autonomic nervous system mostly compensates for scar tissue by isolating or *'walling off'* the pain, but when the nervous system is overrun with stress, this compensation fails and pain results. In each case, circulation and nerve transmissions are impaired.

Take a good look at *'Woody'*. Woody used to be a Super Hero but now he is just Super Stiff. This is a normal situation for the unconscious living. Woody is **malnourished**, dehydrated and bloated as you can tell, due to years of putrefactive waste being backed up in his colon. His muscles are deteriorating due to crystallization and internal scar tissue. Now you know why they call him Woody. You also now understand that neither Woody nor anyone else needs to live this way. **Be The Cure and Become The Super Hero You Were Meant To Be!**

CALCIFICATION OR CRYSTALLIZATION

When internal scar tissue builds up and/or crystallization begins to create blocks in your body, nerve pain will become intermittent or constant until the cause is removed or you have been drugged enough not to feel it. Many health professionals believe that this disorder is due to calcification. Yes, this is true in some conditions such as toxic acidic breasts creating internal scar tissue and becoming fibrotic due to the ongoing signal of inflammation. If this internal scar tissue process, within the breast, is not treated and reversed correctly in a timely fashion then calcium deposits will develop to buffer down the acidity to ward off cancer as long as possible. I have had hundreds of people coming to me believing that calcification was the problem, only to find out that it was mainly internal scar tissue and crystallization with traces of calcium. The body creates this overcompensation of internal scar tissue due to inflammation and infection in an attempt to protect and heal an injured area.

Why do muscular and structural disorders go away only to return again? The cause has never been addressed or dealt with properly. Is it lack of spinal adjustments? No, when it is a muscular problem; ask yourself, "Where is the pain, on or in the bone or in the muscle?" Now ask yourself, "Do bones pull muscles out of place or do shortened, knotted muscles pull bones out of place?" Remember, inflammation and spasms come from deep within the muscle tissue, not the bones.

All answers lie deep within the muscles. Release those invisible bonds and educate yourself on a whole plant based diet, gentle daily cleansing, Structured Water, core exercise and how to achieve a healthy sleep and you will live pain-free. It's not about age, it's all about the internal scar tissue and crystallization build up. Age has nothing to do with pain – unless you're the so-called, average person. When a practitioner has the knowledge of internal scar tissue removal and the ability to teach their patients the foundational keys to vital health on a daily basis, then and only then will permanent healing take place. **Just ask Woody.**

MUSCLE SPASMS FRIEND OR FOE

Muscle spasms are not constant. They spring into action at a certain point in the range of motion to protect arthritic joints, sprained ligaments, inflamed tendons or an injured area from further damage until the true cause is dealt with. Muscle spasms result from a lesion *(internal scar tissue, crystallization)* and their sole purpose is to prevent full extension thus sparing further tearing. Internal scar tissue tears easily due to lack of elasticity, flexibility and circulation, whereas connective tissue has tone, elasticity, flexibility, proper circulation and proper hydration.

Scar tissue in our body can be compared to gristle in a rump roast. It may still have some flavor but it is definitely harder to chew. **Beef Jerky anyone?**

TOXIC & TWISTED

When you experience severe spasms in your body this will cause you to curl up and twist. Imagine these muscle spasms continuing day in and day out in your body for years. Over time these muscle spasms will twist and distort bones, such as in the case of Osteoarthritis or Rheumatoid Arthritis. In these conditions, muscles, tendons and ligaments become burdened with internal scar tissue and crystallization. This causes shortening of these muscles, tendons and ligaments leading to physical distortion and imbalance of bone structures. In both of these conditions, vital minerals and other nutrients are being depleted from the tissues and bones to buffer down the acidity. This symptom is known as osteoporosis. A healthy, nontoxic internal environment would never allow such a debilitating condition to even exist, much less ever get started. How does a patient ever get or even learn how to create a healthy internal environment in their body when most practitioners are taught ineffective techniques when it comes to bodywork and dispense misleading information when it comes to foundational nutrition and detoxification. This is why I developed a professional training course for practitioners and a two- day course for the general public along with a one-on-one training course for couples so that they may learn how to work on each other and live pain free. All our courses have two parts to them, health from the inside out and the outside in. Whole body healing with Whole body results, the way health was meant to be. For training course information go to: www.itioh.com

INVISIBLE BUT DEADLY BREAK THE CHAINS

What makes this internal scar tissue and crystallization formation so frustrating is that it does not show up on X-rays. Ultrasound also does not give a clear picture of this condition, and doctors often diagnose it as psychosomatic. Just because you can't see something doesn't mean that it doesn't exist. Internal scar tissue restricts, chokes and immobilizes joints *(invisible bonds)*. Internal scar tissue is similar to weeds in a garden, in the way that if the garden is not tended to properly, the weeds will overtake the garden, just as internal scar tissue will overtake and choke the tissues of your body. When internal scar tissue spreads long enough, and deep enough, you will prematurely age and lose your flexibility, elasticity and tone and be forced to live in a weakened, restricted state. **Snap, crackle, pop!**

GO DEEP OR GO DOWNHILL

I think I have made things crystal clear. The more acidic you become, the more internal scar tissue and crystallization you form in your body. The vast number of today's chronic muscle disorders, injuries and plain old body pain are reversible. I have proven it and **U** can do the same. To be successful you must first remember what you are capable of and know that you hold the power to make yourself sick or healthy. You must focus on what you want and not what you don't want. Picture yourself the way you wish to be and take charge of your own healing. You will need to drink plenty of Dynamically Structured Water. *Why?* Because we are walking bags of water. You will need to lean to an alkaline lifestyle, along with Gentle Daily Cleansing and Whole Plant Based Nutrition. Start core exercises to mobilize your joints and tissues. Learn proper breathing and relaxation techniques. **One more thing**, the most effective form of body work to reverse scar tissue and crystallization is Wolfe Deep Tissue Restoration. If possible, learn the art of Wolfe Deep Tissue Restoration so you can help yourself and others; or find a therapist who can go deep and release your invisible bonds. Learn to Master your body and you will Live Pain Free.

Get Moving and Be The Cure.

MAKING THE DIFFERENCE

The more acidic you become, the more internal scar tissue and crystallization your body will form to protect you. The vast number of today's chronic muscle disorders, injuries and plain old body pain are reversible and yes, preventable when you take personal action and Master your own well-being. We've proven it and so can you. The body only knows the past. At one time this internal scar tissue protected you from further damage but now you are being crippled by it.

As I have stated, the body only knows the past so you must break up these invisible bonds that no longer serve you, but this is just half the story. If you do not follow up by learning a new way to live, the pain, suffering, crystallization and internal scar tissue will be back. Unless you become the Master of your own health, the scar tissue will return because the body only knows the past. I would like you to take a hard look at the people you love and the people you know.

How successful have they been with keeping their health and restoring their health? To be successful with your health, you must encompass whole body healing: break down and eliminate the internal scar tissue and have a strong foundation in whole body cleansing, nutrition, diet, exercise and emotional processing so that it is never allowed to return. Years ago it became very obvious to me that almost all therapies given and the health information provided to patients only soothed their pain and suffering temporarily; never really removing the true cause of their suffering or personally empowering them with take action information so that they could Master their own health and well-being. This is why I created the *'International Training Institute of Health'* with training courses for professionals, corporations and the general public. For more information go to: www.itioh.com

RELEASE THE THIN WITHIN

"Once you embrace Whole Plant Based Superfoods and Structured Water... You'll never have to embrace another fad or flavor of the month!" Drink Life In

- Dr. Darrell Wolfe, Doc of Detox

TERROR WITHIN

Dieting has become a national obsession. Despite this billion-dollar diet industry, North Americans are more overweight and obese than ever before. An explanation for this phenomenon is the fact that more toxic chemicals than ever are being poured into our food and environment on a daily basis. 74 billion pounds of environmental toxins are produced everyday in the United States. Your body must produce fat cells to store these deadly toxins far enough away from your organs to slow down or prevent cancer and other fatal diseases. Gently Cleanse Daily and live, or become a ticking toxic time bomb.

Another important fact, if you have taken antibiotics for ear aches, sore throats, acne, colds or whatever the reason then you have annihilated a major part of your immune system, mutating your good bacteria to bad and destroying the integrity of the Mother of all organs, the large intestine. After taking antibiotics that same food that never bothered you before now causes you to gain weight. Dr. Blaser, in his book 'Missing Microbes' proves that the more antibiotics we ingest the fatter we can become due to this bacterial war and the loss of integrity we have created in the large intestine. Yes, there are situations where antibiotics are needed to save lives but these should only be taken in life-threatening situations. Antibiotics can cause up to a 15% weight gain due to the adverse effects to the large intestine. Savvy marketers have duped us into buying new and improved when it was really overweight and obese that we bought into. Have you ever noticed the more low fat and diet foods you eat the bigger and sicker you become? The Whole Truth is; there are no watchdogs in the food industry. It's just a dog eat dog world and everybody is running around in circles confused as ever while '***man**-ipulation*' hits a home run because we '*donut*' have a filter for half-truth and deception. It's not bad enough that they totally own most of the adult population as unconscious eaters, but this is also being taught to our children, creating mini-me's, but not so mini. These kids are going to become so sick, not just physically but also emotionally. If you have given up on life and want to eat yourself into a food coma, fine, but don't drag your children along for the ride. They never signed up for the '*give up and eat*' program. Stop buying all that toxic, lifeless GMO food and bringing it home if you want anyone to make it out alive and well. These foods will, and do, make you into half-living, half-breathing **zombies** and the producers of these foods know it oh, so well. They're at home, grinning, as they count your money.

Meanwhile you're at the doctor trying to troubleshoot all these alarm bells going off in your not so happy body, waiting for the next knockout prescription. So here's the skinny; everyone who participates in the processing and the selling of this food does not care what condition you're in, as long as you get in to buy it, even if that means you're using an electric scooter.

This will never be regulated for the health of it because there are too many people making big money in the Health Care Industry when you and your family get sick. The rules to staying slender and healthy have never changed, but we have (*oops*). When you turn your back on Nature you leave your health's greatest protector, healer, and yes, your weight management team on the sidelines, but don't you worry your pretty, little head. When you're all done trying the fads, the quick fixes, the pie in the sky promises and you're truly sick and tired of being sick and tired, Whole Plant Based Superfood Nutrition will be waiting to magically shed the pounds, save your butt and tone it, giving you back the health that you deserve. All will be well again when you finally remember who you are and where you came from. **The Whole Truth** is, we are overweight and struggling with obesity more than ever before... despite all the dieting, weight gain is still on the rise. The percentage of people overweight in 1950 was 25% of the population. Today, just over 70% of the population is overweight. 210 million people are clinically overweight and 114 million are obese in North America as you are reading this.

THE BATTLE OF THE BULGE

At this current rate 75% of the population will be overweight and 41% obese by 2015, unless they have released their '*thin within*' and have embraced Nature to flush the pounds and lighten their load. 1.1 billion adults are overweight on this planet and 300 million are obese. We know we have definitely entered '*the battle of the bulge*', when the slender man is in the minority. No, you're in great shape for the average person of your age, this is quite normal. *Thanks Doc!* **It is definitely normal but in no way, shape or form is this Natural.**

I guess North America takes the cake, so to speak. 20% over your ideal weight will put you in the obese category. A few of the side effects of obesity are, weaker bones, lower levels of vitamin D, loss of brain tissue, dementia, multiple sclerosis, depression, erectile dysfunction, decreased fertility, decreased sperm quality and quantity, increased diabetes, increased birth defects, suicides and lack of self confidence to name a few. Excess fat cannot be viewed as a cosmetic problem if you want it to go away forever.

I know it's not a pleasant situation for most, but if it wasn't for this situation being uncomfortable, we may not be motivated to find the root cause. The rules that we have been taught to live by are not just outdated but downright dangerous in today's environment if healthy living and a slender body is what you desire. There is only one major cause for this epidemic and this is toxicity within the body, which leads to acidosis. When you reduce toxicity, you reduce fat cells, this is simple science. When you restore vital nutrients that have been depleted from your food you turn off the hunger trigger in the brain. It's that simple, you're confused because they make it that way. Life is now sold by the pound. I say to you, **"Be The Cure, an ounce of prevention is worth pounds of fat."**

ARE YOU CURSED OR JUST CONFUSED

In my 35 years of practice there have been two common areas of motivation to lose weight. The first being how people view themselves and the second being how the excess weight makes them feel. Most people who are searching for weight loss have been searching for years and have failed at countless weight loss programs. Most are left feeling helpless and hopeless. Trust me, you're not cursed. If there was a curse it would be called misleading information.

Just a normal day in the office of your average medical doctor. In walks the patient looking 6 months pregnant, but wait! It's a man. *"Doc my feet are swelling, I've got hemorrhoids the size of grapes, heartburn, high blood pressure, low back pain and my diabetes is acting up."*

The doctor says, *"Let's get those hemorrhoids cut off. I'll write you a script for the high blood pressure and heartburn, send you for a blood test for your diabetes and then to a specialist."* Just because someone is well-educated does not mean they use logic.

Where the problem really started is when you went to battle with your weight and allowed others to **man**-ipulate your health with their false promises and cures instead of eating right and Gently Cleansing Daily. Healthy people are not overweight or underweight. Weight loss programs and drugs are only temporary solutions. A healthy lifestyle is a permanent fix to a healthy, slender **U**. To flush the pounds and lighten the load, you must flush the toilet and become conscious of what passes your lips.

All kidding aside, there are physical laws of nature - true laws of Nature. If you want to love your body, then love your body. Give it what it needs and it will give you what you have always wanted. There is a slender body under all those toxins.

When you change the way you look at things then you will change the way you look. Change your mind. Change your body. Take Life In, Take Life On, restore vital nutrients, gently cleanse daily and transform **the real U.**

SICK & FAT OR DEAD

Are you ready to have the body you always dreamed of?

Is your desire to have an awesome body and amazing health?

You cannot have one without the other, they come as a package deal and Nature delivers.

Are you prepared to cleanse the toxins from your body and meet all of its nutritional requirements?

If not, then be prepared to enlarge your closet as your body will do the same. The body cannot break down toxins. They must be eliminated properly and effectively and if not they will be stored in body fat. Toxins and body fat go hand in hand. Your body would rather be **sick** and **fat** than **dead**. It is not by accident that as environmental toxins are on the rise so is body weight.

We are being exposed to enormous amounts of environmental toxins that must be stored in fat cells to protect our vital organs, bones and life itself. **Don't get caught in the trap, your life depends on it!**

PULL THE TRIGGER ON HUNGER

There are two main reasons why the hunger trigger in your body malfunctions and does not turn off, leading to weight problems and obesity. The first reason that I would like to discuss; since our foods have and are being grown in nutrient depleted soil, it stands to reason that our diet is also low in vital nutrients. This is why the hunger trigger in the brain never shuts down. This is why we eat, and eat, and treat ourselves into a food coma, mistaking sugar for nutrients. Although most of the fruits and vegetables eaten today have chemicals and are lower in vital nutrients, never underestimate the power of their healing ability.

Even if they are inorganic, they should always come before any other food choice. We need enzyme rich live foods, they are the spark of life. Let logic prevail though, if you are not restoring the depleted essential nutrients that your fruit and vegetables have been robbed of with Whole Plant Based Superfood Nutrition and cleansing your body of these chemicals and toxins on a daily basis, then your body must take charge and increase fat production in attempts to slow down the inevitable; that being pain, illness, internal scar tissue formation, premature aging, disease and you know the rest of the story. We see this not only in ourselves, but in our children and our pets as well. **Death By Diet.**

In today's society large amounts of toxins are almost impossible to avoid if you buy into the system the way it has been programed for you. North Americans are overweight and fatter than ever; toxic chemical buildup and depleted nutrients are one of the main reasons why. Make no mistake, your body won't change until you do. Some examples of these toxic substances are, artificial sweeteners, trans-fatty acids in processed foods, high consumption of sugar and high fructose corn syrup.

Lots of chemical-laden food with very little nutritional value. What's wrong with this picture? It's exactly opposite to 50 years ago. Get rid of this fairytale idea that you have. There is not, and never will be, a latest, greatest diet that's going to fix this. We have to quit chasing the carrot that they put in front of our noses. You know the one; it's always just beyond your reach, **Doggone' IT!**

THE DOMINO EFFECT TO WEIGHT PROBLEMS AND OBESITY

The second but most important reason for out of control weight gain and obesity is **Metabolic Syndrome.**

1. A diet mainly comprised of refined carbohydrates, animal products, sugars and fatty, greasy foods.

2. Microbes *(bacteria)* become unbalanced in the colon due to foods high in fat and sugar, causing the growth of a family of bad bacteria, which produces and releases a toxic substance called endotoxin from their outer layer.

3. If the endotoxin is allowed to accumulate and stagnate within the colon it will be absorbed into the bloodstream, which will trigger the immune system to react. When this happens your body will conserve energy to gear up for a fight and maybe even a full out battle with these endotoxins.

4. You have now entered what is called Metabolic Syndrome. Your body is now out of balance causing your pancreas to pump out far too much insulin, far too fast. Insulin is used to regulate blood sugar levels. Since the body is out of balance it cannot read the signal from the hormone leptin, which tells the body it has had enough calories, already! The brain does not receive this signal that you are full, so you eat more. However, the lack of the hormone, leptin, is not the main problem that many would wish you to believe.

5. Your fat cells have now become bloated and stressed from storing excess calories and begin emitting a danger signal of low-grade inflammation.

6. Immune activation caused by low vibrational acidic foods, prompts insulin and leptin resistance. Sugar builds up in your blood causing insulin to increase, which causes your liver and pancreas having to strain to keep up to the overload. This is all caused by the danger signal, low-grade inflammation, which blocks your cells' ability to respond to the hormonal signals that are supposed to make you

feel full and shut down the hunger trigger. The next stop is diabetes and/or weight gain.

7. In conclusion, in order to reverse diabetes, lose weight and maintain a toned and slender body, you must eliminate inflammation. To eliminate inflammation you must first eliminate endotoxin from your

SKINNY CAN BE SCARY

In some ways those who are overweight are more protected from toxins than those who are thin, due to their bodies ability to create fat cells. Skinny does not mean healthy unless you are living a healthy lifestyle. You can still be skinny and have a fatty liver, insulin resistance, elevated blood sugar, high blood pressure and low-grade systemic inflammation. It's not how well we fit into our jeans. If you lack the protection that fat cells provide; Skinny can be even more dangerous if you partake in the so-called 'normal' diet. Without fat cells these toxins have a better chance of attacking bones, vital organs and body tissues. Hello, cellulite and internal scar tissue formation. I have worked on countless athletes who have great shaped body's but also have a lot of cellulite. Even runners must replenish essential nutrients that have been burned up, to neutralize the acid created from pounding the pavement.

Whether you are an athlete or the average person, **Whole Plant Based Nutrition and Gentle Daily Cleansing** is an absolute necessity in today's toxic environment. Whether your body tends to be overweight or skinny the same rules apply if a healthy, energetic, pain-free body is your goal.

TOXIC TIME BOMB

Toxic substances and chemicals are minute particles that the body simply cannot break down *(digest)*. Because the body has no ability to metabolize these toxic wastes, the body cannot totally and safely eliminate these harmful toxins, as the manufacturers of these chemicals would lead us to believe. Toxic chemicals are not dangerous at very low levels but where the danger lies is in the body's inability to eliminate them. If we do not understand the importance of daily detox and an Alkaline Superfood Lifestyle, this is where the struggle begins. With every year the planet becomes more toxic and so do we. So it stands to reason, the more toxic chemicals that get trapped in our body, the higher the risk for weight gain and continual pain. The problem is, these toxins if allowed to accumulate have a very nasty effect on your *'waste line'* and your overall well-being.

Biopsies of human fat show that 100% of humans have high levels of carcinogenic PCBs, styrene's and dioxins stored in their fat cells, bringing us just one step closer to cancer and other chronic degenerative diseases. Breaking down the fat will release these toxins into the bloodstream and possibly cause damage to the vital organs and bones if you do not support your body's cleansing and nutritional needs for a quick and effective elimination. Therefore the body's built-in survival mechanism will do all it can, to keep the fat intact until you take proper action to cleanse and restore vital nutrients daily. Toxins, over time, will destroy the body's ability to digest food effectively.

When this happens, the food will putrefy in the intestines and cause infection, inflammation, discomfort and bloating. Some examples of these toxins are pesticides, antibiotics, heavy metals, growth hormone in food, chemicals from our cleaning products, hair care products, make-up, unfiltered shower and drinking water, **PCBs** and other deadly chemicals that leach into food from packaging. You must become your own watchdog. Say, 'No' to that which does not serve your greater good. Say, 'Yes' to the one who loves you. **That would be U.**

REASONS WHY I'M FAT

1. I eat when I'm bored.

2. I'm bored all the time.

FAT WARS

Everywhere you go you see advertising on the latest, greatest breakthrough in the war on fat. Remember earlier when I said you cannot go to war with anything because it will just push back and get bigger. The 'war' train of thought only leads to frustration and a lighter wallet, not a lighter you. You cannot fool the body into losing weight; it seeks balance, it seeks health. When you try to stimulate your body by tricking it into losing weight with the 'flavor of the month' program, you will be left **heavily** disappointed. Everyone wants a balanced life, your body is no different. I want the best for you; stay away from **man**-ipulated food. The more man touches it, talks about it, tries to sell it, the quicker you should run from it. You cannot go to war with your fat and win. Most diets can cause plateaus in weight loss due to an adaptive response in your body. Recently, Dr. Oz stated that a whopping 99% of all

Americans are micronutrient deficient. Embrace Whole Plant Based Food. **Return to your roots.** *It's only Natural.*

INCREASE YOUR CORE REDUCE YOUR WASTE

Your colon *(large intestine)* is the most important organ to detoxify on a daily basis if you wish to lose weight, keep it off or simply not gain it. *Why, do you ask?* Because it is the Mother of all organs. It lives in an area of the body known as the *core (abdomen)*. When your core is strong and healthy, so are you. Give me a person with a strong core and I will show you a healthy, slender, vibrant human being. The colon is a major factor in whether you will be fat and flabby, or slim and toned, throughout your Whole body, throughout your Whole Life. Would you please put your hand on your belly button. Your belly button sits right at the '***waste line***'. No, I did not spell it wrong. Your colon surrounds this area and it's the body's main sewage system. In most people this sewage system becomes a cesspool that eventually leaks deadly toxins into the body's tissues and bloodstream. The first organ to feel the painful side effects of a sluggish toxic colon, as I have stated before, is the liver. *What do you think is one of the major side effects when the liver is overloaded with toxins from a faulty colon?* Pain and weight gain. So begins the **Battle of the Bulge**. Down and out.

Never underestimate the pain of a person, because in all honesty, everyone is struggling. Some people are better at hiding it than others.

- Will Smith

RESCUE MISSION

Let me say this another way. When the body is overloaded with toxins it transfers its energy away from the process of burning calories and uses that energy to try to detoxify a body in crisis. The body can no longer afford the energy to burn calories because the energy is desperately needed elsewhere. It is now on a *rescue mission*. What body tissues are closest to this toxic spillover? **Oops, it's your belly**. Welcome to the belly fat bulge. Why here? Because toxins must be stored quickly and efficiently to protect your bones and vital organs. Why the belly region?

Number 1: The toxins are far enough away when stored in the belly region to keep the bones and vital organs safe.

Number 2: These toxins were leaked mainly into the body tissues from the colon which is only a couple inches away from the belly. The belly is the closest and safest site for toxic storage. The body captures and stores the toxins in fat cells until the Master realizes what's 'growing' on under his/her nose, takes the garbage out and restores the vital nutrients so organ energy and tone is restored. The more toxins that have to be stored, the more belly fat you will accumulate. Do the math.

CELLULAR POWERHOUSE

Another side effect of producing unwanted body fat is damage to your mitochondria. A study done by Pascal Imbealt, concluded that exposure to large amounts of toxins will damage your mitochondria. The mitochondria are known as the powerhouses inside each cell of your body. They are organelles that act like a digestive system breaking down nutrients, thus creating energy for the cell. The process of creating cell energy is known as cellular respiration. Most of the chemical reactions involved in cellular respiration happen in the mitochondria. Mitochondria are the main location where fatty acids eventually undergo beta-oxidation. In the case of damaged mitochondria this may result in impaired fat burning. By avoiding excessive amounts of environmental toxins, Gentle Daily Cleansing, hydrating with Structured Water and restoring vital nutrients through Whole Plant Based Superfood Nutrition, your mitochondria will stay healthy and you decrease the risk of belly fat.

Belly fat has been shown to greatly weaken the immune system according to research done by Alexander Viardot at Garvan Institute of Medical Research. Conclusion: a large waistline will increase the risk of diseases of the immune system. Even when your weight is regarded as normal, studies have shown that waist circumference is almost always an accurate predictor of disease. So, reduce your waist *(waste)* and increase your overall health by getting to the CORE of the issue.

SIX STEPS TO GREAT HEALTH

1. Restore balance with a Whole Plant Based Alkaline Diet and plenty of dynamically Structured Water daily. Read *'Foods and Frequency'* and *'Water - The Structure of Life'* for a deeper understanding.
2. Eliminate toxic substances and EMF from your home.

3. Assist your blood and lymph by exercising 20 minutes minimum a day. Read *'Live Long Core Strong'*.
4. Skin brushing and Salt glows will also support skin, blood and lymph. Read *'Beautiful Skin'*.
5. Get all your body systems working in peak performance with Gentle Daily Cleansing and Whole Plant Based Superfood Nutrition daily. Read *'Superfood Nutrition'* and *'The Scoop On Your Poop'*.
6. Master your mind. You are what you focus on most of the time. Read *'Let's Get Mental'*.

MASTER YOUR BODY

1. **Drink Clean -** *Drink plenty of clean Structured Water. Drink half your body weight in ounces. If you weigh 150 pounds then you would drink 75 ounces or almost 2.5 quarts or 2.5 liters a day. Shower Clean - One of the most dangerous things you can do for your health is shower in chlorinated water. Each shower is equivalent to drinking 10 to 15 glasses of tap water. What do you think this is doing to your skin, lymph system, bloodstream and vital organs? Read 'Water - The Structure Of Life'.*

2. **Complete Elimination of Bowels Twice a Day -** *Cleanse and restore your vital detoxification organs on a daily basis. Castor oil packs on the abdominal area will aid in detox. Read 'The Scoop On Your Poop'.*

3. **Eat Toxin Free Where Possible -** *Organic produce and limit organic animal products this will help you reduce toxins, hormones and antibiotics.*

4. **Eat a Whole Plant Based Alkaline Diet.** *Proper food combining. Eat right for your blood type. Read 'Foods and Frequency'.*

5. **Avoid -** *White flour, white sugar, sugar substitutes and corn syrup. Stevia is your best sugar substitute.*

6. **Eliminate Where Possible -** *Stimulants, sedatives, drugs, caffeine, nicotine, and alcohol.*

7. **Exercising -** *Find an exercise regime you enjoy so you keep doing it. If you like it, you will do it often. Myself, I like to work out on my Core Master and Core Rebounder. I also enjoy yoga and swimming. Find your passion and get moving. Read 'Live Long Core Strong'.*

8. **Get A Sweat On -** *When possible get a good sweat going. To enhance skin detox. See skin brushing and salt glow. Read 'Beautiful Skin'.*

9. **Whole Plant Based Superfood Nutrition -** *Natures most dense phytonutrient plant on the planet. Nutritionally and scientifically backed. Take Life in everyday. Read 'Superfood Nutrition'.*

10. **Find Peace And Joy From Within -** *Meditate, pray, sit in silence, learn to deep breathe or just go for a quiet peaceful walk in Nature. Read 'Let's Get Mental'.*

Create the perfect weight, go to: www.docofdetox.com/consultations

SPOILED ROTTEN

"The All American Meat & Potato Man is now down and out mentally, physically and emotionally because he has allowed others to Spoil him Rotten."

- Dr. Darrell Wolfe, Doc of Detox

HI HONEY, I'M HOME & I'M STARVING

All American Meat and Potato Man. *"Hi honey I'm home! I've had a hard day and I'm starving!"* Well, of course the man is starving, malnourished and toxic; he's only been taught to satisfy his taste buds and fill his stomach, so he's a little grumpy. He has never been taught proper guidelines for eating or the need to cleanse his digestive tract on a daily basis. This is no fault of his or his wife's.

Their nutritional training has been passed down from person to person based on hand me down tips, media advertising and the few hours of nutritional training that doctors receive. As far as health tips go, the rules to the eating game have changed drastically over the last 50 years: environmental toxicity, GMOs, processed foods, plastics and chlorinated drinking and showering water. As far as nutritional facts obtained through the media, make sure you have a great medical plan *(evil plot)*. The average medical doctor is not trained in nutrition or detoxification so it's not fair to make them responsible for something they have never been educated on.

When one is always starving, one is always eating. Here's the dirty little secret: teach the population to eat lots of empty foods with chemical hooks and little nutritional value. What? This makes no sense you may think. Oh grasshopper, it's long past making cents, and onto making **billion$**. Their Master Plan consists of teaching people to eat food deprived of nutrients. This results in making corporations rich while causing the meat and potato man to be sick, frustrated and broke. Not just broke, but actually breaking down both physically and emotionally. The meat and potato man is now Spoiled Rotten. Rotting from the inside out and the bottom up. I love when a plan comes together *(evil plot)*. Now it's off to the doctor to get more chemicals. These are known as pharmaceutical drugs. Because the meat and potato man looks and feels sick, he now needs drugs to suppress the pain and suffering. Have you ever had the feeling you've been played? Do you want to know how the '*Meat and Potato Man*' can mess up this evil plot? By being the Master of his health. You can live by chance or by choice, you decide. The key is the following: always question authority because **U** are the only authority for you. Believe nothing you read, hear or see on TV until you have proven it for yourself. It is also important to learn the art of cleansing and which foods nurture a healthy body.

In order to take correct action it is vital that one:

a. Does not rely on TV information.
b. Shops only the outside aisles of the grocery store.
c. Eats fresh, raw and organic as much as possible.
d. Realizes that the more man touches it the less you want to eat it.
e. Never becomes dehydrated, drink Structured Water.
f. Gets some form of core exercise everyday.
g. Finds that peaceful place within so external chaos does not Master your mind. **Make sure the decisions you are making are actually yours and not unconscious downloads.**

NUTRIENT DEPRIVED AND HURTING

Now let's feed that starving, malnourished, toxic and tired, meat and potato man. Being the loving wife she is, she gives him a large serving of meat and potatoes. The starving meat and potato man gulps down his food, barely tasting or chewing it. We want to chew our food well because we do not have a second set of teeth in our stomach. In addition, the smaller particle size of the food allows a greater surface area for stomach acid and enzymes to digest and assimilate the nutrients captured. Another golden rule for effective digestion is: **NEVER MIX A PROTEIN WITH A STARCH**. Meat requires protein enzymes for digestion and potatoes require starch enzymes. When these enzymes are put together they neutralize one another and allow the ingested food to putrefy (rot). Instead of the food being digested by enzymes, it breaks down and putrefies with bad bacteria. A side effect of this is bloating created by noxious gas. In addition, mixing different types of concentrated cooked foods takes more energy to digest than the actual energy derived from the food itself. This is obvious because after a meal you should feel energized, not sluggish. Another problem arises; not only are the body's internal enzymes neutralized, the cooked foods have had their naturally occurring enzymes destroyed through the heat used in the cooking process. As a result, your food has a greater chance of putrefying. This can lead to gas, ulcers, inflammation, infection, heartburn, bloating, constipation and diarrhea. When we make unhealthy food choices this will be a bumpy ride from the mouth all the way to the rectum. It is always a wise decision to have a salad with every meal where possible. The live enzymes aid in digestion and the fiber supports the cleansing and toning of the digestive tract and also restores the good bacteria in the colon. Is the greater weight and volume of your diet coming from Whole Plant Based Food?

SLOW MOTION TRAIN WRECK

All foods carry a vibrational frequency. Is your diet bringing your frequency *(energy)* up or down? Life breeds Life. The more fresh and raw you eat, the more vibrant *(high vibration)* you will look and feel. Fresh and Raw foods carry a high vibrational frequency that aids in both healing and a strong immune system. The flip side of the coin is, *"The more you cook the worse you look. The more you fry, the sooner you die."* Cooked and processed foods carry a low, or no vibrational frequency, which vibrates at the level of sickness and infectious invaders such as parasites, fungus and bad bacteria. How low will you go? Heads you win, tails you lose your health. Remember when you were younger and could eat a whole pizza? Try that today and see how you look and feel. Our body simply does not produce enzymes like we used to when we were younger. The last time I ate like that I woke up the next morning feeling like I had been hit by a train. No one enjoys a hit and run. Eat live food and stay that way, Nature's way!

FULL BUT RUNNING ON EMPTY

Let's get back to our meat and potato man. He's almost finished eating his meal *('scarfing', to be more accurate)*.

He begins to feel better because his sugar glucose is climbing and he's feeling more energetic. His wife says, *"Honey, do you think you would like to come with me for a walk tonight? We haven't done that for a while."* *"Sure sweetie,"* he agrees. His wife finishes eating and starts cleaning the dishes. Our meat and potato man is just finishing his supper and his wife asks, *"Dear, are you full yet?"* and of course he belches. He is suffering from low hydrochloric acid production in his stomach due to the build-up of mucus congestion created from the constant irritation and inflammation of **The 'All American Die-it'**.

As the meal draws to an end, he grows tired. Poor guy! No matter how much he eats he can't get his energy back, it's been years. Poor eating habits have spoiled him rotten. His food has begun to putrefy due to a broken down digestive tract and poor dietary habits. As mentioned earlier, we either digest our food with enzymes or it breaks down through putrefaction (rotting) with bad bacteria. The purpose of eating; **to feed the body, not fill it.**

"Honey, how about that walk, I'll finish the dishes and we'll go." She says. *"Gee, Dear. I don't know. I just feel too tired to go for a walk right now. I think I'll just sit here for a while and let my food digest (putrefy),"* he replies. You see, our Meat and Potato man has not eaten in an effective way. Blood flow has decreased in his limbs and other organs and has increased in his digestive tract.

This is a protective response coming from his body's system in hopes to reduce the putrefaction (rotting) of his dinner so his toxemia (dirty blood) does not escalate into severe acidosis. The reduced blood flow to his arms, legs, and head has deprived him of the little oxygen he did have. This has made him feel even more tired than when he started to eat.

Where's the Life? This is a story where abnormal becomes normal and now the pressure is starting to build down below and the Meat and Potato man is getting ready to blow.

ACROSS THE ROOM

You guessed it, he has had to loosen his belt a couple of notches. The putrefying food in his stomach strengthens the bad bacteria, which give off gas, blowing him up like a balloon within minutes after the meal. *"Gee, honey,"* he gasps, *"I feel pressure on my chest; I feel like I am having a heart attack."* After a short time a rumbling starts, the dinner table begins to shake; his wife turns in fright to see her husband with one hand on his waistline and the other over his heart with a look of distress on his face. And... **KA- BOOM, across the room!** He lets one go from the back door that shoots him across the kitchen floor. The gas was so fierce it shot him over to the couch. Maybe it's a good thing for three reasons: he may not have moved all night, he can now pull his belt in an extra inch, and the pressure around his heart has been alleviated from the release of gas. Hundreds of people each day visit emergency rooms mistaking a heart attack for a gas attack. As the hot gas rises and puts pressure on the lungs and heart, the absorbed poisons eat up minerals and oxygen needed by these organs, causing undue pressure in the upper chest. It's always better to be safe than sorry, but first lighten the load and flush the pounds to take the pressure off. **It's Tea Time**, not Miller Time. Back to our story, *"Are you okay, Honey?"* She asks from the kitchen. The pressure is gone but not the rotten feeling. *"I think I'll just stay (lay) on the couch and rest for a few minutes (hours),"* he replies (couch potato). Does he remind you of anyone?

BURNT OUT ON ACID

7 million people yearly visit the emergency with Acid Reflux; and yes, he's gripping his chest, the heartburn he is experiencing

now has his full attention. Well, it did. You guessed it, a few minutes later he is sawing logs; snoring to the beat of the band. They're playing Roll Out the Barrel. Do you know why he's snoring? The food did not digest with enzymes, it putrefied with bad bacteria. The bacteria broke the food down leaving behind toxic gas, fungus and waste, causing increased acidity *(pH imbalance)*, decreased oxygen and increased mucus congestion from the irritation. The snoring is caused by his exhausted state, sinus problems *(fungus)* and lack of oxygen. 30 million people suffer from sinus problems today. 20 million people suffer from asthma and 2 million from Emphysema. We become toxic from the bottom up. He is fighting for his life, whether he or his wife realize it or not. Just because this has become a normal way of life, this is in no way a natural way to live. Where's the walk? Where's Romeo?

BEAR BUTT IN A RUTT

It is 11:00 p.m. and time for bed. His wife gently wakes him up but he's grumpy as a bear and has the breath of one too. *Why?* Nobody feels good when they're rotting. One of my teachers told me, *"People aren't grumpy, they're just constipated."* Remember his sewer system has been backed up for years and is now a cesspool that breeds dis-ease. Luckily it's only 11 o'clock, just in time for his daily dose of bad news, like he doesn't feel badly enough already.

He watches the news where all the worst events in the world are condensed to a half hour of even more stomach upset *(evil plot)*. But on the bright side, it makes him feel better on some crazy level, knowing that there's somebody out there worse off than himself. His focus is now on all the world's problems that he cannot solve, instead of focusing on the real problems he can; being The Master of His Health and reviving his relationship with his body and his Honey.

A TRAGIC LOVE STORY

You know how the story ends. Another unfulfilled night with/for his loving wife and, of course, the walk stays on hold. Now he peels himself off the couch and drags his butt to bed. Because the news was the last thing he downloaded to his brain the sweet dreams are on hold too *(evil plot)*.

The cycle continues. You guessed it, it's 3:35 a.m. and our Meat and Potato Man has been to the washroom three times. Just like his bowel, hardly anything comes out and when it does, he has to force it. Drip, drip, drop. His sluggish bowel, his bladder infection and, let us not forget his inflamed prostate have caused his life to become a real struggle.

The *'Domino Effect'* is in full force due to his sluggish colon leaking its toxic waste into the pelvic girdle. This cesspool leads to bladder infection, prostate inflammation, and later, maybe even prostate cancer.

When cells are bathed in toxic waste long enough, inflammation, internal scar tissue formation and mutation become the logical outcome. All his energy is needed to fight the continual inflammation in his body. His life is now in a holding pattern until he takes charge of his health or just burns out. The prostate is located right beside the most toxic section of the colon, this would be the rectum. As I have stated countless times before, the '*Mother*' of all organs is the large intestine. Show her the respect that she deserves or she will back up, you will break down and all cell will break loose.

With the high levels of toxicity in his lifestyle, including toxins from the food he eats, the chlorinated water he drinks and showers in, lack of exercise and government sanctioned diet, this '*Meat and Potato Man*' is in a pickle. Prostate imbalances are illnesses of the digestive tract, primarily the large intestine. Does this have to happen? No! Can you do something about it? Yes! Your body can and will heal itself when you take charge and Master your part of this partnership. Now let's get back to our story.

He wakes up with a sinus headache the next morning, as tired as when he went to bed. 12 million people suffer from sleep apnea. 45 million people today suffer from chronic headaches. His body could not rest, recuperate or restore itself. It's been working overtime all night trying to deal with his toxic state. Oh, and by the way, you better not speak to him until he has had his morning coffee. He feels he needs his daily fix of caffeine to get going; in more ways than one. **Number One:** to alleviate his exhausted state so he can participate in life on some level, and I mean this in the best way. As long as he is being Mastered by others his life will never be his.

Number Two: he will be working on NUMBER TWO for the next twenty to thirty minutes. He must use coffee as a stimulant to go to the washroom as he has done for the last few years because his large intestine is in a state of coma (lacking tone). **He has hemorrhoids the size of grapes and now walks like John Wayne.** *How's that workin' for ya Partner?* He also suffers from a hiatus hernia resulting from the countless years of pushing and grunting, trying to force a bowel movement every morning when he doesn't have diarrhea.

As far as coffee goes it gives neither oxygen nor nutrition to the body. When it hits the liver it increases **metabolism**, giving a false sense of energy that is simply stolen from this organ. If only he realized the best things in life are not found in a line up, on TV, in the newspaper, the tip of the day from his buddies or his medical doctor. Sometimes you have to look under a rock, climb a mountain, swim the river, but the answer will come. If he took XM Plus first thing in the morning followed by SuperMix, which is a Whole Plant Based Superfood, Goodbye, coffee blues and Hello, I love my life, I have energy, I'm losing weight, life looks brighter and I think my wife even likes me more. Go figure.

Eventually, something will have to give if he continues down the same old path. Never put the walk on hold. The next time it may be more than gas for this Master Blaster. Here he sits broken hearted, wished for a movement but only farted. Garbage In Garbage Out. What you put into your body matters.

What stays in matters. What comes out matters even more... If he would just drink Doc of Detox Daily Cleansing Tea and SuperMix, the happier and healthier he and his Honey would surely be. Remember, small steps make big changes. So if you know someone like this let them know they're not cursed, they are the Cure to everything. **Take Control and Be The Cure U** Wish To See!

I AM WOMAN

"God created Man and then he created a MasterPIECE."

- *Dr. Darrell Wolfe, Doc of Detox*

PMS AND PAINFUL PERIODS

Premenstrual Syndrome (PMS) is believed to affect approximately 80% of women at some point in their lives. Some women are mildly affected, experiencing few symptoms, while for others PMS may seriously affect their lives on a monthly basis. The term PMS is used to describe a wide range of symptoms that occur after the middle of the menstrual cycle *(ovulation)* and disappear almost as soon as the period arrives because the toxic pressure in the lower abdomen and pelvic region is now being alleviated. These symptoms can range from bloating, water retention, muscle pain and spasms, breast tenderness, migraines, depression, mood swings, food cravings, etc. So men, be gentle on your partner! Help her to become healthier, it could be you.

Since PMS is so common the general consensus seems to be that this is a condition that you should just put up with each month. This is just another case where abnormal is accepted as normal by the average person. However, our view is quite different. We believe that by having an alkaline lifestyle, mainly comprised of fresh and raw foods, Superfood Nutrition and Gentle Daily Cleansing, along with the proper amount of pure Structured Water, will detoxify and restore these organs; especially the colon and liver, so you can free yourself from this vicious cycle and go with the flow.

> **P.M.S.**
>
> *Punish Men Severely*

BALANCING ACT

Constipation and the health of your intestines may not seem an obvious factor in PMS, but let me assure you, they are. Regular bowel movements are essential in the removal of toxins and processed hormones from your body. If you suffer from constipation or a sluggish colon then toxins and estrogen ready for excretion will be reabsorbed back into your body. These reabsorbed estrogen wastes will add to an already existing hormonal imbalance, which further burdens the liver. In this situation you will also experience increased water retention and bloating. Regular daily bowel movements are a priority to restore balance. Flush the pounds, lighten your load and balance yourself mentally, physically and hormonally.

THE WHOLE POOP ON AND ABOUT THE FEMALE FIBROID

Fibroids are the most frequently seen tumors of the female reproductive system. I will explain what I believe to be the major cause of these fibroids and then let you decide if my theory is based on a foundation of logic and scientific fact. Fibroids are also known as uterine myomas, leiomyomas, or fibromas. These compact, abnormal growths are made of smooth muscle cells and fibrous connective tissue that develop in the uterus. Some studies have shown that up to 77% of women will develop fibroids sometime during their childbearing years, although only about 1/3 of these fibroids are large enough to be detected. In more than 99% of all fibroid cases, the tumors are found to be benign *(non-cancerous)*. Fibroids will range in size, from as small as a pea to as large as a softball or small grapefruit.

When it comes to the cause of fibroids the medical system believes estrogen levels influence them but the true cause still remains unclear to them. I believe that estrogen plays a part, but a much smaller part than they would have us believe. I also believe that the medical system has a tendency to make everything into a mystery that could even boggle the greatest of minds.

For the medical system, fibroids are no longer a symptom of improper self care. They have been labeled a disease that needs a medical specialist, since only they can figure out what is the latest greatest drug to suppress your symptoms because they won't take action until the fibroids are big enough to be cut out (evil plot). Once again we have been given a subconscious download implying that we cannot properly Master our own health. This eliminates the greatest Law of Nature, which assures us that the body heals everything when we follow the Laws of Nature.

Definition of Endometriosis

Endometriosis *(en-doe-me-tree-O-sis)* is an often painful disorder in which tissue that normally lines the inside of the uterus - the endometrium - grows outside the uterus *(endometrial implant)*. Endometriosis most commonly involves the ovaries, bowel or the tissue lining the pelvis. Endometrial tissue may spread beyond the pelvic region, but rarely.

In endometriosis, displaced endometrial tissue continues to act as it normally would - it thickens, breaks down and bleeds with each menstrual cycle. Because this displaced tissue has no way to exit the body, it becomes trapped *(web of destruction)*. When endometriosis involves the ovaries, cysts called endometriomas may form. Surrounding tissue can become irritated, inflamed and eventually develops internal scar tissue and adhesions; both of which are abnormal tissue that binds organs together *(invisible bonds)*. Read 'Web of Destruction' for a deeper understanding.

Endometriosis can cause pain, sometimes severe - especially during menstrual periods. Fertility problems may also develop because basically, it's become a jungle of scar tissue and toxic waste in the pelvic region so life is being choked out.

What are the symptoms of Uterine Fibroids?

- Heavy or prolonged menstrual periods
- Abnormal bleeding between menstrual periods
- Pelvic pain *(caused by the tumor pressing on pelvic organs)*
- Lower back pain
- Pain during intercourse
- A firm mass, often located near the middle of the pelvis, which can be felt by the physician
- Increased urination frequency
- Constipation, gas and/or abdominal bloating
- Pain in the back or legs
- Emotional stress

Definition of Fibroids: Fibroids are benign (non-cancerous) tumors made of muscle and fibrous tissue that grow in a woman's uterus.

Hysterectomy: Hysterectomies involve the surgical removal of the entire uterus. Fibroids remain the #1 reason for hysterectomies in North America. As you're reading forward please keep in mind the above information on Endometriosis, Fibroids and Hysterectomy. You may not be aware of the scientific health fact that your large intestine is not just the bodies sewer system, but also the '*Mother*' of all organs and demands your attention and respect. This is accomplished by Gentle Daily Cleansing.

I believe the most effective method to prevent and reverse endometriosis and pelvic fibroids and to save your uterus, lies within the large intestine. The uterus is sandwiched between the bladder and the last few inches of the large intestine known as the sigmoid colon. How many times have you felt there was just a little more fecal waste to be eliminated but it was caught in the last part of your large intestine. It only stands to reason that as fecal waste becomes stagnant and toxic, the pelvic area will also become toxic and inflamed as the fecal waste is absorbed through the colon wall and into the pelvic girdle. Oh, and by the way, I have patients who have had colon cancer and they pooped regularly, three times a day. It's not what comes out that destroys our health, but what stays in and putrefies. The first step towards health is to create an environment in your large intestine where fecal waste does not stagnate and where invaders, like Endobacteria, cannot exist. Your health rests on you keeping a proper balance of 85% good bacteria and no more than 15% bad bacteria within your large intestine.

As long as your intestinal bacteria are in proper balance, they will keep you in balance physically, mentally and emotionally. For most people the ratio is the exact reverse, or worse: 85% bad bacteria to 15% good bacteria. Your digestive tract makes up 80-85% of your immune system. The greatest percentage of your immune system resides in the Mother of all organs, the large intestine (colon). When kept in balance, the good microbes (bacteria) help break down fibers, harvest calories and protect us from micro invasion. Your gut functions as your body's second brain.

1 out of 4 Americans will eat a high fat, high carbohydrate fast food meal each and every day. 25% of the population participates in this type of eating everyday; it has become widely accepted. These eating habits have a huge negative impact on the abdominal area, but because most of the population eats like this, it is regarded as normal. When your bacteria ratio goes from friendly to unfriendly it will become downright pathogenic, leaking noxious by-products, known as endotoxin into the pelvic area and cause inflammation which leads to the beginning of the web of destruction - the formation of internal scar tissue. Hello, Endo. Prepare for all 'cell' to break loose; this is the beginning of Endometriosis.

When this happens the Domino Effect begins and the trillions of bad bacteria will turn on you and make your life a living hell. This is due to the highly acidic waste known as Endotoxin being excreted by the unfriendly bacteria. Acidosis, inflammation, pain, scar tissue, fibroids, endometriosis, dis-ease, surgery, infertility and even painful lovemaking will be the result for the uninformed. Meals and drinks high in sugar and/or greasy or refined carbohydrate meals will accelerate this inflammation due to the added release of the molecule, known as endotoxin, from the outer walls of certain bad bacteria that now reside in your colon. Endotoxin, if not eliminated from your colon, through Gentle Daily Cleansing, can and will be absorbed into the bloodstream causing inflammation and pain to the weakest and most vulnerable part of the body, which tends to be the pelvis due to the force of gravity.

When this acidic waste enters the body, the circulation in the pelvic region becomes backed up and congested. This waste will settle, stagnate, irritate and inflame tissue cells causing painful contractions. Inflammation is created by the body to warn you of a perceived threat or injury. If left unattended, the body initiates a secondary support system, which starts continual fibrin production (internal scar tissue) to the inflamed area of concern in order to wall off the inflammation overload... Hello, endometriosis and fibroids! To add even more fuel to the fire the majority of women over 40 are suffering from some degree of a fallen transverse colon (prolapsed). This is a condition where the large intestine has fallen down due to weak abdominal muscles thus causing even more unnecessary pressure in the pelvic region. This pressure will decrease circulation to the uterus and ovaries until you learn how to cleanse your digestive tract and tone your core. A good place to start would be to monitor what comes in the front door and what goes out the back door.

This continual fibrin production, if not halted, will drain you of your vital energy, your essential nutrients and will create massive internal scar tissue, which will gradually harden and immobilize, deteriorate, mutate and distort the tissues in and around the pelvic region. This internal scar tissue can and will continue to develop as long as the inflammation is present. Many will suffer massive internal scar tissue formation as if there has been a physical injury to the pelvic area. Hello, 'invisible bonds'. Hello, fibrous mass.

The two groups of women who have the greatest risk for developing fibroids are those approaching menopause and women who are overweight.

Let me first address women who are in or approaching menopause. First of all, let me say that when women come to me with severely painful periods, it usually takes them no more than 4 to 6 weeks to reduce or totally eliminate these painful symptoms. When you reduce the toxic load from the abdominal region and pelvic girdle, you will also eliminate muscle contractions, spasms, inflammation and internal scar tissue formation.

As women enter menopause, the period slows down or becomes nonexistent. The period is a built-in detoxification process that has an added benefit that doctors never talk about. Enormous amounts of toxic waste are eliminated during the period, but when combined with a toxic sluggish large intestine, this overload of toxic waste in the lower abdominal region creates the perfect storm. It brings to the pelvic region severe contractions, over the top spasms, inflammation, fever and high acidic levels, causing internal scar tissue formation.

Another concern can occur when your period completely stops. You have just lost a very effective detoxification process.

What do you think happens to these extra toxins that you are no longer being eliminated on a monthly basis? They are now accumulating in your body and, thanks to a sluggish bowel and the downward force of gravity, we now have chronic tissue inflammation that leads to increased internal scar tissue formation in the pelvic region unless you flush the pounds to lighten the load in your large intestine.

The next group of women who are at a high risk of developing fibroids are those who are overweight. Concern about this very common condition is something, which many women share. For very heavy women, the risk is 2 to 3 times greater than average. For those overweight we usually find 4 problems. The first is the excess weight of the abdomen and the second, a lack of tone in the abdominal muscles and large intestine, so this area has a tendency to fall downward and out ward so everything beneath it in the pelvic area gets choked and squashed. Also overconsumption of greasy or refined carbohydrates, sugar, fatty foods and a lack of Gentle Daily Cleansing of the large intestine.

Whole Plant Based Superfood Nutrition, proper hydration through Structured Water, Gentle Daily Cleansing and core restore exercises must come first and foremost to avoid or reverse this condition. It's what you do daily that forms your life and shapes your body. If you are prepared to make these changes, you could potentially avoid surgery or years of pain and suffering which, for many women, will become their life story.

The effort of taking charge and Mastering your body is a small price to pay to restore joy to your life - and keep it.

If you do not take out the garbage, the bottom line is, the garbage will take you out. Work on that which is sticking out. Instead of getting treatment get training and take control of your health and well being and Be The Cure **U** search for.

HOT FLASH OR FEVER

Hot flashes, a common symptom of menopause, are typically experienced as a feeling of intense heat with sweating and rapid heartbeat. These flashes may last from 2 to 30 minutes for each occurrence. The sensation of heat usually begins in the face or chest, although it may appear elsewhere such as the back of the neck, and it can spread throughout the whole body. Some women feel as if they are going to faint. This is due to a toxic overload *(acidosis)* eating up oxygen and essential minerals, creating a pH imbalance. In addition to being an internal sensation, the surface of the skin, especially on the face, becomes hot to the touch. This is the origin of the alternative term 'hot flush', since the sensation of heat is often accompanied by visible reddening of the face. Excessive flushing can lead to rosacea. The hot flash event may be repeated a few times each week or every few minutes throughout the day.

Hot flashes may begin to appear several years before menopause starts and last for years afterwards. Some women who undergoing menopause never have hot flashes. Others have mild or infrequent flashes. The worst sufferers experience dozens of hot flashes each day. In addition, hot flashes are often more frequent and more intense during hot weather or in an overheated room. The surrounding heat apparently making the hot flashes themselves both more probable and more severe. The number of hot flashes and their length will depend on nutritional support, organ integrity and the amount of toxins the body needs to burn off to accomplish some sense of balance.

I believe this hot flash to be a mini-fever and I will explain why. In a fever you will also experience a hot flash, hot flush, red face, fever and profuse sweating day or night. The hot flash can be compared to boiling water. If you don't want the water to boil then you must turn down the burner to reduce the heat. If you want the hot flash to leave, the toxins must leave. When you follow the Laws of Nature, it's only Natural to feel and look great. It's the law!

CALCIUM DEPOSITS SYMPTOMS OF TOXIC BREASTS

In 2011 breast cancer represented the most common serious cancer of women in the United States, with over 200,000 new cases diagnosed every year, according to the National Cancer Institute. Calcium deposits, or calcifications, in your breast are a common finding on mammograms and can indicate either benign or cancerous changes. Calcium deposits occur in the breasts tissue as a safety mechanism when breast tissue becomes overly acidic *(acidosis)*. These calcium deposits can occur in any part of the body that becomes overly acidic. Due to the acidic nature of our diets, lack of Whole Plant Based Superfood Nutrition and Gentle Daily Cleansing, 44 million people suffer with osteoporosis and another 40 million suffer with arthritis, which is due majorly to the loss of calcium to buffer an acidic condition. Put another way, Osteoporosis can be viewed as a symptom of an acidic body using the calcium to put out the Fire at the expense of your bones. We now know that the main cause of acidity in the body tissues is caused by excess toxins. These being environmental toxins and absorbed toxins from a sluggish colon causing the liver to become over burdened. In the case of breast tissue, when toxins become stored in this area of the body, the tissue becomes acidic and fungal in nature. The body then pulls on calcium as a safety mechanism to help balance and restore pH. Calcium is sent to the breast tissue to buffer down the acidity in the attempt to reduce infection, inflammation, fungal production, cysts, fibroid scar tissue and other abnormal growths. **When abnormal is accepted as normal, this is the sign of a Broken System.**

BREAST MAGNETS

These excess toxins must be stored in fat cells quickly and efficiently to protect damage to your bones and vital organs. *Why the breast region?* **Number 1:** The toxins are far enough away when stored in the breasts region to keep the bones and vital organs safe. **Number 2:** The breast tissue is composed of fatty tissue and when the body becomes toxic this acidic waste must be stored in fat cells. So in a sense your breasts are like magnets for toxins, acidity and then bone calcium. The breasts make ideal ready made storage tanks for acidic overload. To add fuel to the fire, if an antiperspirant is being used, this will compound the problem by shutting down the sweat glands and creating even more acidity within the breast tissue. The more toxins that have to be stored, the higher the acidity, the lower the pH thus greater the risk of calcium deposits in this area to protect you from cancer and other unwanted symptoms. To prevent or reverse this condition one must eat a Whole Plant Based alkaline diet, drink plenty of dynamically Structured Water and cleanse gently on a daily basis. The only way to properly restore balance for whole body healing is with a lifestyle that supports restoring proper pH balance. Eliminate the acidity and leave your bones where they belong...bon appétit.

ELIMINATE BREAST TOXICITY, RAISE YOUR FREQUENCY TAKE LIFE IN.

JUST A SPOONFUL OF SUGAR

"The average American consumes 150 lb. of sugar per year. The average child consumes a whopping 32 teaspoons per day. Gasoline is to Fire as Sugar is to Cancer."

- Dr. Darrell Wolfe, Doc of Detox

FOR THE RIDE OF YOUR LIFE

TYPE 2 - ADULT ONSET Diabetes is an epidemic on fire. As of today there is 26 million plus with diabetes and 79 million with a pre-diabetic condition. At this rate of growth there will be 130 million full blown diabetics by 2050, if the pharmaceutical corporations have their way. This will continue to get even worse due to the increase in environmental toxins, processed packaged foods, processed carbohydrates, sugar intake, chlorinated tap water and plastic bottled water. Where the gas hits the fire is the lack of knowledge, regarding a high vibrational nutrient dense diet and Gentle Daily Cleansing, which will prevent and reverse this life-altering condition. One of the main causes for triggering diabetes is Metabolic Syndrome.

STEPS LEADING TO METABOLIC SYNDROME

1. A diet mainly composed of refined carbohydrates, sugars and fatty, greasy foods.
2. Microbes *(bacteria)* become unbalanced in the colon due to foods high in fat and sugar causing the growth of a family of bad bacteria, which produce and release from their outer layer a toxic substance called endotoxin.
3. If the endotoxin is allowed to accumulate and stagnate within the colon it will be absorbed into the bloodstream, which will trigger the immune system to react. When this happens your body will conserve energy to gear up for a fight and maybe even a full out battle with these endotoxins.
4. You have now entered what is called Metabolic Syndrome. Your body is now out of balance causing your pancreas to pump out far too much insulin far too fast, which is used to

regulate blood sugar levels. Since the body is out of balance it cannot read the signal from the hormone leptin, which tells the body it has had enough calories, already! The brain does not receive this signal that you are full, so you eat more. Lack of the hormone leptin is not the main problem that many would wish you to believe.

5. Your fat cells have now become bloated and stressed from storing excess calories and begin emitting a danger signal of low-grade inflammation.

6. Immune activation caused by low vibrational acidic foods, prompts insulin and leptin resistance. Sugar builds up in your blood causing insulin to increase, which causes your liver and pancreas to strain to keep up to this overload. This is all caused by the danger signal, low- grade inflammation, which blocks your cells' ability to respond to the hormonal signals that are supposed to make you feel full and shut down the hunger trigger. The next stop is diabetes and/or weight gain.

7. In conclusion, to reverse diabetes, lose weight and maintain a toned and slender body you must eliminate inflammation. To eliminate inflammation you must first eliminate endotoxin from your intestines by leaning towards an alkaline lifestyle along with Gentle Daily Cleansing and nutritious Whole Plant Based Food. Many have what I call 'unconscious eating', no fault of theirs. Remember, only **U** are responsible for your body, even though others pretend to be.

When your diet is made up of generous amounts of white processed sugar and refined carbohydrates on a daily basis rising levels of insulin in the blood will be impossible to avoid. Eating processed sugars and refined carbohydrates will create a false chemical high and an endorphin release, which is always followed by a physical and emotional crash. Depression is usually the outcome due to over-stimulation of the brain releasing large amounts of endorphins into the bloodstream. If the consumption of processed sugars and refined carbohydrates continue, essential minerals and micronutrients will be depleted and acidosis will prevail. The body cells will lower in vibrational frequency *(energy)* becoming addicted to sugars and refined carbohydrates in their attempts to get out of a depressed *(low vibration)* state searching for that chemical high.

Whenever large amounts of sugar hit the bloodstream creating this false, acidic high, the body counteracts by sending vast amounts of insulin to the scene of the crime to neutralize the effects, thus creating an emotional and physical downer. This **whiplash effect** is just the body trying to find balance *(rescue mission)*. When you pull on an elastic band too fast and let go, it will whip back to normal and when it does someone always gets hurt. **Better hurt than dead.**

This whiplash effect will cause physical and emotional chaos for *'all'* of those involved. Side effects from the sugar hit will last for about an hour whereas the effects from insulin can last much longer. This up and down roller coaster will deplete the life force from the body on an emotional and physical level, which will weaken the immune system leaving the body vibrating at a very low level and leaving it open to infectious invaders and chronic illness.

When the pancreas becomes chronically fatigued, it will still produce insulin but of a poor quality. This is why the first step of Type 2 diabetes is oral medication to support this ailing insulin situation. In the case of gall bladder problems, due to a diet usually too high in bad fats, gall bladder attacks may result. You would think that logic would prevail and there would be a diet change and Gentle Daily Cleansing implemented. This is not usually the case. Most people will opt to get their gall bladder removed to relieve themselves of the pain but never addressing the cause. With the gall bladder removed there is no longer an alarm system to alert us of bad fat consumption. As a result, most will continue on this path creating a new and worse chronic problem. I shared this story because it's similar to that of Adult Onset Diabetes, which as we know is mainly caused by an unconscious diet resulting in insulin medication. This is usually a ticket to disaster for most because they do not get the educational support they need in getting a new mindset. They use the insulin medications to continue their unconscious eating, thus lowering their vibration, similar to a jet in free fall. This ride will never end unless a high vibrational nutrient dense lifestyle is implemented on a personal level.

Diabetes is a huge money machine where the Whole Truth is easily lost. When acidic wastes accumulate in the pancreas, diabetes can develop due to the lack of quality insulin produced. This delicate process will not return to a healthy state until these pancreatic tissue cells do first. When you work in sync with the Mother Of All Organs and focus on whole body healing with Whole Plant Based Superfood Nutrition, *health will be the only and **Final Outcome**.*

This illness began due to the highs, the lows and the crashes. I guess if you practice something long enough you'll get it right.

SWEET SITUATION

Doctors say that symptoms of diabetes appear mainly in people above 40, with no symptoms of diabetes in their 20's. *How do they differ from each other?* In general, the quantity of accumulated acidic wastes is much greater at the age of 40 because of 20 more years of unconscious living resulting in nutritional bankruptcy. Let logic prevail. When the large intestine becomes sluggish the liver becomes overburdened, toxins will then accumulate in the weakest link *(pancreas)*. If this acidic waste accumulates in the pancreas, Adult Onset Diabetes may very well be the outcome. Just know that you can reverse Adult Onset Diabetes if you take charge and flush out these unwanted toxins and incorporate a nontoxic alkaline nutrient dense lifestyle, Superfood Nutritional support and plenty of Structured Water to reclaim that which was taken away.

When you change the rules, you change the game. Your body is a true miracle, **U** are the game changer. Master these changes and it will do the rest. Once we get out of the way, love and support our body, **SELF HEALING** is the **NATURAL OUTCOME.**

> **If Diabetic Dan has 50 chocolate bars and eats 45, what does he have? Diabetes. Dan has diabetes.**

FOODS & FREQUENCY

"Get a charge out of Life... Plug into Nature and Drink Life In. It's only Natural."

- Dr. Darrell Wolfe, Doc of Detox

TUNE IN & TURN ON

I believed there were only three food groups, these being carbohydrates, fats and proteins. There is a fourth that must be considered in this **New Reality** if a healthy vibrant life is your priority. This fourth food group is known as vibrational frequency. All foods have a high vibrational frequency when left in their natural state. New and improved will usually be found to be depleted of essential nutrients and could possibly contain toxic chemicals and GMOs. These foods will either have a low frequency or none at all. You are what you eat and drink. If your diet has a low vibrational frequency then it stands to reason so will you. If you're sick and tired then it stands to reason so is your diet. If your diet is heavy in toxins then chances are, so are you. When you embrace Nature and avoid **man**-ipulation of the foods you eat, you will be truly blessed with the essential nutrients and the vibrational frequency your body's cells need to communicate for greater health.

Try to view your body as a radio with a built in antenna. Foods all have their own frequency just as all radio stations do. If the heavy metal station brings you down but rock and roll raises your energy level then vibrate to that which makes you happy.

There is common knowledge among science, medicine and metaphysics that certain frequencies can repel disease and certain frequencies can eliminate disease. Here lies the connection between frequency (vibration) and health. This energy vibration is in your body; the foods you eat and in the water you drink. The body eliminates all food and drink we take in; the only thing left behind is the energy and the frequencies within your food and drink.

Albert Einstein is best known for his physics equation E=mc2, that all matter contains waves of light and energy. Everything is frequency and frequency is everything.

Once we become aware of the fact that we are energy bodies and that high vibrational food, water and nutrition are the driving force to a healthy life, we become unstoppable, we become The Cure.

Dr. Robert Becker, MD, the author of The Body Electric, validates that the human body has an electrical frequency and that much about a person's health can be determined by it.

Dr. Otto Warburg was a two-time Nobel Laureate and winner of the Nobel Prize for cancer research, for discovering that human cells have an electrical voltage. Your cells function more like a battery than a pool of chemicals. An acid environment is a diseased environment and an alkaline environment allows the cells to receive 10 to 20 times more oxygen, which is essential for a healthy metabolism. Our goal at the 'Doc of Detox' is to teach you how to become independent from drugs, therapies, specialists and the latest greatest medical or nutritional breakthrough. When you learn to Master your health you will Master your life.

"The living cell is essentially an electrical device..." Albert Szent-Györgyi (1960), 1937 Nobel Prize for Physiology of Medicine. It is important to remember that food provides us with not only nutrients and fiber but also energy and information in the form of frequency. Dr. Kikuo Chishima, Professor of the Nagoya Commercial University, Japan, theorized that the intestinal villi act

like small antennae that absorb both nutrients as well as energetic or frequency information from the food we eat. Phytonutrients give fruits and vegetables their radiant colors and healing ability. Phyto means plant and nutrients being the vitamins, essential minerals, trace minerals, enzymes and anti-oxidants. Doctors Hyman and Gallard say that phytonutrients help *'turn-on'* your body's metabolism at the cellular level and regulate hormones that control appetite. In conclusion phytonutrients turn off the hunger trigger and turn on your electrical Life Force due to the high vibrational frequency they possess.

VIBRATIONAL FREQUENCIES OF THE HUMAN BODY & FOOD

The vibrational frequency of food is typically measured in hertz. 1 hertz is 1 cycle per second of energy flow that is constant between 2 points.

Scientific research has shown that different foods and parts of our bodies have their own sonic signature. In other words, the sound of the cells of your heart differs from the sound of the cells of your kidney.

MHz is the shortened form of the word **megahertz**. It is important to understand the meaning of hertz to understand MHz. The term *'hertz'* is named for Heinrich Hertz, who contributed significantly to the study of electromagnetism.

Frequencies of the Human Body in MHz

Human cells start to mutate when their frequency drops below 62 MHz. Low frequency indicates a pH imbalance due to lack of phytonutrients and proper cleansing. Invading pathogenic frequencies *(including biologicals such as anthrax, plagues, etc)* are low. Positive beneficial bacterial frequencies are higher. The vibrational frequency of your inner terrain will be the deciding factor of who and what comes calling. **U choose,** The Vibrational Frequency! It's always been your choice.

In 1992, Bruce Tainio of Tainio Technology, an independent division of Eastern State University in Cheny, Washington, built the first frequency monitor in the world. Tainio has determined that the average frequency of a healthy human body during the day time is 62 to 68 MHz. When the frequency drops, the immune system is compromised.

If the frequency drops to 58 MHz, cold and flu symptoms appear; at 55 MHz, diseases like Candida take hold; at 52 MHz, Epstein Bar and at 42 MHz, Cancer. Tainio's machine was certified as 100% accurate and is currently being used in the agricultural field today. Frequency information from Tainio Technologies:

HUMAN BODY

Genius Brain Frequency: 80-82 MHz
Brain Frequency Range: 72-90 MHz
Normal Brain Frequency: 72 MHz
Human Body: 62-78 MHz
Human Body from Neck up: 72-78 MHz
Human Body from Neck down: 60-68 MHz
Thyroid & Parathyroid glands : 62-68 MHz
Thymus Gland: 65-68 MHz

Heart: 67-70 MHz
Lungs: 58-65 MHz
Liver: 55-60 MHz
Pancreas: 60-80 MHz
Colds and Flu start at: 57-60 MHz
Disease starts at: 58 MHz
Candida overgrowth starts at: 55 MHz
Receptive to Epstein Barr at: 52 MHz
Receptive to Cancer at: 42 MHz
Death begins at: 25 MHz

FOODS

Fresh foods and herbs can be higher if grown organically and eaten freshly picked

Essential Oils: 52-320 MHz
Fresh Foods: 20-27 MHz
Fresh Herbs: 20-27 MHz
Dried Foods: 15-22 MHz
Dried Herbs: 12-22 MHz
Processed/Canned Food 0 MHZ (the majority of food eaten today)

According to Dr. Royal R. Rife, every disease has a frequency. He found that certain frequencies can prevent the development of disease and that others would destroy disease. Substances with higher frequency will destroy diseases of a lower frequency. The study of frequencies raises an important question, concerning the frequencies of substances we eat, breathe and absorb. Many pollutants lower healthy frequency. American inventor Nikola Tesla (1856 - 1943), a pioneer of electrical technology, said that if you could eliminate certain outside frequencies that interfered in our bodies, we would have greater resistance toward disease. *"In every culture and in every medical tradition before ours, healing was accomplished by moving energy."* - Albert Szent-Györgyi, Nobel Laureate in Medicine (1937).

Your energy follows your thoughts. You create what you expect. Negative thoughts will lower your frequency by 12 MHz and positive thoughts raise your frequency by 10 MHz. We need to raise our body frequency regularly/ daily. We need to eat the right substances that are compatible at the cellular/ energetic level of our being. If you eat low vibrational foods or have low vibrational thoughts on a daily basis you will mentally and physically match this frequency (**zombie**). Why wait until our body frequency has dropped so low that it becomes a host for microscopic invaders and dis-ease. When you make others responsible for your body's well being you have given your power away to be the great creator you were meant to be. **Take Life In & Vibrate High.**

FOOD FREQUENCY CHART

52-320 MHz - Healthy To 100
- 'Doc of Detox' Essential Oils
- Zija® Moringa Oleifera
- 'Doc of Detox' Daily Cleansing Tea
- Structured Water
- Wheat Grass
- Phytoplankton
- Chlorophyll

15-52 MHz
- Raw Cocoa
- Sea Weed
- Almonds
- Goji Berries
- Raw Cacao
- Spirulina
- Mangsteen
- Limes
- Lemons

5-15 MHz
- Blueberries
- Coconut
- Avocado
- Melons
- Raspberries
- Pineapple
- Mango
- Apples
- Strawberries
- Bananas
- Peaches
- Lychee
- Grapes
- Cherries
- Oranges
- "Raw" Nuts
- Dates

0-5 MHz
- Cabbage
- Lettuce
- Spinach
- Cauliflower
- Carrots
- Beets

- Peas
- Kale
- Pumpkin
- Potatoes
- Sweet Potatoes

- Parsnips
- Turnips
- Yams
- Beans
- "Roasted" Nuts

0 Mhz

- Cooked Eggs
- Cheese
- Milk
- Cream
- Whip Cream
- Butter
- Lard
- Cake

- Cookies
- Scones
- Donuts
- Dairy Baked Goods
- Pudding
- Sauces with Dairy
- Dressings with Dairy
- Drinks with Dairy

Negative (-) MHz

- Hot Dogs
- Burgers
- Pizza
- Meat Burrito
- Steak
- Poultry
- Pork
- Dead Animal Tissue

- Lamb
- Duck
- Veil
- Buffalo
- Turkey
- Shrimp
- Lobster & Bottom Feeders

HIGH FREQUENCY FOODS

High frequency foods are those foods that have been left in their natural state, unadulterated, unprocessed, no chemicals, no genetic mutations or alterations. Being energy bodies we are affected greatly by the frequencies *(foods)* we take in. For those who are weight conscious, the more you feed your body what it needs, the more efficient it becomes and the less you need to feed it.

NUTRIENT RICH HIGH VIBRATIONAL FOODS

Phytonutrient Rich Foods should only be eaten if you can handle being ostracized by those who follow Jack and desire limitless energy and clear thought, clear skin and a **Whole Life.**

Tips For Buying High Vibrational Food

1. The most phytonutrient dense plant on the planet is *Moringa Oleifera.*
2. Buy food that is grown organic when possible.
3. Eat locally grown when possible.
4. Eat foods grown in season whenever possible.

Organic Foods can contain 10 times the mineral content of non-organic. If you cannot afford organic then follow the other two rules, in season and locally grown when possible. **Local Produce** has the most nutrients. This ensures they were picked only when ripe not premature.

You also have a better chance at fewer chemicals when they are local. Eating in season keeps us aligned with Nature. Out of season food may be *'force grown'* in artificial conditions.

Fresh and Raw Foods have the highest vibrational frequency of any other food group. What do you think happens when you ingest fresh and raw food? You become what you eat, the highest vibrational frequency.

Whole Foods have the highest frequency. The more they are processed the lower you will vibrate *(immune system depletion)*. If you focus your shopping on the outside isle of the grocery store you will find this the least toxic.

HABITS FOR HIGHER FREQUENCY

- **Chew every mouthful thoroughly -** Drink your solids and chew your liquids.
- **Eat food in moderation -** Overeating kills.
- **Eat an alkaline diet -** See alkaline food chart.
- **Eat in a peaceful calm setting.**
- **Always drink ample pure Structured Water.**
- **Always thank those who made it possible for the food you eat.**

HABITS THAT DECREASE FREQUENCY AND MICRONUTRIENTS

Eating more than your stomach can digest, always leave the table feeling **fed, not full.**

If you must drink at meals *sip your water*. Do not use water to wash food down, it's not a log jam. This will only dilute digestive enzymes and hydrochloric acid.

Eating while emotionally upset or stressed will cause many different digestive problems. Your food will turn on you in this situation. Negative emotions cause lower frequencies, so digestion is interrupted and putrefaction will result.

Eating in a hurry. Without peace at meals your food will never be broken down into small enough pieces for nutrients to be assimilated. Even fresh and raw will turn on you if you're eating in a negative low frequency state.

Low Vibrational Factors - *Noise, EMF, drinking alcohol, smoking, strenuous exercise, dieting, prescription or over-the-counter drugs and last but not least fear, doubt and worry.*

Here's the kicker, I have known many people who eat all organic, follow all the guidelines to healthy living but still are complaining about their health. Negative emotions and dysfunctional **B**elief **S**ystems can sabotage even the perfect diet. ***We are what we think, talk and eat.***

FOODS THAT DECREASE FREQUENCY

- Genetically Modified Organisms *(GMO)*.
- Irradiated
- Microwave
- Refined *(white flour, white rice, all grains that have the germ and the bran removed)*.
- Processed *(all junk food, even most health snacks)*. 75% of all packaged foods are GMO.
- High glycemic. These sugary, starchy foods affect blood sugar levels and weight gain.
- Hydrogenated *(margarine, vegetable shortening, lard)*.
- Foods containing chemicals, hormones, preservatives and color dyes.
- Artificial sweeteners
- Coffee
- Canned foods
- Everyday Micronutrient Depleters can rob the body of additional micronutrients. These include: Drinking

beverages that contain phosphoric acid, caffeine, sugar or high fructose corn sugar. Eating nutrient deficient food.

> **THE MOST IMPORTANT RULE IS TO LEARN WHAT'S GOOD FOR YOU.**
>
> IF YOU TRY TO LEARN WHAT'S NOT GOOD FOR YOU THAT'S INSANITY.
>
> **RAISE YOUR VIBRATION**
>
> **it's only Natural**

EAT WHOLE LOVE LIFE

"Live food gives Life, Dead food gives... You know the rest of the story."

- *Dr. Darrell Wolfe, Doc of Detox*

ALKALINE FOODS

MILDLY ALKALINE	MODERATELY ALKALINE	HIGHLY ALKALINE
DRINK		
Almond Milk	Fresh Young Coconut Water	Structured Water Moringa SuperMix
VEGGIES		
Artichokes	Arugula	Himalayan Salt
Asparagus	Beets	Real Salt
Brussels Sprouts	Basil	Avocado
Cauliflower	Capsicum/Pepper	Broccoli
Comfrey	Cabbage Lettuce	Cabbage
Kohlrabi	Carrot	Celery
Lambs Lettuce	Chives	Cucumber
Leeks	Collard/Spring	Endive
New Baby Potatoes	Greens	Garlic
Peas	Coriander	Grasses
Pumpkin	Endive	(alfalfa, kamut,
Onion	Ginger	wheatgrass etc.)
Rutabaga	Green Beans	Kale
Squash (butternut,	Leeks	Parsley
summer etc.)	Lettuce	Spinach
Watercress	Mustard Greens	Sprouts (alfalfa,
White Cabbage	Okra	bean, pea, soy
	Radish	etc.)
	Red Cabbage	
	Red Onion	
	Turnip	
	Zucchini	
FRUITS		

MILDLY ALKALINE	MODERATELY ALKALINE	HIGHLY ALKALINE
Coconut Grapefruit Pomegranate	Lemon Lime Rhubarb	Tomato
SEEDS, NUTS & LEGUMES		
Almonds Fennel Seeds Lentils Tofu Sesame Seeds Herbs & Spices	Butter Beans Lima Beans Soy Beans (fresh) White (navy beans) Chia/Salba Seeds Hemp Seeds Quinoa (pseudo grain/ seed)	Organic Soy Nuts (soaked soybeans, then air dried)
FATS & OILS		
Avocado Oil Olive Oil Coconut Oil Flax Oil Grape Seed Oil Hemp Oil		Soy Lecithin (pure)

ACID FOODS

HIGHLY ACID	MODERATELY ACID	MILDLY ACID
DRINK		
Alcohol Coffee & Black Tea Fruit Juice (sweetened)	Fresh, Natural Juice	Rice, Soy, & Coconut Milk
Other		
Cocoa Honey Jam Jelly Mustard Miso Rice Syrup Vinegar Yeast Artificial Sweeteners Syrup Mushroom	Ketchup Mayonnaise	Sunflower Oil
FRUITS		
Dried Fruit	Apple Apricot Banana Blackberry Blueberry	Cantaloupe Fresh Dates Nectarine Plum Sweet Cherry Watermelon

HIGHLY ACID	MODERATELY ACID	MILDLY ACID
	Cranberry	
	Grapes	
	Guava	
	Mango	
	Mangosteen	
	Orange	
	Peach	
	Papaya	
	Pineapple	
	Strawberry	
MEAT		
Beef	Ocean Fish	Freshwater Wild Fish
Chicken		
Eggs		
Farmed Fish		
Pork		
Shellfish		
DAIRY		
Cheese	Butter	
Dairy	Goat's Cheese	
	Vegan Cheese	
GRAINS/LEGUMES		
White Rice	Brown Rice	Black Beans
	Rye Bread	Garbanzo Beans
	Wheat	Kidney Beans
	Wholemeal Bread	Seitan

HIGHLY ACID	MODERATELY ACID	MILDLY ACID
	Wild Rice Wholemeal Pasta	Amaranth Buckwheat Groats Buckwheat Pasta Millet Oats/Oatmeal Soybeans Spelt Couscous Rice/Soy Protein**
NUTS/SEEDS		
	Walnuts	Hemp Protein** Brazil Nuts Flax Seeds Hazelnuts Macadamia Nuts Pecans Pumpkin Seeds Sunflower Seeds

PLANT BASED PROTEIN CHART

This information was taken from the USDA Nutrient Database. It will show you the protein content of vegetarian foods.

Amino acids make up protein, you may not be aware of this but there are amino acids in all foods. There are distinct health advantages of a pure vegetarian diet, but the protein question stays with us because animal products have been promoted by the industries that produce them, sell them, and want people to think of them as the best source of protein. This assumption is wrong and can be harmful when we eat too much animal protein. It's important to note that most nutritionists, dietitians and official sources agree that we need only 2.5%-10% of our calories from protein.

Vegetables (cooked)	Protein (g)
Corn (1 large cob)	5
Potato (with skin)	5
Mushroom, Oyster (1 cup)	5
Collard Greens (1 cup)	4
Peas (1/2 cup)	4
Artichoke (medium)	4
Broccoli (1 cup)	4
Brussel Sprouts (1 cup)	4
Mushroom, Shitake (1 cup)	3.5
Fennel (medium)	3
Swiss Chard (1 cup)	3
Sweet Potato (1 cup)	3
Kale (1 cup)	2.5
Asparagus (5 spears)	2
String Beans (1 cup)	2

Vegetables (cooked)	Protein (g)
Beets (1 cup)	2
Cabbage (1 cup)	2
Carrot (1 cup)	2
Cauliflower (1 cup)	2
Rutabaga	2
Squash	2
Celery (1 cup)	2
Spinach (1 cup)	1
Bell Peppers (1 cup)	1
Cucumber (1 cup)	1
Eggplant (1 cup)	1
Leeks (1 cup)	1
Lettuce (1 cup)	1
Okra (1/2 cup)	1
Onion (1/2 cup)	1

Nut/Seed (1/4 cup)	Protein (g)
Chia Seeds	12
Hemp Seeds	10
Flax Seeds	8
Sunflower Seeds	8
Salba	7.4
Almonds	7
Pumpkin Seeds	7
Sesame Seeds	7
Pistachios	6
Walnuts	5
Brazil Nuts	5

Hazelnuts	5
Pine Nuts	4
Cashews	4

Beans (1 cup cooked)	Protein (g)
Lentils	18
Adzuki Beans	17
White Beans	17
Cranberry Beans	17
Navy Beans	16
Split Peas	16
Anasazi	15
Black Beans	15
Garbanzos (Chick Peas)	15
Kidney Beans	15
Great Northern Beans	15
Lima Beans	15
Pink Beans	15
Black-eyed Peas	14
Mung Beans	14
Pinto Beans	14
Green Beans	9

Grains (1 cup cooked)	Protein (g)
Triticale	25
Millet	8.4
Amaranth	7
Oat, bran	7
Wild Rice	7

Rye Berries	7
Whole Wheat Couscous	6
Bulgur Wheat	6
Buckwheat	6
Teff	6
Oat Groats	6
Barely	5
Quinoa	5
Brown Rice	5
Spelt	5

Other Sources	Protein (g)
Sunwarrior Rice Protein (scoop)	17
Cherimoya	7
Egg	6
Sapote (1 medium)	5
Avocado (1 medium)	4
Durian (1 cup)	4

FOOD COMBINING CHART

SANE EATING FOR YOUR ASSEMBLY LINE

FOOD COMBINING FOR YOUR HEALTH

VEGETABLES
Combine Well With Most Foods

SWEET FRUITS
Best Combined With Celery & Lettuce
Do Not Use With Acid Fruits

SUB-ACID FRUITS
Combine With Acid or Sweet Fruit,
Not Both
Good With Lettuce or Celery

ACID FRUITS
Best Combined With Sub-Acid Fruits,
Not Sweet Fruits
Good With Lettuce or Celery

PROTEINS
Best Combined With Salads
Do Not Use With Sugar & Starches

STARCHES
Best Combined With Green Salads
Do Not Use With Proteins & Fruit

MELONS
Do Not Combine With Other Foods
Best Eaten Alone

YOUR GUIDE TO PROPER FOOD COMBINING

The Reason For Proper Food Combining is to bring sanity back to eating

Food Combining is based on the theory that different food groups require different digestion times. In addition, the principles of food combining are dictated by digestive chemistry. Different foods require different digestive enzymes to aid in the digestive process: some acid, some alkaline. For this reason, correct food combinations are important for proper utilization and absorption of the nutrients in our diet.

For example; most protein foods require an acid digestive environment for proper digestion, whereas most carbohydrates will only digest properly in an alkaline environment. The proper combining of foods leads to good digestion and ultimately to better health. Remember, **the simpler the meal the better you feel.**

PROTEINS

Protein foods are those that contain a high percentage of protein in their makeup. Most protein foods require an acid digestive medium. Among these are the following:

- All Animal Protein* *(except fish)* - Animal Protein foods include beef, pork, chicken, lamb, duck, game, etc.
- Dairy products* *(cheese, butter, milk)*
- Nuts, Seeds
- Dry Beans, Dry Peas

- Soy Beans
- Peanuts
- Olives
- Eggs
- Avocados

CARBOHYDRATES

Carbohydrates are starches and sugars. These foods are broken up into three distinct groups or classifications: Starches, Sweet Fruits and Sugars.

STARCHES

- All bread products
- All cereals
- Dry Beans, Dry Peas
- Potatoes
- Pumpkin
- Yams
- Chestnuts
- Squash
- Corn
- Coconut *(Coconuts are a starch/protein combination and also a saturated fat)*

SWEET FRUITS

- Bananas
- Dates
- Fig
- Raisins

- Prunes
- Persimmons
- Dried Fruits

SUGARS

- Pure Maple Syrup*
- Pure Honey*
- Agave*
- Carrots
- Rutabaga
- Beets
- Artichokes
- Parsnips

These foods are not recommended but are included for clarity.

GENERAL PRINCIPLES OF FOOD COMBINING:

MAIN GUIDELINES

1. Avoid eating protein with carbohydrates. Protein foods require an acid medium for digestion, most carbohydrates will only digest properly in an alkaline setting.
2. Salads combine very well with proteins or starches. Non-starchy vegetables may be combined with proteins or starch. Green, leafy vegetables combine very well with most other foods and should form the major part of ones daily diet.
3. Do not consume starch and sugars together.
4. Eat melons alone. They do not combine with other foods.

5. Avoid desserts. Eaten after meals, desserts simply sit in the stomach and ferment. Bacteria turn them into alcohols, acetic acids and vinegars.

6. Sprouts/Grains: The best way to eat grains is as sprouts. When grains are sprouted, they come alive with enzymes and oxygen. They become a pre-digested food. Other seeds and legumes may be sprouted as well.

7. Chew all food until it is close to liquid in consistency. We can easily assimilate foods, which are the most liquefied.

8. Water: Structured Water should be consumed throughout the day. Do not allow your thirst to build up and always avoid dehydration. Water should not be consumed in a large amount at one time. It is better to have a smaller, but continual flow of water throughout the day for proper assimilation and detoxification. Water is important; therefore, make it the best quality you can. Avoid distilled and chlorinated water for health's sake. Use only a chemical free, clean, Structured and alkalizing water.

OTHER IMPORTANT RULES

1. Eat acids and starches during separate meals. Acids neutralize the alkaline medium required for starch digestion resulting in indigestion.

2. Avoid eating carbohydrates with acid fruits. This combination may neutralize the enzymes needed for proper digestion.

3. Eat only one kind of protein food during a meal. Do not consume two proteins of different character and composition *(such as nuts and cheese)* during the same meal.

4. Eat proteins and acid foods during separate meals. The acid foods inhibit the secretion of the digestive acids

required for protein digestion. Undigested proteins putrefy in bacterial decomposition and produce some potent toxins.

5. Do not consume fats with proteins. Our need for fat is small and most protein foods already contain a great amount of fat. Fat has an inhibiting effect on digestive secretions and lessens the amount and activity of pepsin and hydrochloric acid necessary for the digestion of protein.

6. Do not combine sweet fruits with proteins, starches or acid fruits. The sugars in sweet fruits are not apt to ferment if digestion is delayed by mixing with other foods.

7. Use fats sparingly. Fats inhibit the secretion of gastric juice. With the exception of avocado, fats used with starch result in delayed digestion. Though not a high protein food, avocados contain more protein than milk. They are high in fat and the small percentage of protein they contain is of exceptional biological value. They are best used with a salad meal. Avocados should never be eaten with nuts, which are also high in fats.

8. Acid fruits may be used with sub-acid fruits. This combination is best made with less sweet, sub-acid fruits. Never use acid fruits with sweet fruits. Tomatoes should not be combined with sub-acid fruit or with any other kind of fruit.

9. Sub-Acid fruits may be used with sweet fruits. It is best to use the sweeter varieties of sub-acid fruits when making this combination. For people with poor digestion, bananas are best eaten alone.

10. Combine fruit only with lettuce and celery. These uncooked vegetables with a fruit meal may even enhance digestion of the fruit. Avoid over ripe fruit.

11. Eat only one concentrated starch food during a meal.

12. Milk is best consumed alone. Organic is preferred.
13. Do not rush or eat *'on-the-go'*. This will only worsen any digestive problem. Take time with your meals.

SPICES & CONDIMENTS

- Sea Salt, Cinnamon, Cayenne, Cumin, Clove, Turmeric, Ginger, Garlic
- Apple Cider Vinegar
- Cold pressed Extra Virgin Oils *(Grape seed, Olive, Coconut)*
- Whole Grain Mustard

FERMENTED NOT DEMENTED

One of the most important facts that is never talked about is that the fiber from fruits, vegetables and whole grains are not just healthy but critical to human life. The bacteria in your digestive tract ferment these fibers to break them down to become the body's main powerhouse of immune protection. They release acetic acid, butyric acid, B vitamins and K vitamin. The tangy flavor in sauerkraut is an example of the acid by-product of the gorging bacteria on the carbohydrates in cabbage. Fermented foods are an excellent source for building bacteria and should be eaten daily. Try to get this, your friendly bacteria are your body's front line guardians of your immune system. These good bacteria are the greatest detoxifiers and chelators for the body. They help to remove BPAs, heavy metals and other modern day contaminants that we are exposed to. Fermented fruit, vegetables and wholegrain fibers ensure that your bacteria remain your greatest friend and protector whereas sugary fatty foods will turn these same protectors into your worst nightmare. When your bacteria go from friendly to unfriendly they will become downright pathogenic, leaking noxious by-products *(endotoxin)*, which will cause all *'cell'* to break loose; this is the beginning of your demise. When this happens the Domino Effect begins and these trillions of good bacteria will have the potential to turn on you and make your life a living hell.

When **U** truly take care of your body through Superfood Nutrition, a Whole Plant-Based Alkaline Lifestyle along with Gentle Daily Cleansing you will become the Master of your Health.

FERMENTED FOODS FOR LIFE

What are fermented foods you ask? Oh, you're in for a life-saving, butt saving treat. Eating fermented foods will take your health to the next level when you incorporate these on a daily basis. These are foods that have gone through the fermentation process. The seven most popular are Sauerkraut, Kombucha, Tempeh, Kefir, Miso, Seed cheese and Rejuvelac. These are superior foods rich in friendly bacteria *(flora)* and enzymes that support the Mother of all Organs, which is the major part of your body's immune system, **the one and only COLON.**

These are live unpasteurized foods with the power to transform inner health. The fermentation process naturally preserves the food. These foods have life-giving cultures living within them. The word culture comes from the Latin word *'to cultivate'*. Since the beginning of time the fermenting and culturing of foods has existed. As far back as history shows humans were aware of the life preserving qualities of these enzymatic bacteria rich foods. When you make these foods part of your daily life, you will inject more life into every day. *"Humans have been fermenting longer than we've been writing words or cultivating soil."* Sandor Katz. When you cultivate your inner garden you are awakening the true fountain of youth, your immune system. One quarter to half a cup of fermented vegetables is a great addition to the diet. It is always good to rotate different fermented foods in your daily diet. The more varieties of fermented foods that you eat, the stronger you will become and the more you are going to inoculate your colon with different organisms.

This in itself takes your immune system to a higher level. People will also eat fermented grains, nuts, seeds and meats. Even products that once could not be tolerated, if fermented, will be digested usually without negative symptoms. However, some may never be able to digest even fermented grains. This is usually due to antibiotic wipeout. For those it may be best to avoid grains and legumes. **The Whole Truth** is even if you eat fresh, organic veggies, you may still have a problem if you are chronically ill and pathogenic bacteria rule your digestive tract. To shift your health in your favor switch to fermented foods when possible. One quarter to half a cup of fermented vegetables one to three times a day depending how much support you require and what your desired goal is.

You may experience a healing crisis when you begin to crowd out the pathogenic bacteria. Gentle Daily Cleansing and Superfood Nutrition will help alleviate any symptoms of a healing crisis.

BENEFITS OF FERMENTED ENZYME RICH FOODS:

- Supports proper digestion of food.
- Helps in eliminating and preventing Candida albicans. *(fungus)*
- Supports and protects immune system.
- Helps maintain proper pH balance. *(alkalinity)*
- Helps restore balance of friendly bacteria.
- Tones and strengthens colon.
- Helps eliminate cravings.
- Supports detoxification process of the body.

FOUR LITTLE TIPS

1. Steel cut oats are much more nutritious for the friendly bacteria in your colon than rolled oats.
2. Diets such as the Atkins regime that lack fiber, have been shown to cause a dangerously high bad bacterial content in the colon, which may be linked to colon cancer.
3. Pasteurized yogurt is not a cultured live yogurt and it also contains sugar. You want to either make it yourself or find someone who has a raw organic dairy source.
4. The large intestine is called the colon because it has colonies of good bacteria, which is the foundation of a strong immune system and a long, happy, healthy life.

RAW FOOD

Technically, raw foods can be defined as whole food that has not been refined, chemically processed, altered from its natural state or heated above 116°F thereby preserving its natural nutritional content. Raw foods are plant-based foods. That's a textbook definition, but it isn't fully accurate because raw foods represent so much more than that. Most of us know that eating raw fruits and veggies is good for us, right? They have vitamins and minerals and if you want to lose weight, we need to eat more of them. Beyond that, have you ever considered why whole plant based foods are beneficial?

Whole Plant Based Foods are predominantly alkaline; disease cannot exist in an alkaline environment. Reducing your intake of acid-forming foods like sugar, artificial sweeteners, flour, caffeine, red meat and processed foods while increasing alkaline-forming foods is the most effective and efficient way to become more alkaline. An acidic environment and inflammation go hand-in-hand, so as you reduce the acid in your system, you automatically reduce inflammation. Here are just a few reasons to add more raw foods into your diet.

Weight Loss: As you increase your consumption of raw foods you will lose unwanted pounds, especially if you eat raw before other foods at each meal. Your body will naturally find the weight that is perfect for you and the diet roller coaster will end for good.

Balanced Blood Sugar: This is a huge issue and a big part of the diet roller coaster. Why? Because when we eat *"diet"* or *"fat-free"* products, the fat that is removed from them has to be replaced with something - and that something is sugar. Sugar in and of itself is fat-free, however, when you eat it, your body releases insulin to handle the sugar. Insulin is a fat-storage hormone, so, the sugar your body doesn't use immediately for energy is stored as fat.

Eating sugar raises blood-sugar levels and if you don't have an adequate balance of fiber and protein, after a relatively short period of time your blood sugar drops, signaling you to eat again. **Raw foods in their natural state, are balanced foods meaning they come complete with protein, fiber and a balance of vitamins and minerals.**

Energizing: Raw foods do not bog down our digestive system and digestion is what our bodies expend the most amount of energy on. Raw foods are known as *"clean"* foods because they are used quickly, efficiently and actually assist our body in gathering and eliminating waste.

Mental Clarity: Brain fog and sharper mental focus are natural side effects to increasing raw foods. High sugar, high fat processed foods have negative impact on our brains as well as our bodies, leaving in their wake a *"hangover"* type effect. Consuming clean, unprocessed whole foods eliminates that effect, leaving us alert and clear. You get the idea, right?

I could go on and on about the physical health benefits of increasing raw foods in your diet because the list is seemingly endless. *Our bodies are designed to heal themselves and when we give them what they need, not necessarily what the brain is addicted to, magic happens.* However, there is a much bigger picture here, which for me, is the greatest benefit of all. Nature has blessed and gifted us with everything - in total and complete perfection.

All that is required of us is to graciously accept and use these gifts. We are a part of that complete perfection, not separate from it. There has never been, nor will there ever be another *'you'*. You are unique, irreplaceable, and magnificent, worthy of all your heart's desires and in part, here to add beauty and grace to the world. When you remember that, you will naturally choose to honor and respect yourself by taking care of yourself. This is the highest form of self-love and it includes nurturing and nourishing your body and mind with the best foods available. Clean foods that are high in energy, nutrition and frequency keep you healthy and strong in body, mind and spirit, so that you can do what you were put on this planet to do - express your passion by sharing your unique gifts; the world needs what you were divinely created to share. **Be the very best version of U. Be Extraordinary.**

By: Ann Lotwin, Raw Food Chef

FOOD TO LIVE FOR

With Celebrity Chef & Nutrition Expert Janice Skoreyko

When was the last time you leapt out of bed feeling fully rested, before your alarm clock rang; excited and fully in charge, ready to take on the day? For many of us the very thought of this is so far from recent reality that it takes us back to our childhood and Christmas morning. It is time to put the brakes on those energy zappers and recapture your passion for life!

When you join our *'Healthy To 100 Club'* you are privileged to unlimited, mouth-watering, delicious raw food recipes; including deprivation-free dishes that help you feel physically and mentally energized. You will finally have the energy to do all of the things that you love to do!

We are here to share with you how you can put this plan into action; quickly, easily and deliciously. Each recipe is the result of over 20 years of research and development, many of which use less than 5 ingredients, take less than 5 minutes to prepare and will keep you satisfied! Unlike many traditional prescriptions, this is one that you will be looking forward to and you will welcome the side effects with open arms.

The True Rx for Health

When we are feeling sick we have a particular protocol we follow: drink plenty of fluids, eat clean and well, get plenty of rest, take hot baths, watch funny movies, nurture ourselves, allow others to nurture us and for some, revisit our spiritual beliefs and connection.

I invite you to consider that the very same ingredients that we use to restore our health are also those needed daily for optimum health. It is second nature to do these things when we are knocked off of our feet, why not create high energy days and feed a powerful foundation with these ingredients everyday? You have the innate wisdom to make this happen!

While there are things we do when we are under the weather, there are many things we definitely avoid, including: Drinking milk and consuming dairy, as they create even more mucous. Eating processed sugar decreases the immune system. Stimulants such as coffee further dehydrate the body and tax the immune and endocrine systems. Large heavy meals take the body's energy away from healing by prioritizing digestion, so we naturally avoid those and prefer smaller, lighter meals throughout the day.

The same prescription we use for healing is therefore the same prescription for vibrant health. Of course, there are side effects to every prescription. Adopting the principles that feed life daily will result in, greater mental clarity, accelerated learning, sound sleep, clear smooth skin, stable moods, better digestion, low healthcare costs and abundant energy. Overall these side effects can be summarized into an exponentially greater quality of life. No "diet" required.

The "Indulge ME" Philosophy

Indulge: To allow oneself to enjoy the pleasure of. Stop the diet battle! Diets don't work as they are not in alignment with our psychology.

Deprivation increases the stress hormone, cortisol, which as a result increases the acidity level in the body. Diets are irritating, and where we see irritation we see inflammation along with plummeting energy levels.

Overtime, the inflammation increases and manifests into a form of disease. The good news is that disease can only live in an acidic environment.

When we consume alkalizing foods and beverages we are feeding vibrant health. Unfortunately many *'healthy alkaline diets'* are boring, tasteless and impossible to stick with in the long run. I have personally tried every one of these *'diets'* I could get my hands on; and the result was the same every time: **cheating**.

This result produced feelings of guilt, shame, disappointment, disapproval, depression, despair and further destructive behavior. The program running in my head said *"I have fallen off the wagon, so may as well make a weekend re-tox of it. I will start again on Monday."* Can you relate?

In April of 2004, this happened for the last time as a result of a near death experience. I was alone in China at the age of 29, you see for the past 15 years I had been an active participant in my healing journey, traveled to 7 countries, studied medicine in both traditional settings and with village healers, though I had a hard time sticking to the protocols of dull foods and countless supplements and herbs.

I became 100% committed to creating and running a new program in my body; one comprised of the most delicious, decadent nutrition and lifestyle ingredients possible. This led my body to reverse the symptoms of all 5 serious illnesses and enabled me to learn how to indulge without the bulge and make it fun!

When we enjoy whole foods that have not been heated above 116°F, it is not only the easiest for our body to digest but also the most nutrient-dense. DigestComplete enzymes, help break down food into smaller parts that can be absorbed, transported and utilized by every cell in your body.

Dr. Howell's research of 50 years, shows clearly that these enzymes are not present in cooked food. This lack of enzymes causes the food to sit in the digestive system longer than raw food, resulting in decreased capacity for the body to break the foods down and nourish itself. This increases storing of these foods and abdominal bloating. We understand that you may indulge, we suggest taking DigestComplete enzymes with foods that have been cooked above 116°F. These digestive enzymes will help your body to digest cooked foods and keep you on track with your fresh, whole food lifestyle.

5 Ingredient, 5 Minute Gourmet - Your key to more confidence in the kitchen!

Getting started with a new culinary skill-set requires a few things; learning, practice and having confidence in the kitchen. Imagine knowing that your recipes are going to turn out well the first time you try them at home, feels great doesn't it! This is the ultimate form of empowerment.

We have many 5 Ingredient, 5 Minute Gourmet recipes for you in our *'Healthy To 100 Club'*; as well as links to live footage with tips and tricks that will have everyone, from the newbie to seasoned foodie, excited to get into the kitchen and unleash their inner chef!

The *'Healthy To 100 Club'* is the perfect place to start your powerful, health journey; from here you may continue with the 3-Day Raw Food to Live For Immersion or Chef Certification Program. In the Immersion program you will learn more about flavor and taste combining, advanced recipes such as lasagna, pizza, desserts, cheese and chocolate to how to repurpose ingredients efficiently, plan your menu and prepare your food in just 2 hours a week vs. the typical 20 hours per week, along with solid science and nutrition education.

To learn more, visit: www.rawfoundation.ca

FOOD TO LIVE FOR

Delicious Raw Recipes

Watermelon Radish Ravioli

Ingredients:
Gourmet Sweet Chive Cheese
2C cashews (soaked 8 hours)
1/4C extra virgin olive oil
1/2t onion powder
1/4C freshly squeezed lemon juice
1T chives, chopped
1t dill, chopped
2t raw honey/agave nectar
3/4t sea salt
1/4t black pepper

Ravioli
large watermelon radish, peeled
2T extra-virgin olive oil
1T lemon juice
1/4t sea salt

Garnish
1C Enoki mushrooms
1C Pomegranate seeds
20 basil leaves, small

Method:
Gourmet Sweet Chive Cheese
Process all ingredients in a food processor until smooth.

Ravioli

Using a mandolin, slice the radish very thin. In a large bowl, coat the radish slices in lemon juice, oil and salt.

Place a radish slice on your plate and spoon one spoon full of cheese onto it. Next place a second radish slice to top off the ravioli. Repeat for desired serving amount.

Garnish

Finish the plate with a few Enoki mushrooms, pomegranate seeds, a drizzle of olive oil and a basil leaf. Enjoy!

Looking to lighten this recipe up a bit more? Check out our newest savory Cauliflower Cheese recipe in the Healthy To 100 Club!

Candy Cane Beet Salad

Ingredients:
Salad
Candy Cane Beets, sliced thinly
2 Yellow Beets, sliced thinly
1 green apple, chopped into ¼" cubes
1/2C fennel, chopped
1/2C pineapple, chopped into ¼" cubes
2C arugula
2C mixed spring greens

Dressing
1/4C extra virgin olive oil
1/4C coconut aminos
2t lemon juice
1t coconut sugar
1/4t chili flakes

1/4t black pepper
1/4t salt

Garnish
1/4C Gourmet Sweet Chive Cheese
(see Watermelon Radish Ravioli recipe)

Method:
Salad
Toss the beets in 1/4C olive oil and 1/4t salt.
Combine the beets and all remaining ingredients into a large salad bowl. Plate.

Dressing
Combine all ingredients into a medium sized bowl, whisk and spoon onto salad.

Garnish
Chef Tip: Beef this salad up both physically and nutritionally by adding in marinated kale and a sliced avocado. Check out Raw Foundation's Super Bowl Sampler Series in the Healthy To 100 Club!

No-Bake Double Chocolate Brownie Cake

Ingredients:
Cake
3/4C cashews
7 Medjool dates, pitted
1/4C cacao powder
1/2t vanilla bean powder
1/4t cayenne pepper
2t cacao nibs, garnish
Pinch of salt

1 strawberry, fanned (garnish)

Icing
1/4 C raw honey/agave nectar
1/4 C cacao powder
1 T coconut oil, melted

Method:
Cake
Process the cashews in a food processor, until fine.
Add the remaining ingredients and process until smooth.
Place the mixture onto a plate, form into a heart and set aside.

Icing
Process in food processor until smooth.

Assembly:
Ice and garnish the cake.
Place in the freezer for 5 minutes. Enjoy!

New York Style Lemon Cheesecake

Ingredients:
Vanilla Shortbread Cookie Base
2C macadamia nuts
1 pinch of salt
1t vanilla bean

Filling
1C cashews
1C lemon juice
1/2C coconut sugar
1/2C coconut butter

Coulis

3C - berries

2T - raw honey/agave nectar

Method:
Vanilla Shortbread Cookie Base

Place all ingredients in the food processor and process until 70% combined. A light crunch to this cookie will create fabulous finish.

Press the dough into the base of two 4" spring form pans. Set aside.

Filling

Soak the cashews for 6 hours.

Rinse the cashews and continue to soak and repeat rinsing them every 6 hours, for an additional 24 hours.

Combine all ingredients in blender and blend until smooth.

Pour the mixture on top of the cookie crusts, in the 4" spring form pans. Freeze for 6 hours.

Coulis

Reserve 1/4C berries or berry piece.

Pulse remaining ingredients, in a small food processor.

Pour mixture from the processor into a bowl and stir in the pieces that were set aside.

Refrigerate until ready for service. Spoon on top of cake. Enjoy!

Energy Elixir

Ingredients:
Smoothie

4C tightly packed spinach 4 bananas

3C Structured Water 1 pack SuperMix

5 Medjool dates, pitted

Garnish
4 strawberries

Method:
Blend all ingredients.
Garnish your wine glass with a strawberry.
Pour the Elixir into the glass and energize every beautiful cell in your body! For more recipes join our Healthy to 100 Club

Raw Foundation Culinary Arts Institute

The RAW Foundation Culinary Arts Institute is a global, industry leading, raw food culinary school, home of The Raw Food Education Experts and RAW Food Educator Program TM; located in the heart of Vancouver

BC, Canada. We are devoted to educating on the benefits of a plant-based lifestyle, inspiring & empowering foodies, home and professional chefs, health enthusiasts and healthcare professionals from around the world; to prepare delicious, raw meals with ease and successfully share this passion with others while making a positive impact transforming their lives and the lives of those that matter to them most, doing what they love.

Continuing Education / Education Visit: www.rawfoundation.ca
Call 1 855 839 8424 or 778 839 8424

YOUR DAILY DIET REPORT CHART

Log yourself for 30 days!

	Day **1**	Day **2**	Day **3**	Day **4**	Day **5**	Day **6**	Day **7**
Morning *Meal*							
Noon *Meal*							
Evening *Meal*							
Food & Drink *used at other times*							

BE THE MASTER OF YOUR LIFE

LIFE: IT'S IN YOUR BLOOD

"If your Health is a bloody mess - the answers lie within you. Be The Cure."

- Dr. Darrell Wolfe, Doc of Detox

THE BLOOD TYPE DIET

TYPE O

Type O's thrive on intense physical exercise and animal protein. Unlike the other blood types, Type O's muscle tissue should be slightly on the acid side. Type O's can efficiently digest and metabolize meat because they tend to have high stomach-acid content. The success of the Type O Diet depends on the use of lean, chemical-free meats, poultry, and fish. Type O's don't find dairy products and grains quite as user friendly as do most of the other blood types.

The initial weight loss on the Type O Diet is by restricting consumption of grains, breads, legumes, and beans.

The leading factor in weight gain for Type O's is the gluten found in wheat germ and whole wheat products, which interferes with insulin efficiency and slow down metabolic rate. Another factor that contributes to weight gain is certain beans and legumes *(lentils and kidney beans)*, which contain lectins that deposit in the muscle tissues making them less *'charged'* for physical activity. The third factor in Type O weight gain is that Type O's have a tendency to have low levels of thyroid hormone or unstable thyroid functions, which also cause metabolic problems. Therefore it is good to avoid foods that inhibits thyroid hormone *(cabbage, Brussels sprouts, cauliflower, mustard green)* but increase hormone production *(kelp, seafood, iodized salt)*.

Several classes of vegetables can cause big problems for Type O's, such as the Brassica family *(cabbage, cauliflower, etc)* can inhibit the thyroid function. Eat more vegetables that are high in Vitamin K, which helps the clotting factor, which is weak in Type O's. The nightshade vegetables can cause lectin deposit in the tissue surrounding the joints.

Because of the high acidity stomach, Type O's should eat fruits of alkaline nature such as berries and plums. Type O's should severely restrict the use of dairy products. Their system is not designed for the proper metabolism. If you are a Type O of African ancestry, you should eliminate dairy foods and eggs altogether.

Characteristics of Type O - *Best on High Protein Diet*

1. Thrive on intense physical exercise and animal proteins.
2. Do not do well with dairy and grain products.
3. Hardy digestive tract.
4. The leading factor in weight gain for Type O's is the gluten found in wheat germ and whole wheat products.
5. Type O's have a tendency to have low levels of thyroid hormone and unstable thyroid functions, which cause metabolic problems and weight gain.
6. Type O's have high stomach-acid content, can digest meat easily.

TYPE A

Type A's flourish on vegetarian diets. Type A's are predisposed to heart disease, cancer, and diabetes. It is particularly important for sensitive Type A's to get their foods in as natural a state as possible: fresh, pure, and organic. When you get on the Type A Diet, you will naturally be thinner. If you are accustomed to eating meat, you'll lose weight rather rapidly in the beginning as you eliminate the toxic foods from your diet. When you follow the Type diet, you can supercharge your immune system and potentially short-circuit the development of life-threatening diseases. When Type A's eat meat, they experience sluggishness. Type A's have low stomach-acid content, therefore they have a hard time digesting meat. Since Type A's eat very little animal protein, nuts and seeds supply an important protein component.

Type A's also thrive on the vegetable proteins found in beans and legumes, except those mentioned from the 'Avoid' list. These beans can cause a decrease in insulin production, which may cause obesity and diabetes. Tofu should be a staple in the Type A Diet. Dairy foods are also poorly digested by Type A's, and can cause metabolic slowdown. Type A's can tolerate small amounts of fermented dairy products such as yogurt, kefir, sour cream, and cultured dairy products.

Vegetables are vital to the Type A Diet, providing minerals, enzymes and anti-oxidants. Type A's are very sensitive to the lectins in potatoes, sweet potatoes, yams, cabbage, tomatoes and peppers. They aggravate the delicate stomach of Type A. Type A's should eat more fruits that are alkaline, avoid mangoes, papaya and oranges for they are not good for your digestive tract.

TYPE B

The sturdy and alert Type B's are usually able to resist many of the most severe diseases common to modern life, such as heart disease and cancer. In fact, a Type B who carefully follows the recommended diet can often bypass severe disease and live a long and healthy life. Type B's are more prone to immune-system disorders such as multiple sclerosis, lupus, and chronic fatigue syndrome. The Type B Diet is balance and wholesome, including a wide variety of foods.

For Type B's, the biggest factors in weight gain are corn, buckwheat, lentils, peanuts and sesame seeds. These foods have different **lectin** that affect the efficiency of the metabolic process, resulting in fatigue, fluid retention, and hypoglycemia. The gluten lectin in wheat germ and whole wheat products also adds to the problems cause by other metabolism-slowing foods. It is important to leave off chicken for Type B's. Chicken contains a Blood Type B agglutinating lectin in its muscle tissue, which attack the bloodstream and potentially lead to strokes and immune disorders.

Type B's thrive on deep-ocean fish, but should avoid all shellfish. The shellfish contain lectins that are disruptive to the Type B system.

Type B is the only blood type that can fully enjoy a variety of dairy foods. Most nuts and seeds (especially peanuts, sesame seeds and sunflower seeds) are not advised for Type B's, they contain lectins that interfere with Type B insulin production. Wheat is not tolerated well by most Type B's. They contain a lectin that reduce insulin efficiency and failure to stimulate fat 'burning'. Rye contains a lectin that settles in the vascular system, causing blood disorders and potentially strokes. Corn and buckwheat are major factors in Type B weight gain, they contribute to a sluggish metabolism, insulin irregularity, fluid retention, and fatigue. Eliminate tomatoes completely from

Type B diet; it has lectins that irritate the stomach lining. Fruits and vegetables are generally well tolerated and should be taken generously.

TYPE AB

Multiple antigens make Type AB's sometimes A-like with weak stomach acid, and sometimes B-like with genetically programmed for the consumption of meats. Type AB's do best when their muscle tissues are slightly alkaline. Type AB's can't metabolize meat efficiently because of low stomach acid, so it is important to watch the portion size and frequency. Chicken has lectin that irritates the blood and digestive tracts of Type AB's also. Tofu is a good protein supplement for Type AB's. Nuts, seeds, beans and legumes present a mixed picture for Type AB's. Eat nuts and seeds in small amounts and with caution. Type AB's can tolerate dairy foods fairly well, but watch out for excessive mucus production.

Generally Type AB's do well on grains, even wheat, but keep in mind that the inner kernel of the wheat grain is highly acid forming in the muscle for Type AB's. Type AB's benefit from a diet rich in rice rather than pasta. Type AB has a weaker immune system, so you will benefit from the vegetables, which are high in phytochemicals and the more alkaline fruits, which can help to balance the grains that are acid forming in the muscle tissues. Tomatoes do not impose any ill effects on Type AB's. Type AB should begin each day by drinking a glass of warm water with the freshly squeezed juice of half a lemon to cleanse the system of mucus accumulated while sleeping.

THE BLOOD TYPE DIET

SIMPLIFIED CHART

	DIET PROFILE	ALLOWED FOODS	LIMITED FOODS	FOOD TO AVOID (for weight loss purpose)	WEIGHT LOSS SUPPORT FOODS
Type O	High Protein Meat Eaters:	*Grass Fed Meat *Wild Fish *Vegetables *Fruits	*Grains *Beans *Legumes	*Wheat *Corn *Kidney Beans *Navy Beans *Lentils *Cabbage *Brussels Sprouts *Cauliflower *Mustard	*Kelp *Wild Seafood *Salt *Liver *Grass Fed Red Meat *Kale *Spinach *Broccoli
Type A	Vegetarian	*Vegetables *Tofu *Wild Seafood *Grains *Beans *Legumes *Fruit		*Meat *Dairy *Kidney Beans *Lima Beans *Wheat	*Vegetable Oil *Soy Foods *Vegetables *Pineapple

Type B	Balanced **Omnivore**	*Grass Fed Meat (No Chicken) *Organic Dairy *Grains *Beans *Legumes *Vegetables *Fruits		*Corn *Lentil *Peanuts *Sesame Seeds *Buckwheat *Wheat	*Greens *Free Range Organic Eggs *Venison *Liver *Licorice Tea
Type AB	**Mixed Diet** In Moderation	*Meat *Seafood *Organic Dairy *Tofu *Beans *Legumes *Grains *Vegetables *Fruits		*Red Meat *Kidney Beans *Lima Beans *Seeds *Corn *Buckwheat	*Tofu *Wild Seafood *Organic Dairy *Greens *Kelp *Pineapple

WATER: THE STRUCTURE OF LIFE

"U are not a body with water. U are water with a body. Your health will be measured by the life within the water."

- Dr. Darrell Wolfe, Doc of Detox

CHOOSE YOUR WATER WISELY

Water is the most amazing substance on the planet. It is the key to sustaining all life. Water does mysterious and amazing things that even defy the laws of physics. Top scientists today still can't explain some of the characteristics of water and how it actually interacts and communicates with human cells.

Are you the type of person that finds yourself asking these questions:

- Why am I so tired all the time?
- Why am I still thirsty when I drink all of this bottled water?
- Why can I not heal myself?
- Why am I suffering from premature aging?
- Why am I so itchy after showering?
- Why am I bloated?
- Why do I retain water?

The water you drink will either give life or take it away. You can eat a healthy diet, exercise daily and take Whole Plant Based Superfood Nutrition but you must drink high vibrational Structured Water and enough of it to achieve and maintain optimum health, the way Nature intended. Structured Water is the vehicle to nourish, detoxify and restore your body all the way down to the cellular level. Choose your water wisely, your life depends on it.

The cells in your body are surrounded by mostly water. There is a mountain of evidence, which proves the type of water you drink is possibly the most important element of your health. The water you drink will decide how, and how much, your cells absorb nutrients, remove toxins, and how effectively they behave and communicate.

We are told that our body and our planet are comprised of approximately 70% water. What we are not told is that, on a molecular level, the trillions of cells that make up your body are actually composed of 99.9% water. You are not a body containing water; you are a body of water in the form of a human being.

Since water is a nutrient more important than food, the water you are drinking deserves a closer look. If you're drinking tap water, distilled, reverse osmosis, filtered or bottled; I can assure you, you are taking in an inferior product. And guess what? You are slowly but surely depriving yourself of the life you are entitled to and possibly even poisoning yourself. Oh, and by the way, government regulations for drinking water are about the same as a screen door in a submarine *(evil plot)*.

We can discuss the hundreds of toxic materials found in our water, and the ones that are intentionally put there, but that's a whole book in itself. Who really wants to hear about the greed, the negligence and the intentional poisoning of our water systems? Let's get back to real answers and the solution to this internal pollution.

Although drinking water is not the major source of essential nutrients for our body, it is nonetheless an important factor for many reasons. Today the diets of most families lack adequate sources of minerals and micro-elements. The minerals and nutrients in water are present as free ions and therefore more readily absorbed into our body. In food these minerals are mostly bound to other substances; therefore, are not as absorbable on a cellular level.

TIME BOMB IN A TAP

As I stated earlier there are far too many chemicals in our tap water to address. It would be wrong to overlook the one chemical that most have embraced and allowed not just into their life but also into their body.

The drinking and bathing of chlorinated water is fast becoming a serious health problem, not only here in North America but world-wide. Adding chlorine to our water is meant to disinfect the water distribution systems and the water pipes that bring the water to our homes and businesses.

Chlorine is not used because it is safe or healthy. Chlorine is used primarily because it is the cheapest way to disinfect your water. The truth is, in the long run it is the most expensive because it will undermine your precious health.

Side effects of drinking and bathing in chlorinated water:

- Dry, brittle, lusterless hair
- Dry, aging skin
- Skin rashes and irritation
- Acne
- Headache
- Premature aging
- Respiratory problems
- Tissue cell damage
- Cancer
- Cardiovascular disease

THE POWER OF YOUR SHOWER

The two major diseases for some time now, have been heart disease and cancer. Cardiovascular, or heart disease, along with an escalating incidence of bladder, colon, rectal, and breast cancer have all been linked to our continued ingestion of chlorinated tap water.

Many drink, shower, bathe and swim in chlorinated water. Since the majority of the population participates, then it must be safe. There is comfort in numbers.

The results can be very damaging when you put your health in the hands of your government, who's main concern is the bottom line. Would you go to an accountant for health advice?

Studies have shown that when you shower in hot water, the chlorine gas that is formed can be even more damaging to our body than the chlorine found in drinking water.

SWIM AT YOUR OWN RISK

We all know that 'chemical feel and smell' of a pool; stinging, blurry eyes and dry itchy skin.

SALTWATER POOLS

But salt water pools **do** use chlorine - just less of it. The pool owner installs a salt generator which manufactures its own chlorine. Instead of adding chlorine directly to the pool water, salt water chlorinating systems use electrolysis, which releases chlorine gas from the salt into the water. When the chlorine gas mixes with the water, it creates liquid chlorine, which then mixes with the pool water, providing the cleaning component to the system.

Salt systems are more harmful to human health than conventional chlorine, bromine or biguanide chemicals. There are healthy alternatives which will cost you less money and save your health in the long run. Never follow the herd, you will end up at the butcher *(evil plot)*.

Healthy skin is covered in a very thin, slightly acidic film called the 'acid mantle' that is secreted from the skin's sebaceous *(oil)* glands. The pH of bacteria, viruses, and other chemicals are primarily alkaline in nature, so the acid mantle acts as both a physical and chemical barrier to bacteria, viruses, and other potential contaminants penetrating the skin. When we bathe with soap or swim in chlorinated water, the acid mantle is stripped away. Even when conventional lotions are applied, the skin remains too alkaline - leaving the skin and body vulnerable to invasion from harmful chemicals and pathogens.

Side effects of swimming in a chlorinated pool:

- Respiratory Defects
- Neurological Dysfunction
- Cardiovascular Defects
- Skin infection / A Skin Irritant
- Eye infection
- Gastrointestinal Issues
- Kidney Cancer
- Liver infection
- Colorectal cancer

- In hyper-chlorinated pools, dental enamel can become eroded because of increased levels of acidity.

CHILDREN AND POOLS

Children inhale more air per unit of body weight than adults; therefore, children absorb a greater amount of toxins, relatively speaking, than older swimmers. Children with asthma who frequent chlorinated pools, in most cases, will show a worsening of this condition.

Always choose the lake first before a chlorinated or salt water pool. If you do not protect your children then who will? Definitely not our government or all their so called 'health specialists' sanctioned by them. Just because the pool is full does not make it safe. It just shows how naive we are.

WEAR PROTECTION

This is no answer but if you must swim in a chlorinated pool then wear protection. Cover your skin with coconut oil to block chlorine from getting into your skin or, at least, to minimize its exposure. Reapply coconut oil after swimming. It is also better to shower at home if you have a shower purifier. Your skin is your biggest organ. I know you wouldn't knowingly poison yourself or your family.

PHARMACY IN A BOTTLE

Many of our prescription and over-the-counter drugs end up in our waterways and in the water we drink. Discarding prescription medications into the garbage sends them to our landfill systems, where these toxins are leached into the ground and in turn, these toxins find their way into our water systems. Likewise, when you flush these drugs down the toilet they also end up contaminating our water system. Since a lot of bottled water is simply tap water, you are getting a pharmacy in a bottle. Pharmaceutical drugs that were never meant to be combined together because of the toxic reaction they would create inside the body are now mixed together as a poisonous cocktail in your drinking water. People are unknowingly having allergic reactions to an invisible culprit called 'pharmaceutical drugs' within their water. Small and constant exposure to these pharmaceutical cocktails may result in drug allergies.

Millions of people have drug allergies. Are you one of them? If so, how would you know if the unusual symptoms you have been exhibiting are due to ingesting small amounts of drugs from your bottled water?

TICKING TIME BOMB

We have established that drinking bottled water from the shelf can cause serious health risks but the most serious chemical exposure comes from leaving bottled water in the hot sun. Have you ever left your bottle of water in your car on a warm day and noticed that when you took a drink, it tasted like plastic? Just know, that what you tasted was a toxic, chemical, cancer concoction.

Not only did **U** just get ripped off for your money while they fill their pockets in exchange for your precious health as it goes down the drain.

FLUORIDE TRUTHS

A recent study on children in India shows that fluoride doesn't fight cavities. Fluoride is toxic and it actually increases the risk of developing cavities, can cause a weakened immune system and accelerates aging due to cell damage. Young children exposed to fluoridated drinking water are more susceptible to developing Fluorosis. Fluorosis is the developmental disturbance of tooth enamel. It creates stains and streaks on the teeth and may cause a pitted, rough and hard to clean tooth surface.

Bottled water that originates from tap water, in most cases, is loaded with fluoride. A simple and proven remedy for the damaging effects of chlorine, fluoride and other toxic chemicals in our drinking water is the installation of a Structured Water unit. Structured Water units are an effective and inexpensive way to eliminate the negative effects of toxic chemicals in our tap and shower water. These units need no replacement filters, no electricity and have no moving parts, so they remain trouble free. Structured Water interacts with your cells.

ALL FILTRATION IS NOT CREATED EQUAL

DISTILLED WATER AND REVERSE OSMOSIS

Let me say that in my 35 years of practice I have never tried to pass these two sources of water off as being suitable for human consumption. Many health practitioners, however, are often surprised to hear me say that drinking distilled water or reverse osmosis water on a regular, daily basis is potentially dangerous - and here is why. These two water sources are not found in Nature.

Distilled and reverse osmosis water are essentially void of minerals and are acidic. Distillation is the process in which water is boiled, evaporated and the vapor condensed.

While fasting, using distilled water or reverse osmosis can be dangerous to your health because of the rapid loss of electrolytes *(sodium, potassium, chloride)* and trace minerals like magnesium. Deficiencies of these minerals can cause heartbeat irregularities and high blood pressure.

Distilled Water: When it comes in contact with air, it absorbs carbon dioxide, making it acidic. Acidosis is the root cause of all disease.

The more distilled water you drink, the more acidic you will become. Along with this comes inflammation, which leads to pain, suffering, crystallization and internal scar tissue.

Most commercial beverages that people consume are made from distilled water. Studies have consistently shown that regular consumers of soft drinks *(with sugar or sugar free)* spill huge amounts of calcium, magnesium and other trace minerals into their urine due to the acidic nature of these commercial beverages.

Hello, osteoporosis and hormonal imbalance. Let us not forget that these commercial beverages are the king of acidity, which equals inflammation, mutation, pain, suffering, crystallization and internal scar tissue. Hello, again 'Woody'.

The more minerals we lose, the greater the risk for: osteoporosis, osteoarthritis, calcium deposits throughout the body, hypothyroidism, coronary artery disease, high blood pressure and a list of degenerative diseases generally associated with premature aging.

Reverse Osmosis: To fill a 1.5-gallon container of reverse osmosis water you will waste 13.5 gallons down the drain.

Cooking foods in distilled or in reverse osmosis water pulls the minerals out of the food and lowers their nutrient content. So, don't ask yourself why 'you're dead on your feet' (**zombie**).

Cooking with soft water is found to cause substantial loss of all essential elements from vegetables, meat and cereals. Magnesium and calcium mineral loss can reach up to 60%, even higher losses for some other micro- elements such as copper 66%, manganese 70% and cobalt up to 86% loss. In contrast to the above, when hard water is used for cooking the loss of these elements is much lower due to the water being full of minerals.

ACCORDING TO THE WORLD HEALTH ORGANIZATION

Demineralized water *'attacks distribution piping and leaches metals and other materials from the pipes and associated plumbing materials.'* If it does that to pipes just think what it's doing to your internal plumbing system.

Your body contains electrolytes *(e.g., potassium, sodium)* in certain concentrations that are regulated by your body cells. If you drink distilled water your intestine is forced to take electrolytes from body reserves, which in turn, will deplete you of your normal electrical charge and leave you drained - like any other battery.

Drinking distilled water leads to the dilution of electrolytes within body fluids and cells. This in turn, will create an imbalance throughout the body.

Symptoms at the beginning of this condition include:

- Tiredness
- Weakness
- Headaches
- More severe symptoms include muscle spasms and impaired heart rate

We know that Whole Plant Based Foods are the main source of calcium and magnesium for our bodies. So just know that if you lack Whole Plant Based Foods and drink distilled or reverse osmosis water you will increase the chance of running a deficit of these two minerals within your body.

FILTERED WATER

One of the most common types of water purification systems used in our homes today is the carbon filter system. These filters may work for removing many harmful substances but do not remove toxic metals, harmful nitrates, sodium and fluoride that contaminate our water. Other disadvantages of the carbon filter system are that they require frequent filter replacements, may clog and can harbor mold.

CLOGS

Water containing a lot of sediment can clog up your filter thereby greatly reducing the normal lifetime of the filter.

MOLD

Organic substances from water may become trapped in the carbon filter. If left unused for periods of time, this creates an environment for the growth of mold.

pH

Acidic water is common in many households. The minerals that cause your water to be acidic dissolve and pass through the filter, resulting in acidic water remaining acidic.

FILTER REPLACEMENT

Carbon filters require frequent filter changes. To remain at peak performance this is an ongoing expense.

BOTTLED WATER

The bottled water industry really needs an enema for all the manure they pitch (fork) at the general public.

FACTS ABOUT BOTTLED WATER

- It takes an estimated 3 quarts of water to produce 1 quart of bottled water.

- Worldwide, an estimated 2.4 million metric tons of plastic are used to bottle water each year.

ENVIRONMENTAL IMPACT

- Bottled water is destructive to the environment.
- 67 million bottles are thrown away each day.
- Only 10% of bottles are recycled.
- Transporting large amounts of plastic or glass bottled water requires an incredible amount of fuel for it's delivery to you.

There is a lot of conflicting information surrounding bottled water, some positive, some negative. Here is the whole truth to guide you down the path towards healthier water consumption.

What is the true source of your bottled water?

Approximately 40% of bottled water is simply bottled tap water. So now where are those harmful chemicals you were trying to avoid? You are still drinking them along with a list of other chemicals released from the plastic bottles. *(Oops, cancer anyone?*

THE DANGERS OF PLASTIC

You may not realize it, but there are serious health risks to you and your family from drinking water from plastic bottles. If you choose to drink out of plastic water bottles, then you are potentially being exposed to the following chemicals.

BPA (BISPHENOL A)

BPA is commonly used to make polycarbonate plastic and epoxy resins to maintain the 'quality' of canned food and drink. If you are feeding your baby, or older child using plastic bottles or containers, you may be exposing them to harmful chemicals. You may want to change over to a glass or stainless steel container. BPA is an estrogen-mimicking chemical that has been associated with a range of serious health problems such as:

- Prostate and Breast Cancer
- Diabetes
- Obesity
- Early puberty in girls
- Learning and behavioral problems
- Fertility problems in females
- Decreased sperm count
- Altered immune system function

PHTHALATES

Phthalates are widely used to make plastics like polyvinyl chloride *(PVC)* more flexible. These chemicals disrupt natural hormone levels and have been linked to a wide range of developmental and reproductive complications such as:

- Reduced sperm count
- Testicular atrophy or structural abnormality
- Liver cancer
- Studies have shown that exposure to high levels of phthalate in pregnant women increased the chances of their male offspring to have certain demasculinized traits and produce less testosterone.

VITAMIN WATER

Just Another Unhealthy Soda

What's in a name? **U** fell for it. One of the biggest scams brought to us today by soda manufacturers is 'Vitamin Water'. Marketers have worked their magic to disguise this new drink as a 'health drink', and a healthy alternative to soda pop, by promoting the added benefits of vitamins and minerals *(evil plot)*. Don't be fooled! These added vitamins and minerals don't come close to a nutritional drink.

Vitamin Water is one of the worst types of bottled water you can put into your body.

These so called healthy drinks contain health damaging additives such as:
- High fructose corn syrup *(causes obesity and diabetes)*
- Food dyes *(affect physical and emotional health)*
- Just like the phrase Healthcare System, Vitamin Water is also a wolf in sheep's clothes.

Buyer beware... or be dead wrong.

EFFECTS OF DEHYDRATION

Mild-moderate dehydration can cause:

- Dry, sticky mouth
- Sleepiness or tiredness — children are likely to be less active than usual
- Thirst
- False Hunger

- Energy Loss
- Brain Fog
- Decreased urine output
- No wet diapers for three hours for infants
- Few or no tears when crying
- Dry skin
- Headache
- Constipation
- Diarrhea
- Dizziness or lightheaded

Severe dehydration can cause:

- Extreme thirst
- Shriveled and dry skin that lacks elasticity
- Extreme fussiness or sleepiness in infants and children; irritability and confusion in adults
- Very dry mouth, skin and mucous membranes
- Little or no urination — any urine that is produced will be darker than normal
- Sunken eyes
- In infants, sunken fontanels — the soft spots on the top of a baby's head
- Low blood pressure
- Rapid heartbeat
- Rapid breathing
- No tears when crying
- Fever
- Pain and Inflammation
- Muscle cramps
- Insomnia
- In the most serious cases, delirium or unconsciousness

DAILY WATER CONSUMPTION

You are composed of approximately 60 - 80% water. As we age that percentage of water drops but if you are drinking Structured Water, it will remain *(the same)* constant. This is where premature aging gets washed down the drain. Life begins and ends at the cellular level.

Many people follow the 8 by 8 rule: This is where we are told to drink 1, 8 ounce glass of water 8 times a day. *For myself, I like the body weight theory:* take half of your body weight, in pounds, and drink that number of ounces of water. 60% of this amount should be drunk before noon and the remaining amount before 5pm.

Example: A person of 200 pounds would drink 100 ounces before 5 pm.

Drink It, Love It, Live It - Drink Life In

Here are long time, proven advantages of drinking water. *None of these facts have been watered down.*

1. Drink Structured Water to reduce weight safely. Water contains no calories, limits your food intake, removes by-products of fat and reduces your appetite.
2. If you want to look younger, drink plenty of Structured Water every day. Structured Water moisturizes your skin and helps maintain your skin's elasticity. Just from drinking Structured Water, you can say hello to glowing supple, younger looking skin that is free from toxins! Food and beverages like caffeine, chocolate, cola, tea, coffee and alcohol are dehydrating and should be limited - better yet, eliminated.

3. Drinking Structured Water helps to fight against skin conditions such as eczema, dry skin, wrinkles, psoriasis and spots.

4. Since our body is made up of 80% water; drinking plenty of Structured Water is a must to help the body and mind maintain peak performance. The brain communicates with the rest of the body through the cerebrospinal fluid, which is 93% water! Notice your energy levels and your ability to think improve when **U** hydrate - not constipate.

5. Structured Water takes the toxic load and acidic waste out of the body efficiently. We must drink the amount required by our body, weight and lifestyle. When we do not drink enough Structured Water, our bodies run at a deficit when it comes to oxygen and minerals and our hearts pump much harder, due to the increase of acidity.

6. There is absolutely no substitute for Structured Water, whether it is tea, coffee, milk or juice. Studies have shown there is an increased chance of incurring a heart attack when you replace your needed water intake with tea, coffee, milk or juice.

7. Dehydration is a major cause of headaches and back pain. Taking in enough Structured Water can help reduce and prevent these symptoms. Realize before you crystallize. If you wake up stiff like 'Woody' this is a major sign that you are already dehydrated.

8. There are foundational rules to living a happy and healthy life. One of these is to drink enough Structured Water daily. Your life depends on it.

9. Structured Water plays a foundational role in strengthening and preserving your immune system. Drinking plenty of Structured Water will help fight against the flu, kidney

stones, pathogen points and other ailments by promoting healthy aerobic bacteria and eliminating disease- causing anaerobic pathogens.

10. Let logic prevail. The more toxins/ acidity you have within your body the more inflammation, degeneration, internal scar tissue formation and mutation you will experience. When you drink the proper amount of Structured Water for your body weight, each and every day, you are eliminating and greatly reducing cancer causing agents especially in the bladder and colon.

11. Drinking enough Structured Water throughout the day will help your body maintain a proper pH balance. The body requires a neutral pH 7 range in order to remain healthy and vibrant.

Whether you want shinier hair, younger skin, a healthier body, or all three - Structured Water is the world's best beauty elixir.

THE WONDERS OF STRUCTURED WATER

The natural action of water tumbling over rocks, down waterfalls, flowing through twists and turns as it actively descends a mountain actually structures water.

Dr. Gerald Pollack, of the University of Washington, has been one of the leading researchers in this field. His work is absolutely groundbreaking because his main focus is understanding how Structured Water interacts with your cells.

He says that the water in and around your cells is absolutely vital to your health because it makes a big difference in how your cells interact with proteins, which are the building blocks of life. There is great evidence that suggests this type of water increases cellular healing, so it is quite possible that drinking Structured Water is a very important part to healing and longevity.

Cultures that drink Structured Water have been historically known to live longer and healthier. All you have to do is live at the bottom of a mountain by a fast flowing river or purchase a Structure Water Unit.

When the muscles in our bodies are aching, we tend to think that it's the muscle that's in trouble. What Dr. Pollack is saying is that it's actually the type of water and the protein around the muscle cells that are not functioning properly, creating cellular constipation that leads to an acid environment with the end result being inflammation, degeneration and yes even cellular mutation.

HOW MAN HAS DUPLICATED NATURE TO PRODUCE STRUCTURED WATER

They are now able to create a highly tuned environment where water is caused to flow in specific geometrical patterns. The flows and counter flows create an environment of dynamic shear and pressure differentials that turn water into an amazing self-correcting machine. We can now duplicate nature's process within our own lives, any place, any time, when it comes to Structured Water and its life-giving properties.

Gone are the days when you need chemicals or salts, electricity, magnets, moving mechanical parts or filters (although they can be used if the need arises). With the unique and innovative technology of our Structured Water Units, you and your family are now protected and can reap the full benefits of dynamic Structured Water, just as in nature, just as nature intended.

Structured Water devices work at the molecular level altering the structure of the water by activating and retaining the healthful benefits of minerals and life giving characteristics, while at the same time neutralizing the harmful effects.

These amazing Structured Water devices employ the vortex phenomenon, replicating the water of a river, crashing down a mountain side.

If we were a water molecule on the path through this device it would be an exhilarating roller coaster ride. We would come out refreshed and ready to perform our life-given roles. Nature does not clean the water, it allows the water to clean itself. Structured Water devices create an energy environment for water to structure itself. This gives water a lower surface tension and better hydrating properties for the body.

This unique geometric technology breaks up large low energy water molecule clusters into smaller high energy clusters. The innovative technology eliminates negative energy patterns and redefines the water's natural healthy energy pattern. Harmful effects are erased and the water is reprogrammed to do what it was meant to do: **hydrate, heal and restore**. Structured Water allows us to imprint, through our cellular DNA and RNA, the knowledge of its secret blueprint, which helps us to become balanced. The things that are adverse to life are pulled to the inside core of the water molecule and shielded from your body and life itself.

Everything takes less water when it is structured, about 30% less. In most people's homes there are devices that you have to constantly tend, repair and replace filters. We want you to know that there is advanced science and technology out there that is so simple and so powerful that it creates Nature's highest quality water without the worry of any future cost or maintenance. It never wears out, and has no moving parts. The water itself is the moving part; it is the machine, it is the natural action of nature. It is what brings the water to that place of being free to do what it is meant to do, which is to make life absolutely perfect.

As Einstein stated: Everything is Frequency.
Drink - Cleanse - Restore
The Future Is Here - Embrace It!

STRUCTURED WATER AND BRIDGING THE GAP OF AGRICULTURE

What if changing one thing could change everything? For agriculture, it is simple. That one thing is called Structured Water.

Unlike other types of water being used in many agricultural applications, Structured Water contains no energetic toxins, it brings forward a high- oxygenated state, increases the energy and regulates and balances the soil minerals. These characteristics of Structured Water bring forth some truly amazing results in the world of agriculture. Structured Water is the key to bridging the gap of contaminated and mineral deficient soil to create a healthier and stronger foundation for plants, animals and humans.

How does Structured Water benefit food crops?

For many years, the Brix Level has been the scale of measure in the world of agriculture. This was brought forth in the 1800s, when German chemist, Adolf Brix saw the need for a way to tell when grapes were sweet enough for the picking.

An instrument known as the refractometer was developed to measure exactly where the sugar content of the grape stood on any given day. The Brix Level is now known to be an indicator of not only sugar content but nutrient content as well.

A refractometer, measures units called Brix, which is a unit representative of the sugar content of a liquid solution. One degree Brix is equal to 1 gram of sugar in 100 grams of solution. This represents the strength of the solution as a percentage by weight/mass.

True Brix measures a combination of sugar, amino acids, oils, proteins, flavonoids and minerals. Sugar is merely one of the components of Brix. A drop of the liquid from the plant juice is placed on the prism of a refractometer. Then the cover plate is closed so the liquid will spread out on the glass. As you look through the viewing end of the instrument, you see an etched scale calibrated in 0-30 or 0-32 degrees Brix.

For instance, a strawberry crop can then be graded in terms of Brix, with numbers in 4 categories: Poor, Average, Good, Excellent. Most supermarket Brix ratings are in the Poor to Average range. Crops nourished with Structured Water consistently rate in the Good to Excellent range or beyond!

In terms of a plants immune system, a high-Brix plant emits a far superior energetic electromagnetic spectrum than a low-

Brix specimen. Insects are only attracted to a low-Brix range, that's why they only attack plants with the weakest emanations, meaning immune systems. As in all life, the weak become the prey - you are what you eat.

What growers need to understand is the insects serve a great purpose, they are eliminating the food that does not vibrate at the level that is needed for humans to have a healthy immune system. Eliminate the bugs and you reduce the quality of the food. **A Brix reading is merely a way for us to see by proxy what insects see with their eyes.**

BRIX LEVEL CHART

Refractive Index of Crop Juices - Calibrated In % Sucrose Or °Brix

Vegetables	Poor	Average	Good	Excellent
Asparagus	02	04	06	08
Beets	06	08	10	12
Bell Peppers	04	06	08	12
Broccoli	06	08	10	12
Cabbage	06	08	10	12
Carrots	04	06	12	18
Cauliflower	04	06	08	10
Celery	04	06	10	12
Corn Stalks	04	08	14	20
Corn (Young)	06	10	18	24
Cow Peas	04	06	10	12
Cucumbers	04	06	08	12

	Poor	Average	Good	Excellent
Endives	04	06	08	10
English Peas	08	10	12	14
Field Peas	04	06	10	12
Garlic, Cured	28	32	36	40
Green Beans	04	06	08	10
Hot Peppers	04	06	08	10
Kale	08	10	12	16
Kohlrabi	06	08	10	12
Lettuce	04	06	08	10
Onions	04	06	08	10
Parsley	04	06	08	10
Peanuts	04	06	08	10
Potatoes	03	05	07	08
Potatoes, Sweet	06	08	10	14
Romaine	04	06	08	10
Rutabagas	04	06	10	12
Squash	06	08	12	14
Sweet Corn	06	10	18	24
Turnips	04	06	08	10

Fruits

	Poor	Average	Good	Excellent
Apples	06	10	14	18
Avocados	04	06	08	10
Bananas	08	10	12	14
Blueberries	08	12	14	18
Cantaloupe	08	12	14	18
Cherries	06	08	14	16
Coconut	08	10	12	14

Grapes	08	12	16	20
Grapefruit	06	10	14	18
Honeydew	08	10	12	14
Kumquat	04	06	08	10
Lemons	04	06	08	12
Limes	04	06	10	12
Mango	04	06	10	14
Oranges	06	10	16	20
Papayas	06	10	18	22
Peaches	06	10	14	18
Pears	06	10	12	14
Pineapple	12	14	20	22
Raisins	60	70	75	80
Raspberries	06	08	12	14
Strawberries	06	08	12	14

When a plant is out of nutritional balance, internal pressures cause cellular components like simple sugars or incomplete proteins to seep *(bleed)* out to the surface of the leaves and stems. Just as when a shark smells blood he attacks, the same principle applies to insects. Plants are just as susceptible to systemic nutritional imbalances as humans are. Structured Water brings the plant back into the balance of nature by creating an energetic force field.

For more proof and validation read the works of Dr. Carey A. Reams' agricultural methods.

Farm Water Usage

The advent of Structured Water to the farm has left more than one farmer scratching their head wondering why they didn't have to use as much water as they did in the past.

Life is all about energy and frequency. You can't have one without the other. Where there is Structured Water you have the proper balance of frequencies and energy to optimize hydration. When you increase hydration, you decrease the volume of water needed. When farmers begin using Structured Water they find themselves standing in a field of mud surprised that the plant is fully hydrated with smaller amounts of water.

EXPERIENCES OF FLAVOR AND PLANT PRODUCTIVITY

The first time Structured Water was used to grow food, it was an agricultural breakthrough. We had no idea up until this point how good food could really taste.

Soil Health (Calcium Glaze)

There are many other major breakthroughs that farmers experience when they implement the use of Structured Water. The greatest change is the effect of Structured Water on the foundation of the soil. Soil scientists have studied mineral rich soils for years. Very few have studied how Structured Water immediately frees up calcium and makes it available to the plant. All other types of water create a "calcium glaze" on the soil. Structured Water makes all minerals bio-available to plant life.

For pennies a day farmers are able to increase the nutritional value of their crops - Structured Water is Foundational.

There is a saying, *'Just Add Water and Stir.'* We feel this needs to be revised to, *'Just Add Structured Water and Create a Stir!'*

Tangerines

For the first time we truly felt we bridged the gap; real nutrition was a reality. We tested the Brix level of tangerine juice and it checked in at a high 17.8. Good to excellent on the Brix scale.

Lemons

We were able to bite right into the lemons as if they were apples. The normal strong tartness was replaced with a uniquely pleasant and sweet lemon semi- bitter flavor.

Grapes

Grape farmers in Mexico were amazed that their crops were brought to harvest 2 weeks earlier than ever before. The fungal growth that normally happens on grapes never materializes once the vines were nourished with Structured Water.

The normal Brix reading for an excellent grape hits the 20 mark on a refractometer. These grapes were now checking in at 24! Structured Water literally blew the lid off the normal Brix scale.

Strawberries

It was noted that Structured Water had the ability to increase strawberry plant growth from neighboring plants that received no water. Everything is frequency, everything is energy. Just as people, the weather and food can affect your energy, Structured Water can do the same thing to neighboring plants; this is called the ripple effect.

Tomatoes

These pictures were taken in the garden, at the home of Mr. Laphon Puyo's where his amazing tomatoes are watered with Structured Water. He writes: I am retired close to the city of Pau, in France, and let me inform you about the results I have thanks to Structured Water. The pictures I send you are proving the results I had in my garden.

Baths feel better, pH is stabilized to 7, and I don't have to use pH reducer anymore. And these tomatoes are out of this world! The one in the bottom picture is over 2 lb. (1kg) all by itself!

Sprouts

Sprout growers have also seen the amazing growth results from Structured Water. The longevity of sprouts now is much longer. This never-before- seen lasting power has people talking for days, shaking their heads, and saying, *"How can these perishables stay so fresh for so long?!"* Remember, Structured Water increases the frequency, thus increasing the vitality and life force for all concerned.

Roses

We started out with 6-foot high rose bushes. These roses were healthy to begin with. After adding Structured Water from multiple inline structuring units, the rose garden began to truly come to life. The scent produced from the roses was now being experienced everywhere on the property. The rose bushes were now producing sturdy stems with rich, dense leaves and vibrant flowers to match, that had not been seen before.

Neighboring rose bushes paled by comparison. It was clear when we started seeing stems shooting 11 to 13 feet up in the air that there was something very real, if not magical, about Structured Water! The rose bushes now reach to 9 feet high - How sweet it is!

ANIMAL HEALTH

Plants are not the only ones experiencing improved health benefits from Structured Water. Improvements to animal health and production have been enhanced as well.

As we enter into the world of animal agriculture and ranching, this same Quantum Field Effect pertains to all animal studies with Structured Water as well.

Bee colonies have been observed to repeatedly fly away from their hive on a daily basis. They fly 3 feet just to arrive and drink as much Structured Water as possible. Bees are naturally in tune with how the health of Structured Water makes them a far stronger, harmonious, and more productive colony. They must be in tune, because closer water sources are available but are overlooked by the bees!

We even speculate that as beekeepers become educated in the benefits of Structured Water and the effect it has on bees, the dreaded bee colony collapse may become a thing of the past or at least significantly reduced by Structured Water's protective presence.

Dairy

Dairy herds in Chandler, AZ increased and improved their production of butterfat after introducing Structured Water. The cows even began behaving differently, more cohesively.

When the drinking water for the cows was in question by the state because of bacterial levels, a Structuring Unit was placed between the source and the drinking troughs. Within 2 weeks, the water quality exceeded the state's standards and the dairy farm was permitted to remain open.

Chickens

Chicken farms have found greater overall health and an increase in weight when they added Structured Water to the chicken's diet.

Another big insight from using Structured Water was the lowering of overall mortality rates by 50%. The death rate declined from 4,000 birds per house to 2,000 birds per barn in one recent study.

All Animals

All animals from birds and horses to farm animals and house pets are attracted to Structured Water.

When given the choice, dogs naturally choose Structured Water over chlorinated tap water. Structured Water is leading the way in the world of veterinary health.

Farm Machinery

An interesting thing about Structured Water is that its effects are not just with the animals and plants. Even farm machinery operates more efficiently. Engine power and mileage have been shown to increase with the use of Structured Water in the motors.

Structured Water is bringing forth healthier animals and stronger crops. All we have to do now is apply Structured Water, stand back, and enjoy the results!

OTHER BENEFITS OF STRUCTURED WATER

- Fresh tasting invigorating water
- Low surface tension, less than 46 dynes per cubic centimeter.
- Regulates the autonomic nervous system
- More energy and endurance
- Clarity of thought and emotions
- Faster recovery through removal of cellular toxins.
- Greater density
- Increased blood oxygenation
- Wonderful showers and baths – no chlorine smell!
- No more dry, itchy skin!
- Healthier nails, skin, hair & teeth
- Less soap necessary when washing
- Hair and skin rinse cleaner and feel better when washed.
- Healthier mother's milk for breastfeeding newborns.
- Healthier plant growth – green lawns – lower freezing point.
- Reduced chlorine requirements for spas and swimming pools.

- Reduced corrosion and deposits in pipes
- Increased longevity of all systems that use water.
- Reduces odors around water usage facilities.
- Improved growth of crops with increased biomass. *(27% to 40%)*
- Lower freezing point so plants can be sustained at lower temperatures.
- Removal of existing calcium and aragonite deposits.
- Solvency of the water increases profits from sales of coffee & juice.
- Healthier gardens and household plants.
- Healthier farm livestock, domestic pets and fish.
- Structured Water increases absorption of minerals, medications or any other supplement to 100%.
- Elimination of polluting salts, chemicals or corrosive by-products.
- Improved aerobic bacterial activity in septic and sewage systems.
- Structured Water is loaded with negative hydrogen ions... "Hydrogen is the fuel of life."
- Assists in the absorption of healthful vitamins and minerals to all life.
- Structured Water contributes to the solution and well-being of all.
- Structured Water is the ultimate food.
- Structured Water is the Greatest Medicine.
- Structured Water reduces the energy required for hydration.
- Structured Water is the most economical fuel and energy source.

What I have presented here is what we know, however, I am curious about what we still don't know about the amazing life-giving properties of Structured Water. Despite the fact that water is something that has no taste, we still love it! *Who doesn't relish the feeling of a cool drink of water on a sweltering hot day?*

For more information, just click and stir! docofdetox.com/water

16 WAYS TO USE YOUR PORTABLE STRUCTURE WATER UNIT

The Portable Structure Unit is the easiest way to structure not just your water but all liquids at home and on the go. Enjoy the benefits of an energy infusion of Structured Water in your whole life, whether in-town, at a local restaurant or on the road traveling. Also, great for apartment living, where a house product is not an option. Simply pour water through the top and point the small spout into any container to get all the benefits of Structured Water.

1. Run all water through Portable Structure Unit.
2. Make Daily Cleansing Tea using Structured Water. You can also run your tea through the portable unit after it is made to enhance the energy of the Daily Cleansing Tea.
3. Run all liquids through Portable Structure Unit from olive oil to nutritional drinks. Pour 2 oz. of any liquid through Portable Structure Unit and pour back into the bottle to structure the entire liquid. Aftercare: put unit in apple cider vinegar or run it through your dishwasher to clean thoroughly.
4. Protects against hormones and antibiotics in milk making it taste better.

5. Protects against acidity in coffee making it taste smoother and shielding toxic chemicals from the body.

6. Pour 2 oz. from a bottle of wine, beer or liquor through the Portable Structure Unit and then pour the 2 oz. back into the bottle. This will structure the whole bottle, improving taste and protecting you from any toxins, sulfites and nitrates, preventing those nasty hangovers.

7. Pour 1 cup of water into your bath, pool, hot tub or Jacuzzi to structure the entire body of water, this is known as the ripple effect.

8. Spray or run Structured Water over all fruits and vegetables to neutralize pesticides, GMOs and petrochemical fertilizers.

9. Pouring all fruit and vegetables juices through the Portable Structure Unit makes all nutritional drinks more bioavailable but protects against any toxins, giving juice a smoother taste.

10. Put Structured Water into a spray bottle for when out at restaurants. One spray will structure an entire glass of water shielding you from toxins while increasing its hydration value.

11. Using the small end of the structure unit for breathing will balance the brain and autonomic nervous system within minutes when experiencing emotional distress.

12. Fill a Ziploc bag with cold Structured Water to use as a compress when you have inflammation and when you have chronic stiffness fill a Ziploc bag with hot Structured Water and apply to stiff area.

13. Water all plants with Structured Water.

14. Feed your pets Structured Water.

15. These units allow travel to any country in the world to drink and bathe with tap water.

16. Pour 8oz. of Structured Water into your radiator to reduce toxic exhaust and to improve gas mileage.

For more information, just click and stir! docofdetox.com/water

HYDROGEN-ENRICHED WATER

Water is the most common substance on earth. However, it is one of the least understood.

Not a day goes by that water is not a part of our life. We drink it, cook with it, bathe in it, swim in it, give thanks for it when it rains, and play in it when it snows. There is no doubt that water is an integral part of each of us and the world we live in. Water (H2O), which is essential to life, is formed by the combination of oxygen, a powerful oxidizer and essential for life and hydrogen, a powerful reducer and essential for life. Hydrogen (H2) is considered the primordial anti-oxidant. Oxygen (O2) is a well-known oxidant.

Hydrogen was involved in the genesis of life and oxygen is necessary for the existence of life. We breathe in oxygen all of the time, pushing our bodies towards oxidation. Consuming increased hydrogen in your water is the perfect and natural way to balance oxidation. Drinking Hydrogen-Enriched Water is the easiest and most logical method of obtaining the natural H2 anti-oxidant. A large percentage of our bodies are water, most of us simply don't drink enough of it. In my professional and personal opinion, when you combine Hydrogen-Enriched Water with Structured Water you have created the elixir of which great health is the only and final outcome.

Consider the following thoughts:

- It is reported that 75% of all Americans are chronically dehydrated.
- It is said that the thirst mechanism is mistaken for hunger pangs in 37% of Americans.
- Mild dehydration has been shown to slow down metabolism as much as 3%.
- A lack of water is a leading cause of fatigue.
- Staying adequately hydrated can reduce back and joint pain.
- A 2% reduction of water in the body can cause short-term memory loss and difficulty with thinking.
- 5 glasses of water daily decreases the risk of Breast Cancer by 79% and Bladder Cancer by 50%.

Now that you are thinking about how amazing, wonderful, and vitally necessary water is, we will discover how Hydrogen-Enriched Water is better than other drinking water. In short, a Water Ionizer produces Hydrogen-Enriched Water, because of the dissolved molecular hydrogen, which has a powerful anti-oxidant effect. The process starts by filtering the incoming water to remove chlorine, chloramines, 50% fluoride, metals, pesticides, bacteria, viruses, algae, and fungus. After being cleaned, water enters the water cell to receive the amazing H2 gas. The negatively charged electrodes *(cathodes)* in the water cell create hydrogen gas and dissolve it in the water.

There are over 400 studies, 40 human studies, showing the therapeutic benefits of molecular hydrogen on 150 different human diseases and in every organ in the human body.

Why is Hydrogen Important?

The hydrogen molecule, unlike other anti-oxidants, is a selective anti- oxidant that only targets the dangerous free radicals like the hydroxyl radical, converting them instantly to water. It can also prevent oxidative stress by increasing the body's own anti-oxidants such as glutathione. In 2007, it was clearly shown that hydrogen gas can act as a selective anti- oxidant and has the therapeutic properties observed with ionized water. No one had investigated hydrogen gas before. Everyone assumed it was just an inert byproduct of electrolysis - with no biological effect. If we remove hydrogen gas from ionized water the therapeutic effects are lost. When we add additional hydrogen gas to ionized water, via bubbling, the positive benefits are increased. *The biological effects of hydrogen gas have now been confirmed in over 400 studies and on 150 different human diseases and disease models. H2 has been shown to be therapeutic in virtually every organ of the human body.*

Why is Hydrogen-Enriched Water Better?

The majority of people simply don't drink enough water. For this reason, it is believed that a large percentage of the U.S. population is chronically dehydrated. The definition of dehydration is when the body loses more fluid than it takes in. A study conducted by the CDC showed that 54% of children ages 6-19 in the USA are dehydrated.

Why don't people drink enough water?

People don't like the taste of most water and they are worried about the pollutants in water. A study1, released in January

2014, was published in the *Journal of Environmental Pollution*. The study was conducted by the *Environmental Protection Agency (EPA)*. It is the largest study of water coming out of wastewater treatment plants.

The study looked at samples from 50 large-size wastewater treatment plants nationwide and tested for 56 drugs including oxycodone, high blood pressure medications, and over-the-counter drugs like Tylenol and ibuprofen. More than half the samples tested positive for at least 25 of the drugs monitored. High blood pressure medications appeared in the highest concentrations and most frequently.

Another study2 released in January 2014, showed that there were 24,500 chemicals in bottled water that are known to cause cancer, gynecological issues, 90% reduction in estrogenic receptor activity, and 60% androgenic receptor activity. Bottled water companies market bottled water as healthier and cleaner. However, in the processing of the bottles, the water is shown to harm those who drink it, even in amounts as small as .1 oz.

As previously stated tap water can have any number of impurities despite the *"purification"* methods used by city municipalities.

What most people don't know is typically the water we drink, including tap water, bottled water and filtered water has a positive oxidation-reduction potential *(ORP)*, which is not helpful to the body.

Hydrogen-Enriched Water tastes better and has health benefits due to the dissolved H2 gas. Knowing how much healthier

Hydrogen-Enriched Water is can be the first step in changing your life for the better.

Benefits of Hydrogen-Enriched Water

Everyone is talking about how free radicals are damaging our cells. What most people don't know is that many free radicals are beneficial to health. It is only the cell damaging (cytotoxic) radicals that we need to scavenge. Molecular hydrogen converts these free radicals into water molecules in the cells. A Hydrogen-Enriched Water Ionizer converts municipal, well, or reverse osmosis water into Hydrogen-Enriched Water. Once the oxidative burden is reduced in the cells of the body, the body can naturally produce glutathione where needed.

Athletic Performance:

Hydrogen-Enriched Water has increased the performance of many athletes. Elite athletes know that part of keeping their bodies in peak condition is understanding the science of their bodies. Proper hydration is critical for performance, but you don't want to drink just any water. Hydrogen-Enriched Water is the best water for athletes. It better empowers cells to work at optimal efficiency by ridding them of oxidative damage.

Hydrogen-Enriched Water provides a faster rate of gastric emptying. The dissolved hydrogen gas rids the body of hydroxyl radicals *(HO*)* by converting them into water molecules. This improves cell efficiency and increases energy. Athletes can perform significantly better without feeling fatigued. Another huge benefit is their recovery times are cut in half. When a person is properly hydrated on a cellular level with Hydrogen-

Enriched Water, their cells perform at peak levels longer. Athletes who drink Hydrogen-Enriched Water report that they experience increased energy and performance. Many athletes indicate that they were able to get past their plateau after drinking Hydrogen-Enriched Water.

Detoxification & Weight Loss:

Water has been used in purification and cleansing from the beginning of time, after all, water is the "ultimate solvent". Water is used to remove toxins and waste. Hydrogen-Enriched Water is beneficial in supporting healthy cleansing and weight loss. When the toxins and wastes are flushed, the burden on the body is lessened. Many people reported to shed a pound per day initially when drinking Hydrogen-Enriched Water.

The weight loss stems from drinking the appropriate amount of Hydrogen-Enriched Water and letting the body do what it is designed to do. Eating a Whole Plant Based Diet can support a healthy detox and weight loss regime. Hydrogen-Enriched Water helps to support Daily Cleansing Tea in eliminating toxic waste and restoring cellular health. This greatly increases health and immunity. Drinking Hydrogen-Enriched Water will lessen the detoxification burden on your body. People report that they feel more hydrated with Hydrogen-Enriched Water, they experience more productive sleep, wake up more alert, have fewer allergy symptoms, and feel more energy throughout the day.

Immune System Boost:

No one enjoys getting sick because life comes to a screeching halt. The immune system and the digestive system are directly linked to hydration. Being properly hydrated is one of the best decisions you can make to increase the strength of your immune system. Remember, 70-80% of your body is water and it should be no surprise that the type of water you drink directly influences the health of your body. Ionized water is known for supporting the cleansing of the intestines. Keeping the body hydrated is critical for prevention of sickness and disease.

Increased Energy and Hydration:

Everyone wants to live life to the fullest. We have all watched younger children and wished we had half the energy they possess. I have often wished I could bottle this energy. Proper hydration increases the metabolic process.

In his book, *"Your Body's Many Cries for Water"*, Dr. F. Batmanghelidj, M.D., teaches when people are better hydrated their metabolic process increases.

Dr. Batmanghelidj further states, *"Water is a primary nutrient for all brain functions and transmission of information. It gives us power and electrical energy for all brain functions, particularly thinking. As a result, good hydration increases our efficiency at study and work, and expands our attention span."*

We have heard the old adage that 8 glasses of water per day keeps the Doctor away. The rule of thumb is to drink half your body weight in ounces of water daily. A study3 conducted by the University of Utah, showed the more water you drink the better. In the study, subjects consumed either 4, 8 or 12 glasses of water daily. On the fifth day before rising, their hydration status was monitored and a computer measured how many calories they had burned in a resting state. The groups who drank 8 and 12 glasses of water daily were sufficiently hydrated, whereas subjects who drank only 4 showed definite signs of dehydration. Furthermore, the well-hydrated subjects not only reported better concentration and more energy, but they burned more calories at rest than the group who drank only 4 glasses. These results were in line with previous 3 University of Utah findings that the ability to burn calories can decline by about 2% per day when people are dehydrated.

Increased Cognitive Function - Ghrelin:

Molecular Hydrogen has been shown to stimulate ghrelin secretions. Ghrelin is known as the hunger hormone in the body, it affects many things in the body including cognitive function, hunger, weight regulation and anti-inflammatory function. This is accomplished in the hippocampus and hypothalamus in the brain. Specific studies have shown that Hydrogen- Enriched Water can be tremendously beneficial to neurologic pathologies like Parkinson's, Alzheimer's and Autism due to ghrelin secretion stimulation. Water is your first food, you are what you drink.

Water is the most studied material on Earth but it is remarkable to find that the science behind its behavior and function are so poorly understood *(or even ignored)*, not only by people in general, but also by scientists working with it every day.

"The small size of its molecule belies the complexity of its actions and its singular capabilities. Water's unique properties and chameleonic nature seem to fit ideally into the requirements for life as can no other molecule."

- Martin Chaplin, London South Bank University

THE BREATH OF LIFE

"When you harness your breathing, you will Master Your Life."

- Dr. Darrell Wolfe, Doc of Detox

STRUCTURED BREATHING
OXYGEN - THE BREATH OF LIFE

In this chapter we are discussing how it is no longer good enough to just filter our air and water. To maintain or regain optimal health we will personally have to restructure and raise the healing frequency of our water and air. As Einstein stated, *"Frequency is everything and everything is frequency."* The practitioner of the future will practice and teach their patients in the most simple and cost effective way to raise their frequency because frequency is everything. They will use light, frequency and color therapy to restore vital health. In this chapter we will be discussing devices that can and will restructure and add frequency not just to your water but also to your oxygen. It is simple, effective and easy to use. No filters, electricity, maintenance or moving parts. It is portable and long lasting... the way health is meant to be.

There are thousands of people now using and experiencing the life-giving benefits of Structured Water and Breathing devices. These Structuring Units energize and change the quality of your daily water and oxygen intake to its highest potential. Most people are now realizing that oxygen and water are the most important foods for a healthy, vibrant body. The quality of the water and air you take in can be measured by the quality of your health. Many are coming to the realization that these structuring devices provide the body with the highest quality of cleansing and healing water and oxygen today. These two substances that we take for granted are the most important foundational foods for creating a pain-free, disease-free, energized life. Find out and experience how these Structured Water units are also Structured Breathing devices.

Why would a person pursue this? Or, more directly, *what benefit does a person receive from using these devices for Structured Breathing?*

There is a simple principle to all health that brain neurologists and physiologists know. The Autonomic Nervous System must be regulating properly for the brain to control all the functions necessary for human health on a physical and an emotional level.

To quote Wikipedia:

The autonomic nervous system, visceral nervous system or involuntary nervous system is the part of the peripheral nervous system that acts as a control system that functions largely below the level of consciousness to control visceral functions, including heart rate, digestion, respiratory rate, salivation, perspiration, pupillary dilation, micturition *(urination)*, sexual arousal, breathing and swallowing. Most autonomous functions are involuntary but they can often work in conjunction with the somatic nervous system, which provides voluntary control. This means you don't have to think about asking your heart to pump or your lungs to breathe every minute of the day for your body to run. **The autonomic nervous system is divided into three main subsystems:** *the parasympathetic nervous system, sympathetic nervous system, and the enteric nervous system.* Depending on the circumstances, these subsystems may operate independently of each other or interact co-operatively.

The enteric nervous system consists of a mesh-like system of neurons that governs the function of the gastrointestinal system. The sympathetic nervous system is often considered the "fight or flight" system, while the parasympathetic nervous system is often considered the "rest and digest" or "feed and breed" system. In many cases, parasympathetic nervous system and sympathetic nervous system have "opposite" actions where one system activates a physiological response and the other inhibits it. An older definition of the sympathetic and parasympathetic nervous systems were "excitatory" and "inhibitory" was overturned due to the many exceptions found. A more modern characterization is that the sympathetic nervous system is a "quick response mobilizing system" and the parasympathetic is a "more slowly activated dampening system," but even this has exceptions, such as in sexual arousal and orgasm, wherein both play a role.

Without the autonomic nervous system regulating, the body goes into a state known as dis-regulation. The brain starts shutting down its circuit board. As more circuits shutdown, overall body function decreases. Illness and disease begin to occur due to misfiring and blocks created to the body's circuit board. This can be seen with patients that I work with even though they are doing everything right as far as their health goes but something unseen continues to derail their goal of optimum health.

What are some of the factors that blow fuses and cause this shut down?

Negative emotional patterns and worn out **B**elief **S**ystems not dealt with continually cause stress, leading to emotional/physical blocks and increased acidity, crystallization and internal scar tissue formation. Toxins such as chemicals, food additives, sugar, drugs, chlorine, fluoride, PCBs, pesticides, herbicides, fungicides, heavy metals, electromagnetic frequencies, silver fillings in teeth, bacteria, viruses, fungus and worms are all known to be dis- regulators, just to name a few.

When using a structuring unit every person regains balance of their autonomic nervous system regulation within just a few breaths! This is why daily Structured Breathing benefits every person so that they have the ability to open up and maintain a smooth running, regulating nervous system! These structuring units are primary support tools for the body for maintaining and turning your circuit board back on and removing old subconscious thoughts that are undermining and derailing you of a life of bliss! The keys to maintaining vibrant health are baby steps, daily, every day, so just breathe and Take Life In - It's Only Natural!

The following medical and scientific methods have been used to show that this body balancing process is actually occurring:

1. Autonomic Response Testing (ART), the work of Dietrich Klinghardt, M.D. This is advanced biofeedback, known more commonly as, muscle testing.
2. Traditional Chinese Medicine (TCM) Cun Guan Chi pulse testing.
3. Korean Hand Therapy (KHT) Yin Yang Pulse Diagnosis.
4. Gas Discharge Visualization (GDV) High tech computerized biophotonic *(light energy)* analysis developed by Dr. Konstantin Korotkov and a multi-disciplinary team of over 300 top Russian scientists and doctors.
5. Acugraph computerized meridian diagnosis.

We are currently working on providing even more in-depth validation of the structuring process and its health-giving effects by using an acoustic heart monitoring device called the Endo-cardiograph 2, first built in 1937 by Dr. Royal Lee, founder of Standard Process.

We are continually researching and studying to find out what are the main toxic loads that are present in a disease state. We are gaining a better understanding of how these advanced structuring units are assisting the body to remove these toxic burdens so effectively and efficiently. Your water and air becomes the machine when using these structuring units.

Water and air puzzles scientists more than any other topic known to man. The fundamental needs of air and water can now be maintained at higher quality levels than ever before with these simple life-giving devices. This structuring unit instantly and automatically will energize and neutralize toxins from the air, water and your body. Due to your cells now being in a much healthier state the cells are able to carry out their duties much more effectively. The two most valuable nutrients of the body are air and water, through structuring they are now much more available to the cells. In their wake, the other nutrients of the body *(minerals, vitamins, enzymes)* can follow suit: energizing and improving cellular activity.

One of the most important breakthroughs we have found is the release of toxic emotions and subconscious blocks that can hold your organs and the endocrine system in a weakened state. It has become a daily occurrence to watch people's faces change from stressed and in pain to relaxed and open. This may occur even more profoundly as a person focuses on their specific stress complaint as they breathe through the structuring unit. In other words, breathe through what's bothering you. We can live in pain or use this amazing gift to dissolve that which is invisible and keeps us prisoners - subconscious negative emotion. Keep it or release it, it's now your choice.

When proper regulation returns to the autonomic nervous system, old emotions are resolved and brain function becomes balanced. You will still have challenges and hurdles but you have just removed the illusionary drama. You're now in the driver's seat of personal change and awareness.

What can happen with your first Structured Breath?

We hear people tell us consistently,

"I have never been able to breath this deep."

"So this is what its like to feel relaxed and in a calm state."

"My sinuses just opened up for the first time in years!"

"My pain is dissolving with my breath."

"I use my Structured Breathing unit before bed and now for the first time in years I'm finally getting my proper rest."

"My body now feels centered!"

This is an inherent validation and recognition that the two aspects of the

Autonomic Nervous System, Sympathetic and Parasympathetic, are now aligned. See and you thought self-centered was a bad thing. Meanwhile it's everything because you are everything.

Behind these sensational new awarenesses are the fundamental recalibration and regulation of the Autonomic Nervous System - No more brain drain.

Enjoy the **joy** and sense of **peace** it brings, make it part of your daily life and release those invisible bonds that bind **U**. Drink Life In... Breathe Life In. Stay Structured, and live free of that, which does not serve your greater good!

For more information see contact page at the end of the book.

EMF: WHAT THE CELL IS GOING ON

"Everything is Frequency; what you think, what you eat, drink and the environment that you live in, will determine your voltage."

- Dr. Darrell Wolfe, Doc of Detox

PROTECT YOUR HEALTH AND YOUR FAMILY

Practicing Electromagnetic Hygiene In the Home

We live in a virtual **sea of electromagnetic energy**. From the electricity moving through wires connecting to appliances, to the radio frequencies flowing through the air communicating with our wireless phones, baby monitors, smart meters, and computers.

The government tells us the radiation generated by the electromagnetic fields are safe, but a growing number of scientific studies indicate otherwise.

The World Health Organization classifies both radio frequency (RF) and extremely low frequency electromagnetic fields (ELF EMF) as a possible **human carcinogen**. The first is based primarily on brain tumors associated with cell phone use. The second is based on unusually high occurrences of **leukemia in children** who live near power lines.

In addition to cancer, electro smog *(the term commonly associated with various forms of electromagnetic pollution)* has been shown to adversely **affect sperm and contributes to miscarriages.** As levels of electro smog continue to increase and become omnipresent in our environment, a growing population is complaining about a handful of symptoms that have been classified as electro hypersensitivity (EHS), although this illness goes by various names including: electromagnetic sensitivity, EMF intolerance syndrome, idiopathic environmental intolerance-EMF, microwave syndrome, and radio wave sickness.

The Most Common Symptoms Include:

- Headaches
- Poor Sleep
- Depression
- Skin Irritation
- Heart Palpitations
- Nose Bleeds
- Altered Blood Sugar
- Chronic Pain
- Impaired Short-Term Memory
- Anxiety
- Nausea
- Seizures
- Bed Wetting
- Tremors
- Chronic Fatigue
- Difficulty Concentrating
- Tinnitus
- Dizziness
- Loss of Consciousness
- Frequent Urination
- Cold Extremities
- Spatial Disorientation
- Asthma
- Flu-like Symptoms

The Austrian Medical Association recently released guidelines on how to diagnose and treat those who have electro sensitivity. The Women's College Hospital in Toronto has an **increasing caseload** of those affected by EMF with a waiting list that exceeds 10 months.

What Are the Different Types of Electro Smog In My Home?

Scientists classify electromagnetic energy according to its frequency. For example, electricity in North America has a frequency of 60 cycles per second *(or 60 Hertz)*. Electronic devices that are not properly filtered generate frequencies thousands of cycles per second and our wireless devices rely on radio frequencies and microwaves at millions to billions of cycles per second.

The lower frequencies–technically referred to as extremely low frequency (ELF)–need a wire for transmission. The higher frequencies can radiated through the air and can travel for kilometers. The intermediate frequencies flow through wire and radiate short distances from the wire.

What Are the Sources of Electro Smog In My Home?

Sources of electro smog include those that are generated within the home and those that come from the neighborhood as electromagnetic radiation. Magnetic fields are able to penetrate most types of building material.

All electric appliances *(those that are plugged into an electric outlet)* generate an ELF electromagnetic field. Appliances that generate heat tend to have the highest magnetic fields *(electric stove, hair dryer, vacuum cleaner, electric blanket, water bed, in-floor electric heating)* but electric shavers, can openers, clock radios, computers, entertainment units as well as wiring in the home all produce ELF electro smog.

People who live within **50 meters of power lines, transformers, or substations** may be exposed to elevated levels of magnetic fields. Electric fields outside the home may also be elevated, especially near high voltage transmission lines, but fortunately these electric fields are readily shielded by buildings so levels within the home are not necessarily elevated.

The good news is that these fields *(both electric and magnetic)* decrease with distance and sometimes just a few feet can significantly reduce exposure.

Intermediate frequencies or dirty electricity are generated by electronic devices such as **computers, plasma television sets, energy efficient compact fluorescent light (CFL) bulbs and dimmer switches**. Neighbors on the same transformer often share dirty electricity and a neighbor turning their dimmer switch up or down can affect the dirty electricity in your home.

The best way to reduce dirty electricity is to not have some of the devices that generate it *(such as **CFL light bulbs**)* although it is difficult to know which devices are worse than others. Specially tuned capacitors or filters that reduce dirty electricity when plugged into electrical outlets are now available for home use. So it is possible to still enjoy our electronic gadgets and not be exposed to this form of electro smog.

The high frequencies that include radio frequencies and microwaves are generated by **wireless technology** and **microwave ovens**. The most common and offensive in North America include **cordless phones, Wi-Fi monitors**, and wireless **baby monitors**. These devices are **constantly emitting radiation**, even when they are not being used.

Other major sources in some homes are **smart meters** and **smart appliances**. Some smart meters emit short bursts of radiation a few times each hour, while others emit radiation continuously. These continuous emitters **are making people ill**.

In apartment buildings, condominiums or row houses, the **Wi-Fi router** and **cordless phone radiation** in one unit is often strong enough to penetrate and be picked up in nearby apartments. Similarly radiation from **cell phone antennas** on top of towers or on nearby buildings, **radar** at airports or seaports and TV or radio broadcast antennas can penetrate walls and ceilings. Products are available to shield against this form of electro smog but careful monitoring is required when these products are installed to ensure that the radiation is reduced and not magnified.

A fourth type of electro smog is contact current. If there is a current flowing through metal water pipes, touching a tap or faucet can result in contact current flowing through the body. This is a concern in areas that have a ground current problem and in areas where the wiring and grounding are faulty or inadequate. Hiring an electrician who is knowledgeable about ground current *(also referred to as stray voltage)* is the best way to deal with this form of electro smog.

How Do I Practice Good Electromagnetic Hygiene?

The most important room in the house is where you spend a lot of time and in most homes this is the bedroom. During the night your body is healing and cleansing. If the bedroom is contaminated with electro smog the body is unable to properly heal.

For this reason, **turning off** wireless devices at night or better yet, **replacing them** with wired technology, is the ideal solution. Keeping the **electric clock radio** at least 2 meters away from the bed or better still out of the bedroom. Avoid using **electric blankets** or sleeping on a **heated waterbed**. It is the duration of exposure that is important from a health perspective.

Companies produce on-demand switches that **disconnect** the electricity to your bedroom, this is one way to reduce the magnetic field and the dirty electricity at night. Alternatively, installing tuned filters around the home is another way to reduce both your daytime and nighttime exposure to dirty power.

Radio frequencies coming from outside the home can be shielded by special carbon based paint, silver lined fabric, and special film placed on windows. Triple E glass is another way of reducing the radiation that penetrates windows. If the sources are from multiple directions then placing a canopy around the bed (*covering the top, sides and bottom of the bed*) may be the best solution to reduce nighttime exposure.

Our government is mandating that we use energy efficient light bulbs but not all of these light bulbs are the same. Most compact fluorescent bulbs generate poor power quality, magnetic fields, and radio frequency radiation. So the best bulb is still the old fashion **incandescent bulb.**

Some light manufacturers are producing LED bulbs and **some** of these are better than others in terms of electro smog emissions. Unfortunately it is not possible to tell from the package whether the bulb is electromagnetically clean or not. Labeling is needed if the government continues to insist we use these energy efficient bulb. In the meantime the best bet is the **incandescent bulb**. One bulb I do recommend is the **Philips dim-able LED**. We tested this light bulb and it is as clean as an incandescent bulb.

How Can I Tell If My Microwave Oven Leaks?

Try this simple test to determine if your microwave oven leaks microwaves.

If you are able to get cell phone reception in your kitchen, then place your cell phone into the microwave oven. Do NOT turn the microwave oven on, as this will destroy your cell phone. Call your phone. If your cell phones rings then your microwave oven is leaking microwaves. In this case, **leave the kitchen** when you turn on your microwave oven and definitely do not stand in front of it watching your food heating. Your eyes are extremely sensitive to microwave radiation, causing **cataracts** to form. The microwave can also **denature** the nutritional value of food so you may want to limit your use of your microwave oven for that reason as well.

What Are the Health Effects of Electro smog?

Extremely **low** frequency (ELF) electromagnetic fields have been associated with **childhood leukemia** at levels at or above 2 milli Gauss *(mG - this is the strength of the magnetic field).* These fields have been associated with **adult cancers (leukemia, brain tumors, and breast cancer)** with occupational exposure at values between 2 and 12 mG. **Miscarriages** have also been linked to high magnetic field exposure during the first trimester of pregnancy *(above 16 mG).* For this reason it is important to keep magnetic fields as weak as possible and definitely below 2 mG.

INTERMEDIATE frequencies, in the form of dirty electricity, have been linked to **asthma, higher blood sugar among diabetics, tremors among those with multiple sclerosis, and a broad range of symptoms collectively called electrohypersensitivity (EHS).** Dirty electricity has also been associated with a greater risk of developing cancer from exposures above 2000 GS units. Values should be less than 40 GS units. **high** frequencies *(radio frequency radiation, microwaves and radar)* produced by wireless technology have been associated with hypersensitivity symptoms mentioned above as well as **various types of cancer, especially leukemia** for those living near antennas. Use of cell phones and cordless phones has been linked to **various tumors of the head *(including brain tumors, tumors of the acoustic nerve, eye, and salivary gland.)* Children are particularly vulnerable.**

The only way to determine if electro smog is present in your home is to measure it. Ideally professionals trained in this area should do this. However, since electro smog is not recognized as an environmental pollutant there are few agencies that conduct these tests as part of their environmental assessment.

How Can I Tell If I'm Electrically Sensitive?

If you have any of the symptoms mentioned above that get worse when you are near **fluorescent bulbs, using a mobile phone, or in a shopping center then you might be electrically sensitive**. Another way to find out is to turn off the power to your bedroom every night for a week and unplug all your wireless devices. If your symptoms diminish you are probably **electrically sensitive**. People more likely to become sensitive to electro smog are those who have been electrocuted, have had physical trauma to their spinal cord (whiplash), have been exposed to toxic chemicals especially neurotoxic pesticides or mercury, have had infections or have a compromised immune system. **All who have had cancer or have a family history of cancer need to minimize their daily exposure to electro smog.**

What Can I Do If I'm Sensitive to Electro Smog?

If you think you are sensitive then the first step is to practice electromagnetic hygiene (i.e. reduce your exposure to electro smog). Have your home measured and remediated by someone with proper credentials. **Healing cannot take place if you continue to be exposed**. You need to fortify your immune system with a Whole Plant Based Superfood Nutrition, Quality Structured Water and reduce other types of stressors in your life. This involves Gentle Daily Cleansing, rest and core exercises.

Often the **adrenals are exhausted** and they need to be supported nutritionally.

Getting rid of mercury in your diet and from your body is critical, including mercury fillings. Removal of mercury fillings should be done by a biologic dentist as removal–if done improperly–will increase your mercury load. Other helpful steps include colon and liver cleanses and low EMF saunas. Also, to remove toxic metals, IV chelation can be performed by a health care professional. People can and do recover from EHS but it does take time.

Magda Havas, BSc, PhD. *Environmental & Resource Studies, Trent University, Peterborough, ON*

FREQUENCY MATTERS

Be Energy Wise - Choose Frequencies Fit for Life

"Many indications tell us we are about to experience a rapid transition to a new world that will change the essential nature of who we are and how we understand reality. Transcending the coming chaos is possible with the toolset provided here. Understanding frequency matters is an unprecedented gift for the person who is ready to evolve." Seeing ourselves as energy beings is the most important breakthrough of our times. Profound implications in life have been generally unacknowledged, but now we can intentionally reduce and avoid exposure to harmful frequencies and use helpful frequencies to keep ourselves healthy and improve the realities we live in. We are not going back to living in caves, trees and simple dwellings but we must use the gifts that we are given in a conscious, mindful and meaningful way. Without the ability to harness some of the many frequencies available we would still be in the dark. We now need to push forward the knowledge of frequency and it's potential to center stage bringing more light and hope to our present health and energy crisis.

The Responsibility and Obligation For Staying Healthy.

We have been given the gift of life; it's up to us to give ourselves the gift of living well. Health isn't everything, but without it everything else is nothing.

Bioelectrically what in the cell is going on?

All matter, each individual cell—as well as the entire organism—is made up of magnetic resonant field and bio-field patterns of varying strengths and frequencies, which become dependent and charged with external sources of magnetic resonance. Outside disruptive frequencies can have an influence on any disease process by displacing ions *(electrical charges)*, pulsating magnetic fields can lead to an abnormal membrane potential. **Ultimately, every illness is the consequence of impaired cell metabolism.** Diseased cells have different amplitudes of oscillation due to their reduced potential, their frequency remains the same, and their oscillation becomes weaker.

MY OWN EXPERIENCE

In 1986 I was closing down my Mexican food restaurant business called *Zoro's* where I had 5 microwave ovens, not feeling 100% certain about their safety I asked my bother, Darrell whether or not I should keep a unit for myself. He knew enough at that time to tell me that they not only destroyed the life force, the enzymes, but also caused free radicals. Today of course we now know more. Measurably there is no such thing as a healthy microwave oven.

Then in 1987 my father as a result of having veins pulled out of his leg to be used for his triple bypass surgery became uncomfortably cold at night. So he decided that he would use the convenient warmth of an electrical blanket. We told him at the time it was not a good idea having that form of energy so close in proximity to the body and it would not be conducive to his overall health and well-being. He then said, *"They wouldn't sell it if it wasn't safe."*

Pure air, water, organic food and safe EMF levels of exposure are what constitutes a healthy environment. These are regulated by governments and other authorities and are based on:

1. Level of recognized awareness on said subject.
2. Level of motivation or willingness to serve the common good.
3. Level of what is considered by society as being acceptable in the cost versus harm ratio.

Do not allow your thinking to be overclouded by the general acceptance or conveyance factor of this technology. Also do not become overwhelmed by the complexity of the subject.

Even Nikola Tesla, the greatest inventor of all time, and the person Albert Einstein called, 'The World's Most Intelligent Person Of His Time', admitted to not understanding exactly what electricity is. But he knew the benefits as well as the potential for harm these various frequency fields represented better than anyone in his day and arguably even today.

You will want to eventually have the ability to see for yourself whether or not you and your family are safe from your present and future environments. Here is a helpful acronym to remind you of the steps you need to follow (DPPE) Detect any hidden problems with an accurate AC magnetic/electric meter and a RF radio frequency meter. Protect by putting in place the necessary measures to create a safe environment. Prevention by taking the necessary precautionary approach. Enhance your immune system by exposing yourself to high frequency foods and supportive PEMF technologies. Remember when the Fukushima disaster occurred and the government was reporting that the effected area was much safer than it really was? Then an unknown female with a simple meter, showed the world with her smart phone that **they were not telling the truth**. Some things in life are just too important to leave in the hands of others.

"A foolish faith in authority is the worst enemy of the truth."

- Albert Einstein

EMF SAFETY TIPS

SO WHAT IS AN INDIVIDUAL SUPPOSED TO DO?

We are surrounded by these frequencies 24-7, there is no escape! The first step in the **Green** approach is to **reduce**, yes reduce your exposure, and here is how.

How safe is your living environment from an EMF perspective?

- Reducing your EMF exposure can benefit your overall health and wellness. In some cases, avoidance is essential to rebuilding health. Here are some suggestions that could change your life:
- Use cell phones as little as possible. When using a cell phone put it on speaker phone when possible. Studies have demonstrated that biological effects occur when holding the device against your ear 30 seconds into making or receiving a call. Use your cell phone to take messages and use a corded land-line to make calls.
- Cell phones emit radiation even when you are not making a call. For this reason wireless communication devices should

not be carried against your body. Cell phones kept in pockets should be turned off.

• Do not let young children use cell phones at all, or restrict their use to emergency situations only. This is not a toy.

THIS IS ONE OF THE MOST HELPFUL TIPS TO BE REMEMBERED

FIND THE POSSIBLE THREAT:

F is for frequency; identify whether it is a RF (radio frequency); AC magnetic or AC electric?

I is for intensity, measure how strong is it?

N is for nearness; measure how close in proximity the frequency is to living things?

D is for duration; measure how much time exposure there is to the frequency?

• Do not let a child use a cordless home phone. These can be replaced with a hard-wired corded land-line phone. We had 3 of them; they were convenient but deadly!

• Replace all DECT/digital cordless phones, which emit high levels of RF radiation even when they're idle, with corded land-line telephones. We are back to the land-line with a 50-foot cord. Corded land-line telephones have low EMF emissions and are a good alternative.

• Avoid cell phone use in a car unless you are using a roof mounted external antenna. Without this, the RF signals from your cell phone will intensify because of multiple reflections from the metal surfaces of the car creates a similar environment to that of faraday cage. Remember that cell phones emit RF radiation even when they are not being used to make a call.

- Many children's games use wireless technology. Disable the wireless component if possible and replace it with a cable. Verify that RF emissions have ceased with an RF detector or RF Meter.
- All microwave ovens leak RF radiation when they are in use. Replace microwave ovens with safer appliances such as a convection toaster oven or a conventional electric or gas range oven.
- Do not use your laptop on your lap, the frequencies emitted have been proven to cause hormonal disruption and cellular dysfunction, especially in the pelvic area. When using a notebook/laptop or a computer use a hard wired network connection. Settings to disable the wireless connection are found in Network Settings on a PC or AirPort on a Mac. Once disabled, verify that the device has ceased emitting RF by using a RF detector or RF Meter. You can also use a secondary keyboard so that your hands are exposed to a lower safer field.
- Replace wireless Internet routers with hard-wired units. Some wireless router models allow the user to shut off the wireless component and convert it to a hard-wired unit, check with your provider.

You will need:

- D-Link - 1 Power line AV+ Mini Adapter (DHP-308AV) that attaches to your router.
- D-Link - 1 Power line AV+ 3-Port Switch w/ Pass through (DHP- P338AV) for every computer in your home. *(Found at places like BestBuy and Future Shop)*
- Now your Internet is traveling through the electrical wiring in your home, therefore; there is no need for long cords just plug into the closest outlet to your computer and you are off and running. **Make sure that you call your Internet provider to disable the Wi-Fi to protect your family.**
- Restore analog utility meters. **Avoid smart meters and smart appliances.**
- **Do not use compact fluorescent or any low voltage lighting technologies.** CFLs emit high levels of electric fields and magnetic fields. Incandescent light bulbs or 120-volt halogen bulbs are a safer alternative. We now have an effective meter for measuring light photons. Helping us distinguish healthy and unhealthy light.
- **DVDs / VCRs, electric clock radios/ alarm clocks, stereo systems, heating pads, electric blankets, and water beds must be unplugged to cease electric and magnetic field emissions. During sleeping hours, remove or unplug electronic devices located in the sleeping areas.** Clearing your sleep area is your first priority. Sleep in an electricity free bedroom. Shut down all of the flow of electricity in the walls of your bedroom. Power off by using a remote and demand switch at the breaker box. Put cell phones on airplane mode or turn them off completely while sleeping. Your bedroom should be as dark as possible, as quiet as possible and as close to zero EMFs as possible.

- Electrical appliances produce toxic electromagnetic fields (EMFs). These fields can layer, one upon the other, creating a harmful soup of radiation. That's why the kitchen is a hotspot for harmful EMFs, but other rooms are affected, too. **The harder an appliance works the larger the electromagnetic field**. Examples treadmills, fans, blenders, hairdryers etc.
- Consider sleeping an all-natural bed without metal or synthetics. If possible head facing north, feet facing south.
- This is your most critical and your most vulnerable time of the day for your environment to be safe and supportive.
- In some extreme cases it may be necessary to move, especially if your home has high EMF sources that are out of your control. *(Power lines, cell towers, banks of smart meters)*
- Work with policy makers to create responsible public policy to reduce EMF and RF in the environment.
- See also many other holistic lifestyle choices to clean, support, and shield you from EMFs such as PEMF technologies, radiation- protective foods and other protective solutions.

Written by: Marcel Wolfe
Bio Ed., Certified PEMF Consultant and Building Biologist

THE FUTURE OF HEALTH: ENERGY MEDICINE

"We are light beings living in matter. Plug in and turn life on."

- Dr. Darrell Wolfe, Doc of Detox

THEBODYGUARD™

This is an active not a passive energy product.

It is up to **100 times more powerful** than other passive scalar products, pendants and bracelets. This is the first of its kind, it is a groundbreaking, revolutionary energy medicine device. It protects you from negative EMFs *(Electromagnetic Fields)*, but our device goes much further than that, it continually balances your body's frequency for optimum vitality.

The frequencies in TheBodyGuard™ run from 0 to 18,000 hertz and then back to 0 in 2 seconds.

TheBodyGuard™ has an electro-optical signal generator and an electromagnetic signal generator with biofeedback means and there is an electromagnetic emitter in the same vibration range of 0-18,000Hz. TheBodyGuard™ has built-in biofeedback, which helps to regulate and balance internal and external body frequencies. TheBodyGuard™ continually monitors and effectively balances all body frequencies.

TheBodyGuard™ is a protective, life- enhancing device that can be worn or plugged into your computer and any other USB port, even in your car! It creates balance throughout the mind, body, emotions, and 'etheric' body, it is the most powerful personal tool to facilitate balancing and healing.

Think of your body bathing in the complete spectrum of sound, color and life- enhancing PEMF *(Pulsed Electromagnetic Fields)* frequencies. Every cell of the body benefits from 'bathing' in these sounds. TheBodyGuard™ is a one of a kind device that has a gold plated pyramid shaped tuning fork, which has the ability to sense and invert the negative frequency of your environment into positive frequencies. It also comes with a self-contained battery. TheBodyGuard™ is an international patent circuitry, its lights, and its coils are all designed to bring balance not only within your environment but also within the physical body. All of this in a small, convenient size, approximately 2x2 inches that can be worn or plugged in.

Many indications tell us we are about to experience a rapid transition to a new understanding that will change the essential nature of who we think we are and how we process reality. Seeing ourselves as energy beings is the most important breakthrough of our time.

Profound implications in life have been generally unacknowledged, but now we can reduce and avoid exposure to harmful frequencies and use helpful frequencies to keep ourselves vitally healthy. These are exciting times!

Types of Electromagnetic Energy

Natural EMFs: Everything that lives, from the earth to ourselves, has a pulse. The earth produces an electromagnetic field *(EMF)* and so does the human body. Scientific research has demonstrated that every cell in your body has its own built-in EMF regulator, helping to regulate important functions and keep you healthy. Natural EMFs or ELFs *(extremely low frequencies)* are low in intensity; for example, a healthy human body resonates with the earth's magnetic field at around 10 hertz.

Artificial EMFs: Human technologies - from high voltage wires to appliances like hairdryers, which are alternating current electric and magnetic fields (AC) and cell phones, which are radio frequencies (RF) create powerful measurable EMFs. These strong EMFs have been shown to disturb the human body's natural energetic field, lowering the immune system and also causing weight gain.

It's estimated we are now being exposed to a trillion times more harmful negative frequencies than our grandparents. Enough is now known about EMF pollution to make it a real topic for immediate concern.

"The only safe exposure level to negative frequencies is zero, this level has been confirmed by dose-response trends in epidemiological studies. Electromagnetic fields and radiation damage DNA and enhance the rate of cell death; therefore, artificial EMFs are carcinogenic and enhance the rates of Cancer, Cardiac, Reproductive and Neurological diseases and mortality in the human population." - Dr. Neil, Cherry Associate Professor of Environmental Health Lincoln University, New Zealand

It is a well-known scientific fact that it is frequency that turns the cancer gene on and it is frequency that turns the cancer gene off. It is also frequency that determines whether a bacteria is good or bad and whether fungus can grow within the human body, oh, and by the way, cancer is a fungus. We now have more control on the frequencies that affect our cells, which means that we now have more control on our day-to-day health, no matter where we are or where we work because Wi-Fi is everywhere, it is an epidemic.

We must now use technology mindfully. Everyone who is in range of a cell phone, computer, electrical wiring, microwave, television, any electrical appliance or Wi-Fi needs

394   www.docofdetox.com

TheBodyGuard™ protective device to enhance his or her own energetic field for overall health and well-being.

How Does It Work?

TheBodyGuard™ projects light waves and signals in and all around your body, helping to override and making man-made EMFs and radiation more harmonious to your cells.

What Does EMF Stand For?

EMF stands for Electromagnetic Fields, which are often called EMFs, they are invisible, electrical, magnetic forces. EMFs are a type of radiation that takes the form of waves. There are waves *(frequencies)* that support and build your immune system, such as TheBodyGuard™ and then there are waves that tear down your immune system, such as Wi-Fi, cell phones, computers, tablets, microwaves, smart meters, negative emotions and any electrical appliance, creating disease.

How Does TheBodyGuard™ Work For Your Body?

Somewhat like a musical piano, the law of resonance, sweeping back and forth up and down the musical scale. Every split second you are taking in a frequency or a harmonic of that frequency, which your body is needing to create balance. Like superfood nutrition, your body will only absorb the nutrients *(frequencies)* that it needs. Like a musical piano you have 12 steps on the keyboard, then it repeats itself. For example, start with a low C and as you go up the scale 12 steps, what happens when you hit the 13th key? It returns to the key of C, but it's a higher octave. Octaves *(frequencies)* on the musical scale continue to go higher and then beyond the hearing range into the megahertz and gigahertz, this is the law of resonance, this is universal law.

Another example is that you can hold down the low C without making it ring and hit a high C, which will cause both Cs to oscillate. A tuning fork works the same way, if you had a low C tuning fork and had another high C tuning fork, when you hit either one of the tuning forks and hold them close together, they will both oscillate because of the law of resonance.

The same thing happens with TheBodyGuard™, causing the meridians to oscillate like strings on the musical piano bringing back balance, harmony and wholeness in the body as well as the environment. This is all accomplished through lights, magnetic coils and scalar waves. As the frequencies are oscillating through the lights, it causes the iris of the eyes to oscillate bringing balance to the body. What is amazing is that the light waves are bouncing off the walls bringing harmony to the environment. Scalar waves are known to open and release higher energies into the physical dimension for balance and restoration.

With TheBodyGuard™ you can do the protocol of Emotional Freedom Technique *(EFT)* is a form of counseling intervention therapy. It draws on various theories of alternative medicine such as: acupuncture, neurolinguistic programming *(NLP)*, energy medicine, and Thought Field Therapy *(TFT)*. Looking at the lights for around 1 minute will produce the same benefits as doing EFT tapping on the body. TheBodyGuard™ is a science-based device, it taps all the acupuncture points, meridians and centers in the body at the same time for the emotional balance that we all need and search for.

Frequency is the medium for transferring energy and information and the means for all of us to get closer to vital health.

The main part of the multifrequency oscillator, is a quartz crystal controlled circuit. This produces a absolutely pure and ultra-clear perfect signal for the next stage of the circuitry. The next stage has a series of cascading frequency dividers that are perfectly harmonic in nature.

There are thousands of healing frequencies functioning together at the same time from TheBodyGuard™. They create a minimum 15 foot invisible barrier around the body that can be seen with a digital measurement instrument called an Oscilloscope, which can measure and indicate their shape, amplitude and frequency.

As long as you follow the herd, you will always believe that you are only human.

The transistor within TheBodyGuard™ serves many purposes, first of all, it isolates, selects and amplifies the perfect signal from the rest. In other words, the input current going into the transistor is less than the current going out, this phenomenon is also called *'gain'* because the current increases or is amplified by the transistor. The gain of this amplifier *(transistor)* is known as hFE or Beta. One reason why we want to amplify the signal is because it will enable us to drive the multi-colored LEDs. There is a unique and revolutionary feature to this invention, a very small gold tuning fork. This gold tuning fork acts as an antenna to allow healing signals in and around the user.

"Change the energy, change the manifestation of the mass."

- Albert Einstein

When TheBodyGuard™ is used as a healing tool, the vibrations create the healing. A healthy body is always in perfect harmonic balance, when the body is out of balance, TheBodyGuard™ can bring about positive shifts in your energy patterns in and around you to facilitate this harmonic balance.

Sound, resonance and harmonic therapies will equalize brainwaves, increase the depth of breathing, slow the heart-beat and pulse, lower blood pressure, reduce muscle tension, increase circulation and endorphin production, balance hormones, boost immune function, improve memory and learning, increase endurance and productivity, strengthen digestion, decrease depression and restore balance which we will call joy.

The Miracle of Solfeggio Frequencies and Fibonacci Numbers

Solfeggio Frequencies and Fibonacci Numbers are constantly emitted from TheBodyGuard™. As we have stated before, everything is frequency and frequency is everything. I wish to discuss just a few of these amazingly powerful frequencies that you will experience when you use TheBodyGuard™.

Six original notes called Solfeggio frequencies make up the ancient 6-tone scale used in sacred music, these frequencies were used in over 150 well- known and beautiful Gregorian Chants.

The great hymn written for John the Baptist was called the most spiritually uplifting hymn of all time. Listen here

Each Solfeggio tone is comprised of a frequency required to balance your energy and keep your body, mind and spirit in perfect harmony. Church authorities led people to believe that they were lost centuries ago. It was a transparent attempt to hide these incredibly powerful chants so that the masses would not benefit from these life-altering frequencies. When sung in harmony during mass, these chants would create frequencies that were able to heal.

The original Solfeggio scale was created by a Benedictine monk, Guido d'Arezzo *(c. 991 AD – c. 1050 AD)*. It was used by singers to learn chants and songs more easily. Today we know the Solfeggio scale as seven ascending notes assigned to the syllables Do-Re-Mi-Fa-So-La-Ti.

What do you feel when a favorite song comes on? Joy. The Solfeggio frequencies represent sound frequencies that assist you in your own healing and consciousness. David Hulse, a sound therapy pioneer with over 40 years of experience, described the tones as the following:

UT - 396 Hz: Liberate guilt and fear.

RE - 417 Hz: Undo situations and facilitate change and expand consciousness.

MI - 528 Hz: Repairs DNA and initiates transformation and is known as the love frequency. **Solfeggio frequencies are guaranteed to work. It is this exact frequency that is used by genetic biochemists to repair DNA.**

FA - 639 Hz: Connecting with family.

SOL - 741 Hz: Helping one to express themselves and creating solutions. Cleansing and restoring on a physical, mental and emotional basis.

LA - 852 Hz: Restoring balance.

The original scale was six ascending notes, which were Ut-Re-Mi-Fa-Sol-La. In the mid-1970's Dr. Joseph Puleo, a physician and America's leading herbalist, found six electro- magnetic sound frequencies that corresponded to the syllables from the hymn to St. John the Baptist.

How were the frequencies discovered?

According to the documentation provided in "Healing Codes for the Biological Apocalypse", Dr. Joseph Puleo was introduced to the Pythagorean method of numeral reduction. Using this method, he discovered the pattern of six repeating codes in the Book of Numbers, Chapter 7, verses 12 through 83.

Solfeggio notes open up a channel of communication and balance right down to the DNA within in your cells. Each syllable has been thoroughly studied by Dr. Puleo and other professional researchers.

The tuning practice adopted for western cultures from about the 16th century and used today is known as "Twelve-Tone Equal Temperament". According to Joachim Ernst-Berendt, the Twelve-Tone Equal Temperament mistunes all consonant intervals except the octave. Our modern scale can create situations such as 'boxed-in' thinking, stuffed and suppressed emotions, fear-based or lack consciousness, all of which then tend to manifest into physical symptoms called 'dis-ease' or disease.

Our modern day musical scale is out of sync when compared with the original Solfeggio scale. If we want to bring harmony in our lives, we need to replace the dissonant western scale with

Solfeggio music for balance and joy to be more permanent. Let the music tones and frequencies of TheBodyGuard™ raise, balance and protect your frequency, 24/7.

Tune yourself back into perfect vibration. Nikola Tesla, the great genius and father of electromagnetic engineering, had once said, the 3, 6, and 9 are the fundamental root vibrations of the Solfeggio frequencies.

"If you only knew the magnificence of the 3, 6 and 9, then you would hold the key to the universe." - Albert Einstein

"Concerning matter, we have been all wrong. What we have called matter is energy, whose vibration has been so lowered as to be perceptible to the senses. There is no matter, just frequency." - Albert Einstein

All matter-beings vibrate at specific rates and everything has its own melody. The musical nature of nuclear matter from atoms to galaxies is recognized by science and is now being embraced by the masses when welcoming TheBodyGuard™ into their lives.

Light & Energy Beings

It doesn't matter whether it is a cell belonging to the muscular, skeletal, nervous, endocrine or circulatory system; they are all primarily directed by light, sound, color and electromagnetic frequencies. Many of life's physical, mental and emotional challenges, even mental illness is a reflection of a vibratory imbalance or impurity at the quantum level of our human energy field. Einstein never said chemistry is everything but what he did say was, *"Frequency trumps chemistry, frequency is everything."*

85% of all physical disorders have an emotional vibrational attachment. You cannot be physically out of balance without being out of balance vibrationally.

Cell Health

The human body is one of the most exquisite, dynamic, profound, beautiful and still mysterious forms in all of nature.

The cell functions more like a battery than a pool of chemicals. The cell is self-regulating and aware. The electromagnetic forces bind atoms and molecules together which gives shape, form and function to matter. Proteins *(amino acids)* are the building blocks of life. There are two sets of proteins in the membranes of the cell called receptors and channels.

Receptors are antennas that receive all of the information from the outside environment. The receptor proteins represent awareness of their environment. Frequency or energy waves are a more efficient and effective medium for information and energy transmission than the lock and key physical approach of matter. The majority of the activity that occurs in nature happens at the speed of light. The constant flow of energy in our environment both informs and creates our physical world.

"The living cell is essentially an electrical device." - Dr. Albert von Szent-Gyorgyi

Cancer by definition is abnormal cell generation. In his later years, Dr. Albert von Szent-Györgyi , The Father of Modern Biochemistry, focused his research on cancer in what he termed quantum biology. In 1978, he published *"The Living State and Cancer"* in which he outlined his theory that cancer is a sub-molecular, electronic disturbance, just as frequency can turn cancer cells on, they can also turn cancer cells off.

If a part of the body is out of balance, it will energetically resonate 'out of tune'. By wearing or being within range of the TheBodyGuard™, the correct frequency is created that entrains the part that is out of balance back to its correct frequency. The body will only take in and absorb the vibrational frequencies needed.

A series of 8 colors sweeping from side-to- side represent the different frequencies that align with the energetic distribution centers in the body also referred to as acupuncture meridians, bio-fields or chakras.

Benefits of TheBodyGuard™

1. Energizes and strengthens your body.
2. Overrides disruptive effects of man- made pollutions found in radiation from computers, tablets, cell phones, WiFi, florescent lights, smart meters, etc.
3. Helps to neutralize geopathic stress like underground streams.
4. Reduces muscle pain, inflammation, internal scar tissue formation and mutation due to lowering the acidity within the body.
5. Soothes and balances the nervous system.
6. Lifts the spirit.
7. Promotes a deep state of relaxation.
8. Promotes a long-lasting, deep sleep.
9. Promotes a meditative state.
10. Improves mental clarity.
11. Enhances brain function.

12. Increases mental concentration.

13. Enhances all therapies.

14. Balances and integrates both sides of the brain.

15. Balances the body's cells.

16. Balances and realigns the chakras.

17. Clears and charges the aura.

18. Balances and raises energy levels in the body.

19. Enhances detoxification of organs and tissue cells.

20. Helps in the reduction of excessive weight and helps increase weight when underweight.

21. Eliminates hair loss due to EMF.

22. Reduces headaches and migraines.

23. Helps to protect and restore your immune system.

24. Improves digestion, assimilation and waste elimination.

25. Gives a sense of joy and peace on an emotional and physical level.

Simply wear TheBodyGuard™ wherever you go to continually protect yourself from negative EMFs and feel the amazing health benefits.

This is the most important breakthrough we have had in the last 30 years in the world of EMF and healing frequencies. Nothing in the world compares to TheBodyGuard™!

See how just a few minutes on a computer or a cordless phone will alter your blood cells, interfering with the natural processes causing the blood cells to stick together, reducing normal blood flow, lowering oxygen transportation and causing poor circulation, blocking nutritional uptake and a backup of cellular waste creating low level frequency within the cells. Symptoms from negative EMF toxicity are headaches, fatigue, difficulty concentrating, numbness, cold extremities, heart and blood pressure problems including risk of stroke. As science has proven, it's frequency that turns the cancer gene on and it's frequency that turns the cancer gene off. TheBodyGuard™ is putting people in the drivers seat for the first time in creating not just a healthy environment but a healing one!

Click here to view online demonstration by Dr. Magda Havas.

Live Blood Analysis & Rouleaux Blood Test: *Rouleaux is the French term for "cells in a row." Rouleaux or rolls, is the tendency of red blood cells to aggregate or stick together and form long rows that look like stacked coins.*

Live blood analysis is a method to investigate the quality of blood. Ideally the shape of the cells should be all round and even, they should be separated from each other and reside in their own space.

Oxidative stress, caused by acidic lifestyle, junk food, smoking, etc deforms the cells and leads them to stick to each other, sometimes creating long chains *(rouleaux formations)*. Rouleaux is a nonspecific indicator of the presence of disease.

TheBodyGuard™ protects the body from the harmful effects of EMF (Electromagnetic Fields)

WE ARE LIGHT BEINGS

"We know today that man, essentially, is a being of light."

- Prof. Fritz-Albert Popp

Photobiology is a proven science, showing that humans are light beings and light is our main source of life. When healing with light, the results are incredible and life changing. We now know that the rays from polarized light create a domino effect of positive healing reactions within the cells and that genetic cellular damage can be repaired within hours by beams of light - frequency is everything.

"We are still on the threshold of fully understanding the complex relationship between light and life, but we can now say emphatically that the function of our entire metabolism is dependent on light."
- Prof. Fritz-Albert Popp

Fritz-Albert Popp was born in 1938 in Frankfurt. His first diploma was in Experimental Physics *(1966, University Würzburg)*, followed by the Röntgen-Prize of the University Würzburg, Ph.D. in Theoretical Physics *(1969 , University Mainz)* . Habilitation in Biophysics and Medicine *(1973, University Marburg)*. Prof. Popp rediscovered and made the first extensive physical analysis of "Biophotons". He was awarded Professorship *(H2)* by the Senate of Marburg University, and lectured at Marburg University from 1973 to 1980. He was Head of a research group in the Pharmaceutical Industry in Worms from 1981 to 1983 and Head of a research group at the Institute of Cell Biology (University Kaiserslautern) from 1983 to 1986 and of another research group at the Technology Center in Kaiserslautern.

Through his extensive research, Dr. Fritz-Albert Popp has scientifically confirmed the existence of biophotons. Biophotons *(from the Greek meaning "life" and meaning "light")* are photons of light in the ultraviolet and low visible light range, which are produced by a biological system. These particles of light have no mass and transmit information within and between cells. Dr. Fritz-Albert Popp's work shows that DNA in a living cell stores and releases photons creating *"biophotonic emissions"* which is proving to be one of the greatest health breakthroughs for reversing illness and sustaining vital health.

In 1996, Dr. Popp founded the International Institute of Biophysics in Neuss, Germany. He invented biophoton theory and has coined the term *'biophotons'* which refers to coherent photons emitted from biological organisms. In biophoton theory, DNA is the most probable source of biophoton emission.

The biological emission of photons *(biophotons)* is a term used to describe the permanent ultra- weak emission of coherent photons from living systems. *(Fritz-Albert Popp, 1976)*

The coherent emission of biophotons is responsible for transferring energy and information in the biological organisms, and has been linked to the function of DNA and to gene regulation. Biophotons directly effect metabolic and homeostatic processes and cell growth.

Furthermore, this phenomenon has been experimentally verified independently by many governmental and university research laboratories. These verified experiments were on unicellular organisms, tissues, organs, plants, animals, humans and tumor cells. These experiments showed that tumor cells exhibited characteristic photon emission patterns different from that of normal cells.

Further experimental studies have shown that ultra-weak photon emission from the surface of the human skin is emitted in the visual and in the infrared spectrum and is also strongly correlated to electrodermal activity *(Popp et al, 2006)*.

Polarized Light Enhances:

- Cellular Metabolism
- Oxygenation of Cells
- Antioxidant Protection
- Mitochondrial Energy (ATP) Production

We conclude that the future of medicine, will be energy medicine and the future of energy medicine will be frequency and light therapy. We are light beings and when we finally embrace this idea, then we will take in high vibrational healing light and frequencies, not just to energize but to heal ourselves right down to the cellular level. Gentle Daily Cleansing, Whole Plant Based Superfoods, Structured Water and advanced light and frequency therapies will help light up your life. **So lighten up and let life and light in**

ADVANCED LIGHT THERAPY

Thanks to advanced energy medicine: burns, leg ulcers, pressure sores, psoriasis, aches and pains, arthritis conditions, acne, seasonal affective disorders, atopic dermatitis in children and skin rashes in babies are all treatable with polarized, incoherent, polychromatic and low energy light at the Doc of Detox Clinic and in the comfort of your home.

Current technologies are offering us the latest in medical-care and equipment but more than ever, people wish to further their understanding of the knowledge and wisdom used by their ancestors. More people are discovering and relying on holistic approaches such as Light Therapy and Color Therapy as an alternative and addition to health-care medicine.

Light Therapy already has a long history going back thousands of years. The first source of light used for medical treatment was the sunlight, which is known as heliotherapy and dates from about 1400 BC. In 1903, The Danish Physician, Niels Ryberg Finsen, was awarded one of the earliest noble prizes for his *'Finsen Light Therapy'* for infectious diseases. Dr. Finsen is considered to be the founder of modern light therapy.

The therapeutic effects of light prompted many researchers and scientists to develop and use filtered solar and artificial light sources; phototherapy techniques became an alternative to heliotherapy. Further studies by other researchers and scientists resulted in the creation of advanced polarized light that works with almost the whole range of the visible and part of the infrared light. This was a huge development, and Advanced Light Therapy became an effective and viable additional treatment for various conditions and illnesses affecting both adults and children.

Studies of the effects of phototherapy using polarized, incoherent, low energy light therapy showed that polarized light helps speed up the healing process in cases such as venous leg ulcers, pressure sores and burns.

A quote from a paper by the University Hospital of Gent that was submitted to the British Journal of Plastic Surgery states:

"In conclusion, the results of this clinical study demonstrate that polarized-light therapy reduces the need for surgery in the treatment of deep dermal burns. In this group of patients, the use of polarized light accelerated wound healing and allowed very early pressure therapy, thus reducing hypertrophic scarring and contracture. No extension of the hospital stay was required.

Because of the better aesthetic and functional results (especially in burns of hands), polarized-light therapy has become the therapy of choice for deep dermal burns in our University Hospital."

The term 'light' refers to the visible part of the electromagnetic radiation spectrum. The light used in the submitted clinical trials consists of the visible and part of the infrared light measuring between 480 nanometers and up to 3000 nanometers. This advanced range ensures the exclusion of any UV light thus avoiding any UV radiation and poses no risk to the patient.

Today, it is known that the human organism transforms light into electrochemical energy, which activates a chain of biochemical reactions within cells, stimulating metabolism and reinforcing the immune response of the entire human body.

Advanced Light Therapy can be beneficial to people of all ages including children and babies. Advanced Light Therapy can be used in children as a complementary therapy to reduce pain and promote healing in various types of conditions such as: skin disorders, infections of the upper airways *(common cold, sinus infection, tonsillitis)* and conditions affecting muscles, joints and bones.

Advanced Light Therapy can be used as mono-therapy and/or as complementary therapy for pain treatment in the following indications: rheumatology *(osteoarthritis, rheumatoid arthritis and chronic arthritis)*, physiotherapy *(low back pain, shoulder and neck pain, carpal tunnel syndrome, scar tissue, musculoskeletal injuries)* and soft tissue injuries *(soft tissue injuries of muscles, tendons and ligaments, muscle spasm, sprains, strains, tendinitis, tennis elbow)*.

General Benefits

Advanced Light Therapy can be used both as a complementary treatment to support conventional medical methods and as mono-therapy for certain indications.

Advanced Light Therapy can:

- Improve microcirculation
- Harmonize metabolic processes
- Reinforce the human defense system
- Stimulate regenerative and reparative processes of the entire organism
- Promote wound healing
- Relieve pain or decrease its intensity

The outstanding characteristics of Advanced Light Therapy enable the light to penetrate not only the skin, but also the underlying tissues. Thus, the positive effect of Advanced Light Therapy is not limited to the treated skin area but also has a beneficial effect on the entire organism. **Advanced Light Therapy has bio-stimulative effects when applied to the skin:**

- It stimulates light-sensitive intracellular structures and molecules. This initiates cellular chain reactions and triggers so-called secondary responses which are not only limited to the treated skin area, but can involve the whole body.
- Stimulates and modulates reparative and regenerative processes as well as the processes of the human defense system.
- Acts in a natural way by supporting the regenerative capacity of the body and therefore, helps the body to release its healing potential.

Wound Healing

- Wounds after trauma (injuries)
- Burns
- Wounds after operations
- Leg ulcers
- Decubitus (pressure sores, bed sores)

Pain Treatment

Rheumatology:

- Osteoarthritis
- Rheumatoid arthritis (chronic)
- Arthrosis

Physiotherapy:

- Low back pain
- Shoulder and neck pain
- Carpal tunnel syndrome
- Scar tissue
- Musculoskeletal injuries

Sports Medicine - Soft tissue injuries of muscles, tendons and ligaments including:

- Muscle spasm
- Sprains
- Strains
- Tendinitis
- Ligament and muscle tears
- Dislocations
- Contusions
- Tennis elbow

Color Therapy

Health is contingent upon balancing not only our physical needs but our emotional, mental and spiritual needs as well. The color chakra therapy principle is based on the assumption that colors are associated with seven main chakras, which are energy centers in our bodies located along the spine. These chakras are like spirals of energy, each one relating to the specific area.

Chakra is the Sanskrit word for 'wheel'. It is assumed that chakras store and distribute energy. There are seven of these chakras and each is associated with a particular organ or system in the body. Each chakra has a dominant color which may become imbalanced. If this happens, it can cause a disorder and physical ramifications. Introducing the appropriate color, the disorder will not just improve but heal. Light and Color are essential for balancing our body's physical and emotional state.

Color is Light, and Light is Color. The sun emits light at different frequencies, and a process called refraction can separate these frequencies. When the light goes through a crystal prism, it refracts and divides into the seven colors of the spectrum. Each color has its frequency. If the separated colors go through another prism, they will form white light.

Here are just a few conditions that Color Therapy aids in:

Poor Concentration - Yellow or Violet

Shortness of Breath - Blue

Indigestion - Yellow

Feeling Cold - Red

Emotional/Sentimental Problems - Orange

Bereavement - Pink or Green

Stress - Green

Persistent headache - Blue or Violet

To learn about the most advanced light and color therapy available, go to www.docofdetox.com/lighttherapy and/or call 1 855 900 4544 for questions or training.

THE AMAZING MICROCIRCULATION SOLUTION

Understanding Microcirculation

Did you know that the underlying problem of many chronic conditions is poor microcirculation?

What is microcirculation? It is an incredible network of small arterioles, venules and little capillaries that distributes blood throughout the body - about 60,000 to 70,000 miles. This system delivers oxygen and nutrients to the cells and transports all waste products away from the tissues. It is one of the most important aspects, if not the most important aspect of well-being. Our macro-vessels, which are our arteries and veins, in contrast, make up only 26% of the vessel system. Only they receive blood due to the heart pumping.

If microcirculation is impaired, it will lead to impairment of cell function, where all disease and mutation starts. Chronic diseases usually develop over many years. That means, the break-down in circulation has been going on unnoticed. Extensive research in the field of Information Medicine in Europe has led to a new cutting edge approach to regulate and positively influence microcirculation. When you experience impaired blood flow throughout the capillary system, your tissues will not receive the required amount of oxygen and nutrients needed for cellular function. Oxygen is necessary for the production of ATP (Adenosine Tri-Phosphate). Without ATP, the cell is not able to maintain itself.

Why is ATP so important?

ATP is our energy source and is required in large amount. A human body needs about its own body weight of ATP daily. Unfortunately, the body does not store it somewhere. It is used up within seconds to maintain cell membrane potential (a voltage charge on the cell membrane) and protein synthesis (repair proteins, enzymes, hormones, information proteins, etc).

An optimal level of cell membrane potential assures that oxygen and nutrients can enter easily and wastes can exit the cell. That means the cell will perform well. If ATP is lacking, the cell membrane potential is disrupted and the cellular function diminishes; therefore, if a body lacks ATP, the origin can be found in inadequate oxygen supply and impaired micro-circulation. A prolonged condition will lead to chronic ATP deficiencies and then to chronic conditions. By the time symptoms manifest, the underlying issues have been going on unnoticed. Micro- circulatory blood flow can be improved substantially. It depends on a specific physiological process called Vasomotion; the rhythmic contraction and relaxation action in pre and post-capillary small blood vessels. Stimulating vasomotion is the key to increase blood flow into the capillary beds. Vasomotion occurs in larger calibered arterioles due to superior regulated mechanisms, but in small calibered arterioles, it functions completely autonomous. Up until now, western medicine lacked an effective method for this area of our cardio-vascular system. However, a promising technology from Europe shows through scientific research that it can be done. It may change the course of medicine.

For more information, go to www.docofdetox.com/ microcirculation or call us at: 1 855 900 4544

NATURE'S WAY

"We are what we repeatedly do. Excellence then, is not an act, but a habit."

- Aristotle

THE RULES HAVE CHANGED

These are very toxic times that we live in. No longer will the 2-3 week spring cleanse, supplementation and filtered water even come close to pulling you out of this toxic fire. It will be very challenging for those who do not recognize or have the understanding that the environment concerning health and well-being has drastically changed over the last 25 years. You will need to pay more attention to the health choices that you are making on a daily basis. No longer will supplements and a few health tips, in any way, protect you from this unhealthy climate that the average person is immersed in on a daily basis.

The climate concerning the health of the environment has and is changing rapidly and not in your favor. It has been common practice in the past, for those who strive to be healthy and stay healthy, to deep cleanse every few months from 3 days to 3 weeks long. 3 days is not long enough to do the job. 3 weeks of a deep cleanse will definitely remove many toxins but it can be very hard on your body because our detox organs are already severely overburdened and backed up due to this toxic environment we call Home. Safer and long lasting results can and are accomplished through Gentle Daily Cleansing and simple guidelines when followed daily without the ' *no pain, no gain theory*'. Some practitioners promote what I call, 'The Spring Cleanse'.

Why would you pile up toxic waste in your body that causes most of the pain, suffering, disease, and yes, even premature death that many experience?

Incorrect information given to patients and ineffective training has caused most health practitioners to practice the same way as the medical system does. Allowing the patient to go into a health crisis and then come to their rescue, because they have been educated in the same manner. 75 years ago our environment was not in this toxic state.

Should we gently cleanse daily for prevention or should we stay with the old rules and pile up that which does not serve us, and then do a cleanse every few months that only delivers temporary relief?

This attitude of 'create the problem and rush to the rescue' must end if you wish to make a permanent difference in our health. Let logic prevail. Unless your practitioner is empowering you to Master your own well-being with gentle baby steps on a daily basis, they are keeping you from the health that you truly deserve.

Nature does not just cleanse in the spring, she does it on a daily basis. If Nature were to let toxic waste pile up and did not cleanse and nourish on a daily basis, then humankind would become extinct. Your body is no different. Yes, deep cleanses have benefits but only if your organs are not backed up and in a state of fatigue.

The majority of the population will never experience long-term benefit from deep cleanses, nor the vibrant health they seek, because permanent health only comes with gentle steps done daily each and every day.

The rules to having and maintaining a healthy body have changed, but the proper training and guidance has not come with it, as we see with our family and friends. Our immune systems are now under attack 24/7 in this new toxic reality and health care today has mistreated and guided most into an unhealthy state of being.

When it comes to natural health people have been taught to dive into a deep cleanse when they feel they're in trouble and then fall out during or right after the deep cleanse, going back to the bad habits and symptoms they were trying to rid themselves of in the first place. At the *'Doc of Detox'* we have created the most effective, simplistic program to guide, protect and empower you step-by-step and day-by-day, because the rules have changed, and as therapists we must teach this new reality if we wish to make a permanent difference in the health and well-being of our patients.

It is a much wiser practitioner that teaches their patients to do a little each and every day to ensure that they stay vibrant, happy, healthy and disease- free on a continual basis, than one who continually runs to their rescue pretending to save them. Our success as practitioners is only measured by the success of our patients. Our patients will only be successful when they become Masters of their own health and well-being. **Be The Cure U Wish To See!**

We are burdened with toxins because our foods are, because our soil is. *Where does this leave us?*

Deficient of vital nutrients and burdened by toxins. It's much wiser to do a little each and every day to ensure that you stay vibrant, happy, healthy and disease-free on a permanent basis. An ounce of prevention is worth a pound of cure. Small baby steps daily prevent us from needing the pound of cure - Be The Cure!

KISS THEORY KEEP IT SIMPLE SAFE

We tend to do things in an *'extreme'* way but there is usually a price to be paid. This is known as the whiplash effect. Here's the kicker. Deep cleansing programs release many chemical toxins and acidic waste all at once that have been stored in fat and tissue cells. 75 years ago, many of these toxins were never in the environment or in our bodies. These toxins cannot be broken down by the body. When released and not eliminated effectively and efficiently the toxins will naturally settle in the weaker parts of the body where they are free to do more harm. A deep cleanse, in most cases, can cause the body to detoxify too much too fast, very similar to a dam. If you open the flood gates all at once and the rivers were never meant to handle this amount of water what do you think would happen?

The water will overflow and flood unprotected areas causing unnecessary damage and destruction because the release was not Nature's Way; this being gentle and gradual, in harmony with all. Today's truth; 50 years ago the toxicity in the environment and in the average person was minuscule compared to the new toxic reality that is around us, in us and a part of us today. We must all learn to detoxify gently and daily, hydrate with Structured Water and nourish our bodies with Whole Plant Based Nutrition or we will never experience that for which we search. If we play by their rules medically or nutritionally, we will not have the health we deserve because these rules are neither simple nor safe. Let us return to our roots, Nature's Way. From which we came we shall return, it's only Natural.

RISE AND THRIVE

How long should you keep drinking *'Doc of Detox'* Daily Cleansing Tea and SuperMix Superfood Nutrition? As long as you will be breathing, eating, drinking and wish to release your thin within. The greater the buildup of toxic waste, the longer it will take to restore balance. Once balance is restored you will want to keep it. Just like a garden, you must weed it daily so that the vegetables will thrive and not be choked out. Your body is no different.

Every one of your trillions of cells is a breathing, life-giving miracle that vibrates at the frequency of the food, water and air you ingest on a daily basis, no compromise. Rise and Thrive, you are Everything. For some this may sound absurd, but for me absurd is never questioning taking prescription drugs every day, wine every night, or 3 beers or 10 cigarettes a day. All choices have consequences; hopefully your choices are not from unconscious living. **Rise and Thrive.**

SMALL STEPS BIG CHANGE

As we get older, we produce less and less stomach acid and digestive enzymes, which means we may not fully digest our food or eliminate our waste effectively. The more you lean to a Whole Plant Based Superfood Lifestyle the more enzyme rich and cleansed you will feel and look. Small steps make big change. *'Doc of Detox'* Daily Cleansing Tea should be used on a daily basis for prevention, proper pH balance and to maintain excellent health throughout your life.

The objective is to regulate bowel movements 2-3 times daily to keep the waste moving through the digestive tract for complete elimination. This will stop any build-up and prolonged exposure to the fecal waste and poisons which would be absorbed by cells in intestine walls, creating a burden on the blood, bones and vital organs. Master your greatest gift one day at a time with baby steps, that would be **U.**

DOC OF DETOX DAILY CLEANSING TEA

Cleansing gently each and every day is the most powerful and important step in reclaiming and keeping your immune system strong. Be the cure you wish to see – flush the pounds to lighten the load!

DOC OF DETOX DAILY CLEANSING TEA FORMULA

'Doc of Detox' Daily Cleansing Tea does NOT contain: stimulants, caffeine, cascara, senna, sugar, harmful chemicals, or pesticides. *'Doc of Detox' Daily Cleansing Tea has been infused with vibrational frequencies.*

Made from the finest quality organic ingredients: Milk Thistle (Silybum Marianum), Blessed Thistle (Cnicus Benedictus), Malva Leaves (Chinese Mallow and Dong Kui), Persimmon Leaves (Diospyros Kaki) and Marsh Mallow Leaves (Sweetweed)

DETOXIFICATION IS FOUNDATIONAL

For All True Healing

70% of your body's immune system is in your digestive tract, the majority of this 70% is in your large intestine. You must have a compromised immune system if you suffer from pain, inflammation, premature aging, diseases and yes, cancer. We live in the most toxic times this planet has ever experienced, the Royal Society of Medicine did a major study and proved conclusively that 85% of all illness begins in the large intestine. In Natural Health, detoxification is foundational for all healing. In The Medical System, detoxification is never mentioned. Why? Because detoxification eliminates the need for most pharmaceuticals. Let logic prevail, should we do a cleanse every few months and allow the toxic waste to pile up? Should we wait until we're sick? Or, should we **gently cleanse daily** and relieve ourselves of at least **85% of the pain and suffering** that the majority of the population experiences on a daily basis? Baby Steps Daily is the only true way to live Happy and 'Healthy To 100'.

DAILY CLEANSING TEA INSTRUCTIONS

- Bring 1 gallon (4 liters/quarts or 16 cups) of (structured) water to a boil then remove from heat.
- Let the boiling stop before adding the tea bags - this will preserve the natural enzymes and the effectiveness of the herbal ingredients.
- Add 2 bags of 'Doc of Detox' Daily Cleansing Tea.
- Cover and let steep for 8 hours to bring the herbs to full potency.

- Leave tea bags in container and refrigerate until finished.
- You may reheat the tea but do not bring to a boil.
- Never microwave the tea bags or the water used to make the tea.
- Used tea bags can be saved, the herbs dried and added to food.
- This batch with last for eight days.
- Drink 4 ounces twice a day for 3 days then 8 ounces twice a day.
- Make new batch of tea when 1 liter of tea is remaining, with Structured Water for best results.

Call **1 855 900 4544** before you start the tea to get personal instructions from the 'Doc of Detox'.

DAILY CLEANSING TEA DIRECTIONS

Start 'Doc of Detox' Daily Cleansing Tea with half a dose (4 ounces) twice a day for the first 3 days. Then increase the amount, gradually working your way up to 8 ounces twice a day. You can increase or decrease as needed. Some may need a 4 ounce booster or more in between the two 8 ounce glasses where lack of abdominal tone, back up of old fecal waste, build up of old mucus or when you're above normal weight. You may drink more but follow guidelines at the beginning. There are those that may need to add 3 bags to a gallon to get the desired effects.

You can drink Daily Cleansing Tea at any time but drinking it just before meals may help to reduce heartburn and acid reflux. Drinking Daily Cleansing Tea protects esophagus and intestinal lining, soothes irritation and helps eliminate and prevent parasites, viruses, bad bacteria, heavy metals and acidosis (low pH) from environmental toxins.

Drinking 'Doc of Detox' Daily Cleansing Tea on an empty stomach or twenty to thirty minutes before a meal is best.

Some of the following may occur when beginning 'Doc of Detox' Daily Cleansing Tea:

- Gas and cramping are symptoms of loosening of old mucus, bad bacteria, fungus and fecal waste off of the intestinal walls. This is a normal occurrence and the waste can be 20-30 years old.
- This can occur for 3 to 14 days in people who lack tone and bacterial integrity. These symptoms will not last - there is light at the end of this tunnel I guarantee it.
- If extreme cramping occurs, decrease the amount of the tea taken, but do not stop the cleanse. This is due to the break down of scar tissue in the colon. Don't hesitate to call if you have any questions.
- Loose stool is normal when starting 'Doc of Detox' Daily Cleansing Tea.
- If the stool is watery, decrease the amount of tea taken, but do not stop the cleanse. You should maintain 2 bowel movements per day, slightly on the loose side but of good volume for the first few weeks then it should hang together.
- Your rectum may feel warm. This is due to the acidity and ammonia that is being dumped from your tissues from extreme putrefaction.
- Feces that is extremely dark in color (black) is very old waste that is being expelled.

- Weight loss will occur only if the body needs it.
- 'Doc of Detox' Daily Cleansing Tea acts as a body balancer and purifier.

If you wish to save thousands of dollars, eliminate needless pain and suffering for your pets - it's tea time! Dogs are people too!

CLEANSE BUILD & RESTORE

Stool may be soft and foul smelling when you start to cleanse and may last for some time depending on the back up in the small and large intestine. If you feel your stool is too loose then reduce amount as much as you need to and drink 'Doc of Detox' Daily Cleansing Tea after meals and do not stop unless necessary. Do not hesitate to call us. Do not mistake mushy, soft stools for diarrhea - Diarrhea is very watery, very light brown or yellowish in color, and floats. Real diarrhea can be caused by many things such as stress, a change in diet, certain foods, consuming too large a meal or too much fat in a meal, certain parasites and bacteria and by at least 600 pharmaceutical drugs which list diarrhea as a side effect. Using Daily Cleansing Tea on a regular basis will provide you with so many important health benefits. If you experience soft stools, just reduce the amount you are drinking for a day or two, drink it before a meal, and stay with the program, and you will soon see how great you will feel!

Contact your medical doctor if pregnant, if you've had a recent major surgery on the digestive tract.

DAILY CLEANSING TEA

For Children

Children have worse bowel problems than any other sector except for seniors. They must be taught at an early age what a good bowel movement looks like, feels like and that they should have two to three a day. If your desire is to have happy, healthy children that don't suffer like you did, then proper bowel management is foundational for vital health and prevention of disease for these little one's. Help teach your children to answer Nature's call it's only Natural. Why not end needless pain and suffering and increase their vitality. Don't let your children pile their poop up like we did. Lighten their load one pooh at a time.

Under 75 pounds

Start with 1 ounce twice a day for three days and gradually work up to 2 ounces twice a day. Increase or decrease as needed.

75 pounds and greater

Start with 2 ounces twice a day for three days and gradually work up to 4 ounces twice a day. Increase or decrease as needed

DAILY CLEANSING TEA

For Pets

Constipation is a constant problem with pets. Diarrhea is a recurring problem caused by constipation with your pets. Do not underestimate gentle daily cleansing for your pets. Keep your pets healthy for cents a day and save thousands.

'Doc of Detox' Daily Cleansing Tea will help eliminate and prevent:

- Parasites
- Bad Bacteria
- Worms
- Viruses
- Toxic Waste Build Up

Dosage for pets:

One ounce for every twenty pounds once a day.

Can be given to your pets straight or mixed with water or food.

GENTLE DAILY CLEANSING

The Key To Longevity

The longer you drink 'Doc of Detox' Daily Cleansing Tea the deeper the cleanse and the greater the effect on the body's self healing process. Just to cleanse the small and large intestine can take 3 to 9 months. Your liver will always need this type of support in this environment. All organs and systems will benefit from Daily Cleansing Tea. You will know by the way you look and feel. As long as your breathing, eating and drinking there will always be toxic build up. So as long as you wish to protect your vital health it will be Tea Time. If you are a person that smokes, drinks or has any other toxic addiction do not forget your life jacket - 'Doc of Detox' Daily Cleansing Tea. We will maintain our car, house and vacuum but what about the most important vehicle of all?!

Iced Tea anyone? The objective is to regulate bowel movements 2-3 times per day to keep the waste moving through the digestive tract for complete elimination. This will stop any buildup and prolonged exposure of the fecal waste and poisons that would be absorbed creating a burden to the blood, tissues, bones and vital organs.

REVIVE THE ELDERLY

A wise elderly woman once told me "We're not grumpy, we're constipated." Thanks grandma. Bowel mismanagement is the worst when it comes to this age group. The pharmaceuticals being ingested due to the pain and discomfort of a stagnated bowel is epidemic. Those responsible for the care and health of our elderly lean towards the quick fix and not the cause. The elderly deserve our respect and attention as they are shown in other cultures. Shame on us. I assure you that once you lighten this toxic load the body will do what it was created to do at any age. Heal you. If you must start your day with toast and tea make it Daily Cleansing Tea. So lighten your load and be happy and healthy.

DAILY CLEANSING TEA USES

- Acid Reflux Disease (GERD) or Heartburn
- Excess Gas / Foul Flatulence / Stomach Cramps
- Indigestion / Stomach Ache
- Belching / Bloating / Water Retention
- Enlarged Abdomen / Protruding Belly / Midriff Bulge

- Irregularity / Chronic constipation / Hard Stools / Hemorrhoids
- Irritability and anxiety
- Irritable Bowel Syndrome (IBS) / Crohn's Disease
- Abdominal Pain / Inflammatory Bowel Diseases (IBDs)
- Spastic Colon / Colitis / Ileitis / Enterocolitis / Leaky Gut Syndrome
- Candidiasis / Yeast Overgrowth / Parasites / Worms
- Bad Breath / Bad Body Odor
- Excess Stored Fat / Excess Weight / Obesity
- Skin Conditions / acne / Itchy, flaky skin or scalp / Dandruff
- Inflamed Skin / Dermatitis / Eczema / Psoriasis / Acne
- Allergies and Hay Fever / Food Allergies
- Chronic Fatigue / Fibromyalgia / Sciatica
- Joint Pain / Back Pain / Sciatica / Arthritis / Migraine Headaches / Headaches
- Insomnia / Restless sleep
- Low Energy / Chronic fatigue
- Loss of Mental Clarity and Concentration / "Brain Fog" / Forgetfulness
- Clearing out pharmaceutical / recreational / chemical drug residues
- Clearing out aspartame and its byproducts
- Decrease in sex drive

'Doc of Detox' Daily Cleansing Tea is a very special blend with infused frequency that allows the gentle cleansing of the whole body with continued use.

Thousands have lost weight and kept it off due to its cleansing action.

Over the years, thousands of clients from around the world have taken Daily Cleansing Tea to cleanse their colon, liver, detox their body, lose weight, and feel great.

Note: The information provided is "for educational purposes only" and is not intended in any way to be considered as medical advice or a consultation about the diagnosis, treatment, cure, or prevention of any disease. Consult your medical doctor or professional health care provider if you have a medical condition.

If pregnant, recent major surgery on the digestive tract consult a medical doctor before using 'Doc of Detox' Daily Cleansing Tea.

WHOLE PLANT BASED SUPERFOOD NUTRITION

Moringa Oleifera: The most dense phytonutrient plant on Earth. (Scientific Fact)

BRIDGING THE GAP

The food chain is and has been broken for 50 years. Most have come to realize that it is impossible to get the nutrients needed from our foods to have a healthy, vibrant body. The *'Doc of Detox'* is about bridging that gap and delivering the most effective techniques, training and foundational nutrition in the most simplistic and cost effective way, so that you can regain and keep that which has always been your universal right - **GREAT HEALTH!**

Give a man a fish and he will be healthy for a day. Teach a man how to fish and he will be healthy for life. There has been almost a generation of deception, selling off nature and our health, one piece at a time, favoring the new and improved and the latest and greatest medical or nutritional supplement breakthrough. When you strip away the commercial health that most receive and return to foundational nutrition and detoxification, you will no longer be patients, you will be Masters of your own well-being.

Although fruits and vegetables should always be your first choice, they have been absent of the foundational nutrients to create or sustain a healthy body since the 1940s. You now need roughly 10 servings of vegetables and fruits just to obtain the nutritional equivalent of 1 serving from 50 years ago. We are not cows, and I am not about to believe that anyone is going to eat 10 servings of any one thing in a given day only to find out that they're still nutritionally depleted. You will never be depleted nutritionally when you know the truth and how to take personal action. You're either being taught how to regain your health or you're being left powerless like many patients today. You cannot do better until you have been taught better. If you're not taking personal action by taking gentle baby steps on a day-to-day basis, you will eventually end up on your back, broke, sick and in pain.

As long as you remain an average, normal person, satisfied with handout health, willing to cut corners and make your health choices secondary, or put it in the hands of others, do not complain or explain. The answer can only be found in real, raw, organic Whole Plant Based Superfood Nutrition. Unless you're willing to purchase the fuel needed for the human body to repair, rebuild and restore, then sit back and try to get comfortable because, well, you know the rest of the story by now.

In this chapter, I will show you that almost 90% of the nutritional supplements on store shelves are filled with empty promises that fall short with their delivery and may even cause negative side effects. We will also take a look at the most potent form of food and the process that has enhanced the world's most dense phytonutrient superfood on the Planet. I also challenge you to find a better, Whole Plant Based Food that is a healthy, nutritional, scientifically proven and let us not forget, financially more rewarding product. Let us begin. First I would like to touch on a topic that is rarely discussed. In my 35 years in practice I have seen thousands of people with many different beliefs. The most common dysfunctional belief that is learned from our peers, parents, government and society is that we should never be self-centered or selfish. This is a fear-based belief that comes from a foundation of lack. "*There is just not enough to go around.*" is a crippling thought that is driven into us at a very young age, and can leave us with little self-worth or otherwise never being true to ourselves and our individual needs.

Your first need should always be to put your health and happiness first. If you don't you will become bitter and out of alignment with your true purpose. You must come first. When your main focus and attention is on the external world and trying to please it first, you will always be gravely disappointed. The most precious thing is lost and forgotten - that would be you. Even if your spirit has been or is broken, don't pass it on - rise.

You are the end all be all, invest in **U** wisely, lead the way. Without good health, we are left to have very little. Unless we change this program that has been passed down from generation to generation, we will keep teaching our children these programs which sow the seeds of fear, lack and sickness. Please take the time to start observing not just of yourself, but others. One example, in North America we will spend roughly double on our pets than we will our own children. Most people's 'nutritional value point' for themselves hovers around the zero mark, some are worth $1 a day and some are worth $10 a day. The truth be known, the majority of the population has downloaded a program of little self-worth when it comes to investing in that which would truly make a difference - a healthy body. The $10 pack of cigarettes comes first, the case of beer, the junk food, dumping thousands of dollars into their hobbies and vices, while living in fear as all Hell-th breaks loose in their bodies. Somewhere deep down inside they have signed up for the **zombie nation** and are now crying, *"Why me!"* I'll tell you why, because they're feeding into a **B**roken **S**ystem... The Health Care System, not your own Immune System.

Your body is like a credit card. When you use it continually without making regular payments, eventually it will be cut into pieces. Just like the Visa card, when you replenish your body with counterfeit nutrition and not with Whole Plant Based Nutrition, you will pay piece by piece, in this case with your health. You have just bought a ticket for a ride on a slow motion train wreck; malnourished and drugged until you reach your final destination; Mentally, Physically, Emotionally and Financially broken, just like the system you signed up for. I can tell you with certainty that your lifestyle now is more costly for you than it needs to be, on many levels. One of these levels being that the level of your health will always affect the tone of your relationships with the ones dearest to you and will remain that way until **U** sign up for the greatest health care plan on this planet, this being the most dense phytonutrient Whole Plant Based Superfood: **Moringa Oleifera.**

Zija® Nation, or **zombie** occupation? Remember that health and happiness are one in the same. You truly cannot have one without the other. Are you someone who has been living a lifestyle unconscious of your health choices and wish to erase potential seeds of sickness that have been sown, unknowingly to you? Have you been searching for the real **U**?

"Medical debts are the number one cause of bankruptcy in America. "

- Barbara Ehrenreich

Are you suffering from a chronic or degenerative disease and seek complete health restoration? Do you fall into the, *'This is normal for your age'* category, when you are experiencing muscle aches and pains, signs of disease, wrinkles and sagging skin, loss of memory and generally poor vitality? Do you yearn to regain your youth so you may look and feel, not older, but much younger than your chronological age? Or, are you someone, like myself, in good health but wish to become the fountain of youth to slow down the aging process and live a full and fruitful life - and die healthy?

If you want predictability and stability then you want The Whole Truth about Health. If you want total health then your body needs the total package: Whole Plant Based Superfood Nutrition. It has no boundaries when it comes to health conditions, gender, age groups or nationalities.

This is a one size fits all program, the way Nature created it, the way Nature intended it, unstoppable and predictable. If you give the body what it needs, the body self-corrects. Just relax and get out of its way and let your body do what it was born to do, heal **U**. This is where all true healing begins and ends. Wellness is a derivative of you making correct decisions; meaning giving your body Whole Plant Based, Life-Giving raw materials that make miracles happen... **Drink Life In.**

WHY SUPPLEMENTS CAN SUCK THE MONEY AND LIFE RIGHT OUT OF YOU

"Taking multivitamins does not solve the problem, it is impossible to capture all of the vitamins, minerals Disease fighting nutrients in a pill."

- National Cancer Institute

The saying; "The whole is greater than the sum of its parts," is nowhere more important than in the food we eat.

I would like to address one of the greatest planned and **man**-ipulated nutritional stings orchestrated by the supplement industry. Just so you understand, I spent the first 20 years of my career in the health business down the rabbit hole of confusion. In life, it seems, we always need a good guy and a bad guy. Because I was a natural health practitioner it was only natural that the bad guy was the pharmaceutical corporation and the good guy was the supplement industry. Ohhh, no, grasshopper, you are young and naive. It took me 20 years to realize that a little bit of truth mixed with a bunch of B.S., provides enough fertilizer to grow the Grand Illusion, which, when neatly packaged, can be sold to the trusting public. 68% of the population takes some form of nutritional supplement, 52% on a regular basis. The majority of these people are in the *'one a day'* supplement group. They are flushing their money literally down the toilet.

This is so because most fragmented supplements are nutritionally useless and some even downright dangerous because they are **man**-ipulated and are viewed as *'alien'* by your body.

Many of these fragmented man-made supplements that are labeled natural are a complete waste of money and can be reclaimed at your local sewage treatment plant (recycle, reuse). Inferior nutrition = an Inferior body. The supplement industry knows very well how the propaganda machine operates, Big Pharma has been a great teacher along the way. They will do whatever it takes to distract you from The Whole Truth About

Health because once you realize that Whole Plant Based Superfood Nutrition is the answer, the only answer; their involvement in your life will cease to exist. We can say that a specific nutrient has the ability to eliminate a disease or perform a specific function but what is not disclosed by the manufacturers is that this only occurs when this nutrient is found in its Whole form, this being in the form of Whole Plant Based Food.

The supplement industry leads you to believe that they can take a single active ingredient from Whole Plant Based Foods and sell us the same nutritional results as if it were a whole food. Limited science will always give us limited results and fall short with their *'nutritional promises'*, known as single supplements. Most natural health practitioners are trained in this manner or should I say programmed in this manner. Teaching their patients the best they know how, but continually missing the mark to helping their patients Master their own health.

The food chain broke when the *'parts'* became more profitable to the corporations controlling our food source. Here at the *'Doc of Detox'* we promise to provide you with correct information and the support that you deserve to ensure that we are helping you bridge the gap to your permanent success.

The food chain broke when the PARTS became more profitable to the CORPORATIONS controlling our FOOD SOURCE.

FAD OF THE WEEK

Almost all nutrients cannot function properly alone. It is an 'all for one and one for all' mission. As in the case of enzymes, they cannot function properly without minerals. In the absence of minerals, vitamins have no function. Lacking vitamins, the system can make use of the minerals, but lacking minerals, vitamins are useless. For every fragmented nutrient breakthrough they have more products to sell, resulting in more profit. Problems arise when we think a nutrient breakthrough is actually a health breakthrough. This year it's vitamin A; next year it's vitamin C, the following, Calcium. You get the picture. When you sell just the nutrient and not the whole food, you are only telling, oh, I mean *'selling'* a piece of the truth, not The Whole Truth.

When you sell just the nutrient and not the whole package, you are only selling a piece of the truth, not the whole truth. Most commercially sold, so- called Superfood supplements contain 15-71 ingredients or more, but many of these Superfoods are in trace amounts, too small to deliver any real health benefits. It is not just the layperson that buys into this savvy marketing but many health practitioners do the same, when all they want to do is help. But an empty promise is an empty promise, no matter how good their intentions are. Most health practitioners end up going through this learning curve, I know I did. Invest is short for investigate. I did my research; make sure that you do yours. Your body is depending on it.

If the majority of the population had a Whole Plant Based Superfood Lifestyle there would be a financial disaster for a time because our nation revolves around making money from the sick. **How sick is that?!** *How's that working for you?* Big Pharma and the supplement industry will ignore and discredit scientific research on Whole Plant Based Superfood Nutrition in order to fortify their industries based on empty promises and empty nutrition because their survival depends on it. Whole Plant Based Superfood Nutrition creates balance and restores life. Single nutrient therapy (pills) has fallen short of its promises and will continue to do so because it's not 'Only Natural'.

Today's western diet has double the calories of a consumer in 1965 and we are receiving 75% less nutrient value for the current calories consumed. Quality whole plant based nutrient supplementation on a daily basis is not an option but a necessity for a pain-free, disease-free body.

The average American consumes over 3200 calories per day but they are receiving 75% less in nutrient value than they did in the mid '60s with 1500 calories a day. Today, we are over consuming, yet we're still undernourished. It's not a mystery that there is a pandemic of obesity in America today. As you read this, 34.8% of the US population is medically diagnosed as morbidly obese, and another 32% are diagnosed as obese. More than two-thirds of America's population today is overweight! At the 'Doc of Detox' we feel you will know better because we have taught you to know better. Instead of getting treatment, get the proper training and take control and be the cure you search for.

THE MORINGA IT'S NOT A DANCE!

Real Food Real Nutrition

Nature has, and always will, provide everything that our bodies need to live an amazing life. Nature has already put a backup plan in place for when we deplete the soil and our food. That time would be now! Something so simple as a tree, can change your life forever. You may not have heard of the Moringa tree, but it has been called a miracle tree. Once you understand about this miracle, I hope you will share it with everyone.

The definition of a Superfood is a food with a high concentration of various nutrients and phytochemical content that delivers exceptional health benefits. The best Superfoods are scientifically proven to be functional foods for whole body healing and exceptional health.

What if I told you that a pharmaceutical corporation has developed a pill that meets all your body's nutritional needs and prevents or reverses most of the illnesses we suffer from today?

Firstly, I believe many would buy into this due to the pharmaceutical propaganda and fairytale advertising that we are accustomed to on the latest, greatest cure. The Pharmaceutical Industry tried for over 6 generations to create a synthetic form of Moringa Oleifera, but they failed. When they tried to synthesize Moringa to patent it, it lost its essence, this being the amino acid sequencings. Another reason they were desperate to patent this amazing Superfood was for its naturally occurring anti-inflammatories. Ibuprofen is 1 anti-inflammatory whereas Moringa Oleifera has 36 naturally occurring anti- inflammatories.

Secondly, nature has already created and perfected these thousands of years ago and with the expertise of Russ Bianche, a world class formulator and his team of caring brilliant minds, after 140 trials, enhanced not only the taste but also the delivery system and nutritional benefits of this most dense phytonutrient plant on Earth. This had never been accomplished before. Yes, a scientific breakthrough can actually be a nutritional breakthrough when you work in harmony with Nature and not around her. Man in all his wisdom will always fall short when he tries to **man**-ipulate a million years of evolution. You can work alongside Nature but when you try to go around her you will be gravely disappointed.

JUST IMAGINE

- How much healthier you'd be if you drank the most dense whole plant based phytonutrient on Planet Earth on a daily basis.
- How fast your body might heal itself of diseases, aches and pains. For only the body heals.
- How much younger you'd look and feel.
- How much more energy you would have to do the things you love.
- What would it mean to **U** to go to the doctor and not have him say, "That's normal for your age."

You can live that 'abnormal life' that others only dream of when you make Whole Plant Based Superfood Nutrition a way of life. You have only one thing to do, get out of the way and let your body do the thinking. Moringa is known and prized for its medicinal purposes in 82 countries, by 210 different names. Indigenous and ancient peoples, including the Roman, Greek, Egyptian, and Indian (Ayurvedic), have used this plant for thousands of years, with known writings dating back to 150 A.D. Life is full of magic in the way that when you hit the wall and wonder what now, the answer pops up just like a 'miracle tree'.

The Discovery Channel was so impressed with the Moringa tree that it created a multi-million dollar documentary on the tree. A first in the National Institutes of HealthTV industry.

National Institutes of Health (NIH): The March 2008 issue of the NIH "Record" praises Moringa Oleifera and states that;

"...perhaps like no other single species, this plant has the potential to help reverse multiple major environmental problems and provide for many unmet human needs."

It was also recognized by the National Institutes of Health as the Botanical of the Year for 2007, and praised again in 2011 and 2012. It is valued worldwide for its ability to treat over 300 diseases. It has the ability to retain high concentrations of electrolyte minerals, allowing it to stay internally hydrated in the driest of conditions. Africans have honored it with names that translate as: *"Never Die,"* and *"The Only Thing that Grows in the Dry Season," "Manna Tree"* and *"Mother's Milk."* The Moringa tree is helping to rid hunger and malnutrition and has saved more lives in Third World countries than any other food or substance.

A November 2012 feature in the *National Geographic* noted that, gram for gram, dried Moringa leaves have 25 times the iron of spinach, 17 times the calcium of milk, 15 times the potassium of bananas, 10 times the vitamin A in carrots and nine times the protein of yogurt. Dr. Oz has helped bring Moringa into the mainstream by including it in his *'5 Ways to Reenergize Your Day'.*

"A whopping 99% of all Americans are micronutrient deficient."

-Dr. Mehmet Oz, MD

Moringa has the highest protein ratio of any plant identified so far. Food scientists once believed that only soy had protein comparable to meat, dairy or eggs. Now they have added Moringa to the top of that very short list. Many consider Moringa's protein superior to soy, as it is more digestible and non-allergenic. Amadou Ba, director of a Senegalese African village health post, concurs:

"We were all trained in the Western solutions for treating malnutrition with whole-milk powder, sugar, vegetable oil, and peanut butter. But these ingredients are expensive and inefficient. The recovery of malnourished infants can take months. We now nourish them with Moringa, and we start seeing great improvements within 10 days." **Moringa has no known impurities, and no adverse reactions have ever been recorded.**

The Moringa oil has more impressive attributes than olive oil. It is used in cooking and to moisturize the skin. Because it won't spoil or turn rancid, it is used as a preservative, and as a machine lubricant even for fine watches. What's left after the oil has been extracted from the seeds is called seed cake, and is used worldwide as feed to increase milk production in cows.

Lack of drinkable water is one of the world's most serious threats. Roughly 1.2 billion people in developing countries simply do not have access to clean, safe water, leaving them with little choice but to drink and wash with contaminated water. This accounts for 80% of the world's diseases! An estimated 25,000 people die from water-borne diseases every day. Yet, a dash of Moringa can make dirty water drinkable.

When Moringa seeds are crushed and added to dirty, bacteria-laden water, they absorb the impurities. This action is replicated within our bodies as the seed cake binds to toxins in the organs and intestines.

Professor S. A. Muyibi, of the International Islamic University of Malaysia, believes that Moringa seeds could potentially provide a renewable, sustainable, and biodegradable material for treating global water supplies. International aid organizations now produce and/ or promote the use of Moringa in poverty-stricken areas. The World Health Organization (WHO) estimates that 80% of the world's population relies on traditional medicine (i.e., plants rather than drugs) for their primary healthcare needs. L. Fuglie, director of the Church World Service in West Africa, found that powdered Moringa leaves were more readily embraced by rural villagers than other dietary aids or pharmaceuticals, and decided to put it to the test. After a 2 year pilot project in the villages of Senegal, his organization recently convinced the government to promote Moringa as part of the national diet. Lack of Vitamin A, due to malnutrition, causes 70% of all childhood blindness. That translates to 500,000 children going blind around the world every year. The Bethesda, Maryland-based "International Eye Foundation" is now using Moringa, with its high content of beta-carotene converting to Vitamin A in the body, to combat childhood blindness.

Doctors are using Moringa to treat diabetes in West Africa and high blood pressure in India. It can staunch a skin infection, feed livestock, and enrich the soil, increasing the nutritional value and growth of other crops. Dozens of humanitarian organizations, including the Church World Service, the

Educational Concerns for Hunger Organizations, Trees for Life, and the National Science Foundation are pursuing research on the use of Moringa Oleifera to combat health challenges.

In addition to its high nutritional value, Moringa boasts an impressive list of traditional medicinal uses by various cultures around the world. Moringa has fought child death and disease due to malnutrition in Africa. Moringa, a near perfect food, has a niche in staving off the current food crisis threatening more than 100 million people worldwide.

- Endorsement by Wanda Dyson, MD

Moringa Oleifera - *With its 90 nutrients, 46 anti-oxidants, 36 anti-inflammatories, and more, Moringa has proven to be the most nutrient-dense and enzymatically active botanical on planet earth.*

Moringa Oleifera Beverages Contain Over 90 Verified Nutrients

1. Protein constituents or amino acids *(the building blocks of protein)*. There are 20 amino acids necessary, and found in human proteins, of which 9 are essential. All 9 are found in Moringa, properly sequenced and in the optimal ratios.
2. Minerals such as Calcium, Chloride, Chromium, Copper, Fluorine, Iron, Manganese, Magnesium, Molybdenum, Phosphorus, Potassium, Sodium, Selenium, Sulfur, and Zinc.
3. Fats, as vegetable oils: Beneficial Omega (3,6,9) oils.
4. Vitamins, many of which have anti-oxidant properties: Vitamins C, D, E, F, and K, provitamin A *(Beta-carotene)*, Vitamin B *(Choline)*, Vitamin B1 *(Thiamin)*, Vitamin B2 (Riboflavin), Vitamin B3 *(Niacin)*, Vitamins B5, B6, and B12.

5. Other phytonutrients and anti-oxidants such as Alanine, Alpha- Carotene, Arginine, Beta-sitosterol, Caffeoylquinic Acid, Campesterol, Carotenoids, Chlorophyll, Delta-5-Avenasterol, Delta-7-Avenasterol, Glutathione, Histidine, Indole Acetic Acid, Indoleacetonitrile, Kaempferal, Leucine, Lutein, Methionine, Myristic-Acid, Palmitic-Acid, Prolamine, Proline, Quercetin, Rutin, Selenium, Threonine, Tryptophan, Xanthins, Xanthophyll, Zeaxanthin, Zinc.

6. Plant hormones with anti-aging properties in humans: Cytokinins such as Zeatin. Moringa Leaves are a healthy anti-aging powerhouse because they contain several thousand times more of the powerful nutrient Zeatin than any other known plant. The Zeatin in Moringa creates new cells at a faster rate then that of old skin cells that die.

7. In total, there are over 46 anti-oxidants and 36 anti-inflammatory compounds all naturally occurring in the Moringa plant.

Here are the currently verified nutrients, by category, found in Zija® Moringa—all in the bioavailable, synergistic blend that Nature intended:

Zija® Moringa is an organically grown, 100% Bioavailable, FULLY ABSORBABLE Whole Plant Based Superfood.

Dr. Russ Bianchi, one of the world's top formulation food scientists, managing director and founder of Adept Solutions Inc. of Monterey, California, is the scientist (MD, PhD, neurosurgeon) who developed Zija's® wholesome nutritional products.

After more than 140 trials on his way to perfecting this supplement, he now calls it his greatest achievement: The USDA, researchers, botanists, nutritional scientists, and Zija®

International health experts have all put the Moringa through extensive analysis. The Zija® beverages, such as SuperMix, contain the Moringa tree's most beneficial parts: leaf, fruit and seed. They deliver full-spectrum nutritional value, along with a documented 539 medicinal activities. No berry juice or other single plant botanical compares with what Zija® Moringa beverages have to offer.

"This organic, whole-food beverage *(now available i n raw powder form as "SmartMix" and "SuperMix")* is the most bioavailable and nutritionally dense formula I have ever seen—bar none! For long-term health, there is nothing on the market globally that gets anywhere near Zija® quality and overall benefit."

- 28-Isoavenasterol
- 4-(Alpha -L-Rhamnosyloxy)-Sen
- 4-(Alpha-L-Rhamnosyloxy)-Ben
- Alanine
- Alpha-Carotene
- Arginine
- Arschidic-Acid
- Aspartic-Acid
- Behenic-Acid
- Beta-Carotene
- Beta-Sitosterol
- Biotin
- Caffeoylquinic Acid
- Calcium
- Campestanol
- Campesterol
- Carotenoids
- Chlorophyll
- Cholesterol
- Choline
- Chromium
- Clerosterol
- Cobalt
- Copper
- Cystine
- Delta-7 & 14-Stigmastanol
- Delta-5-Avenasterol
- Delta-7-Avenasterol
- EFA Omega 3
- EFA Omega 6
- EFA Omega 9
- Ergos tadienol
- Fiber
- Flavonoids
- Flavonols
- Fluorine
- Folate (Folic Acid)
- Gadoleic-Acid

- Glucosinolates
- Glutamine (Glutamic-Acid) Glutathione
- Glycine
- Histidine
- Indole Acetic Acid
- Indoleacetonitrile
- Iodine
- Iron
- Isoleucine
- Kaernpferal
- Leucine
- Lignoceric-Acid
- Lithium
- Lutein
- Lysine
- Magnesium
- Manganese
- Methionine
- Molybdenum
- Myristtc-Acid
- Neoxanthin
- Niazimicin
- Niaziminins A & B
- Niazinin A
- Niazinin B
- Oleic-Acid
- Omega 3
- Omega 6
- Omega 9
- Palmitic Acid
- Palrnitoleic Acid
- Phenylalanine
- Phosphorus
- Potassium
- Prolamine
- Proline
- Protein
- Quercetin
- Rutin
- Selenium
- Serine
- Silicon
- Sodium
- Stearic-Acid
- Stigrnasterol
- Sulfur
- Superoxide
- Dismutase
- Threonine
- Tryptophan
- Tyrosine
- Valine
- Vanadium
- Violaxanthin
- Vitamin A
- Vitamin B (Choline)
- Vitamin B1 (Thiamin)
- Vitamin B12
- Vitamin B2 (Riboflavin)
- Vitamin B3 (Niacin)
- Vitamin B6 (Pyridoxine)
- Vitamin C (Ascorbic-Acid)
- Vitamin D
- Vitamin E
- Vitamin E (Alpha Tocopherol
- Vitamin E (Delta Tocopherol)
- Vitamin E (Gamma Tocopherol)
- Xanthins
- Xanthophylls
- Zeatin
- Zeaxanthin
- Zinc
- Zirconium

Amino Acids

- Alanine, Arginine, Aspartic Acid, Cystine, Glutamine Glutamic Acid, Glycine, Histidine, Isoleucine, Leucine, Lysine, Methionine, Phenylalanine, Proline, Serine, Threonine, Tryptophan, Tyrosine, Valine

Anti-inflammatories

- Arginine, Beta-sitosterol, Caffeoylquinic Acid, Calcium, Chlorophyll, Copper, Cystine, Essential Fatty Acid (EFA) Omega 3, EFA Omega 6, EFA Omega 9, Fiber, Glutathione, Histidine, Indole Acetic Acid, Indoleacetonitrile, Isoleucine, Kaempferal, Leucine, Magnesium, Oleic Acid, Phenylalanine, Potassium, Quercetin, Rutin, Selenium, StigMasterol, Sulfur, Superoxide Dismutase, Tryptophan, Tyrosine, Vitamin A, Vitamin B1 *(Thiamin)*, Vitamin C *(Ascorbic Acid)*, Vitamin E *(Alpha Tocopherol)*, Vitamin E *(Delta Tocopherol)*, Vitamin E *(Gamma Tocopherol)*, Zeatin, Zinc

Vitamins & Anti-Oxidants

- Alanine, Alpha-Carotene, Arginine, Beta-Carotene, Beta-sitosterol, Caffeoylquinic Acid, Campesterol, Carotenoids, Chlorophyll, Cholesterol, Chromium, Delta 5-Avenasterol, Delta 7-Avenasterol, Glutathione, Histidine, Indole Acetic Acid, Indoleacetonitrile, Kaempferal, Leucine, Lutein, Methionine, Myristic Acid, Palmitic Acid, Prolamine, Proline, Quercetin, Rutin, Selenium, Superoxide Dismutase, Threonine, Tryptophan, Vitamin A, Vitamin B (Choline), Vitamin B1 (Thiamin), Vitamin B2 (Riboflavin), Vitamin B 3 *(Niacin)*, Vitamin B 6 *(Pyridoxine)*, Vitamin C *(Ascorbic Acid)*, Vitamin E *(Alpha Tocopherol)*, Vitamin E, *(Delta Tocopherol)*,

Vitamin E *(Gamma Tocopherol)*, Vitamin K, Xanthins, Xanthophyll, Zeatin, Zeaxanthin, Zinc, Vitamin E *(Alpha-Tocopherol)*

Carotenoids

- Apha-Carotene, Beta-Carotene, Chlorophyll, Lutein, Neoxanthin, Violaxanthin, Xanthophyll, Zeaxanthin

Cox-2 Inhibitors

- Caffeoylquinic Acid, Flavonoids Kaempferol & Quercetin, EFA Omega 3

Essential Nutrients

- Alpha-Carotene, Beta-Carotene, Biotin, Calcium, Carotenoids, Choline, Copper, Cystine, EFA Omega 3, EFA Omega 6, EFA Omega 8, Fiber, Flavonoids, Folate *(Folic Acid)*, Glutamine Glutamic Acid, Iodine, Iron, Isoleucine, Leucine, Lutein, Lysine, Magnesium, Manganese, Methionine, Molybdenum, Phenylalanine, Phosphorus, Potassium, Protein, Threonine, Tryptophan, Valine, Vitamin A, Vitamin B *(Choline)*, Vitamin B1 *(Thiamin)*, Vitamin B2 *(Riboflavin)*, Vitamin B3 *(Niacin)*, Vitamin B6 *(Pyridoxine)*, Vitamin B12, Vitamin C *(Ascorbic Acid)*, Vitamin D, Vitamin E, Zeaxanthin, Zinc, Vitamin E *(Alpha-Tocopherol)*

Fatty Acids

- Arachidic-Acid, Behenic-Acid, Gadoleic Acid, Lignoceric Acid, Myristic Acid, EFA Omega 3, EFA Omega 6, EFA Omega 9, Palmitic-Acid, Palrnitoleic Acid, Stearic-Acid, Flavonoids Kaempferol & Quercetin, Selenium

Glycosides & Glucosinolates

- 4-(Alpha -L- Rhamnosyloxy)-Benzylglucosinolate, 4-(Alpha -L-Rhamnosyloxy), Senzylisothiocyanate; Niazinin A, Niazinin B, Niaziminins A & B, Niazimicin, Rutin

Isoflavones and Sterols

- 28-Isoavenasterol, Beta-Sitosterol, Brassicasterol, Campestanol, Campesterol, Cholesterol, Clerosterol, Delta-5-Avenasterol, Delta-7, 14-Stigmastanol, Delta-7-Avenasterol, Ergostadienol, Stigmastanol, StigMasterol

Minerals

- Calcium, Chromium, Cobalt, Copper, Fluorine, Iron, Lithium, Manganese, Magnesium, Molybdenum, Phosphorus, Potassium, Selenium, Silicon, Sodium, Sulfur, Vanadium, Zinc, Zirconium

Plant Phenols

- Caffeoylquinic Acid and Fat-Soluble Vitamins: Alpha-Carotene, Beta-Carotene, Vitamin A, Vitamin D, Vitamin E (Alpha Tocopherol), Vitamin E (Delta Tocopherol), Vitamin E (Gamma Tocopherol), Vitamin K. Water-Soluble Vitamins: Biotin, Vitamin B (Choline), Vitamin B1 (Thiamin), Vitamin B2 (Riboflavin), Vitamin B3 (Niacin), Vitamin B6 (Pyridoxine), Vitamin C (Ascorbic Acid), Folate (Folic Acid) and many others.

Moringa's Medicinal Biochemical Activities - *Here are a just a few of the 539 medicinal chemical actions that Moringa provides to the body:*

- Antiulcer (9)
- Vasodilator (9)
- Hypocholesterolemic (14)
- Antitumor (10)
- Cancer-preventive (19)
- Pesticide (13)
- Antiviral (9)
- Hypotensive (9)
- Diuretic (8)
- Fungicide (8)
- Antiseptic (7)
- Hepatoprotective (7)
- Antiasthmatic (6)
- Antiparkinsonian (7)
- Laxative (5)
- Antiatherosclerotic (6)
- Anxiolytic (6)
- Hypoglycemic (5)
- Antiherpetic (6)
- Antihistaminic (5)
- Antirheumatic (5)
- Antifatigue (5)
- Antimenopausal (4)
- Sedative (4)
- Antiprostatitic (4)
- Antidepressant (8)
- Cardioprotective (8)
- Antiosteoporotic (5)
- and 345 more!*

---

*For the full list of Moringa's 539 medicinal biochemical activities, see "Dr. Duke's Phytochemical and Ethnobotanical Database" on the Moringa.

*For more in-depth information see: Moringa Oleifera: Magic, Myth, or Miracle book By: Dr. Howard Fisher.

---

docofdetox.myzija.com

BRIDGING THE GAP BETWEEN SCIENCE AND NATURE

Zija® is the first available nutritional health beverage *(100% natural liquid dietary supplement)* from the nutrient-rich

Moringa Oleifera. Unadulterated Moringa Oleifera delivers nutrition that has systematically been removed from our food chain. That's why I'm thrilled to be able to share with you about Zija® Moringa. Here are a few reasons why:

WHY ZIJA® SETS THE STANDARDS?

Most Superfoods are not certified organic Zija®. Most Superfood Supplements contain ingredients that are not raw, but highly processed. There are so many differences in what may be made available in health food stores or anywhere else and the Moringa Oleifera in Zija® products. Let us start with the fact that Zija® moringa is: The correct varietal *(there are 58 varietals)* and the Zija® varietal is the most potent.

Organically grown *(and they control all the farms in the district so no windblown pesticides and fertilizers)* whereas most are grown anywhere. Zija® controls all the plantations in the district to ensure that no one is using any pesticides or fertilizers in the district. Handpicked and sorted. Most growers buzz down the tree and mix all the parts together bark and all.

Zija® Proprietary formula is comprised of five different Moringa components and does not include bark or roots *(which can be toxic)*.

Zija® plants are shade-dried. Most other growers save money by putting plants into driers causing loss of enzymatic activity due to temperatures above 104 F.

Also UV light degrades enzymatic activity and growers who use these techniques have plants with far less nutrient value.

Zija® plants are vacuum packed and shipped to United States for processing in an FDA approved facility that manufactures at pharmaceutical grade quality.

Food grade processing is all that is required for most other brands. Their criteria is the same as your local restaurant, on some table in a back room, not in a sterile facility.

> **Dollar for dollar nothing compares to Whole Plant Based Superfood Nutrition. Do your research, your life depends on it.**

ZIJA® SCIENCE - NOT SCIENCE FICTION

ZIJA® TRULY SETS THE BAR. Zija® is made to the highest standards, offering nutrients from five parts of the Moringa plant. To get these many nutrients in a totally bioavailable form from any other dietary supplement, food, beverage, combination of herbs, fruit, vegetable, other botanical, over-the-counter brand, or even a prescription medication is simply impossible.

SUPPORTED BY MODERN SCIENTIFIC FINDINGS.
Among these institutions are Johns Hopkins School of Medicine, the World Health Organization, the Center For Disease Control, and the National Institutes of Health.

100% BIOAVAILABLE. Unlike many popular fruit juice blends that are heavily pasteurized, artificially modified, colored or flavored, Zija® uses only all-natural, organic, non-GMO ingredients. No compromise.

ENZYMATICALLY ALIVE. Increased nutrient uptake due to increased hydration, high enzyme activity, and a balance of amino acids which are unmodified, as Nature intended.

PROMOTES HEALTHY CIRCULATION. Normalizes blood pressure with nutrient hydrators and vasodilators. Also contains antihistamine and antispasmodic activities for better respiratory circulation. Promotes natural serum cholesterol for heart and artery health.

SUPPORTS NORMAL BLOOD GLUCOSE. Today's standard diet is the main contributor to the explosion of diabetes. Zija® Moringa provides nutrients that help support and normalize blood glucose levels for hypoglycemia and diabetes.

NOURISHES THE BODY'S IMMUNE SYSTEM. Zija® Moringa Oleifera provides all nutrients needed for maximum immunity. Better overall cellular hydration, perfect electrolyte balance of potassium, magnesium and calcium and improved cell structure.

PROMOTES INTESTINAL FORTITUDE. Better digestion (high enzyme activity, high mucous cleansing, less burping, bloating and acid reflux) and elimination (promotes intestinal flora). Effective in reduction of harmful bacteria and harmful microorganisms (parasites, yeast, fungus, etc.)

DELIVERS ANTI-INFLAMMATORY SUPPORT. Inflammation is the primary contributor to today's most common diseases, including cancers, cardiovascular disease, dementia, depression, arthritis, attention deficit disorders, diabetes, obesity, and many more. Several compounds in the Moringa plant, include Quercetin and Caffeoylquinic Acid, are known to support normal anti-inflammatory activity in the body.

PROVIDES NATURAL ANTI-AGING BENEFITS. Zija® wide array of anti-oxidant nutrients, which include Zeatin, Quercetin, Omega-3,6,9 Fatty Acids (naturally occurring), which are 100% absorbable, as opposed to such things as fish oil and flax oil which are partially or non absorbable.

IMPROVES OVERALL BRAIN FUNCTION. Zija® Moringa provides mental and cognitive clarity. Restores the needed nutrients for the brains neurotransmitters, which relay, amplify and modulate brain functions.

KOSHER AND NONALLERGENIC There are no harmful ingredients in Zija®. Zija® is also Circle U Kosher & Parve, Hasidic Approved, and hypo *(non)* allergenic. Zija® Moringa is grown to the highest standards available for assured, consistent and empirical quality.

IMPROVES OVERALL METABOLISM. Zija® Moringa triggers the metabolism for fat burning and energy production due to its complete nutritional content.

PROMOTES DEEPER REM SLEEP. A perfect blend of serotonin precursors, which reduces sleep apnea *(breathing interruption during sleep)*.

PROMOTES ALKALINITY. Produces far lower lactic acid levels than eating animal protein. Zija® Moringa promotes an alkaline system whereas animal protein promotes acidity in body cells.

There are 58 different varieties Moringa Oleifera. Zija® is the only grower of the most potent variety of Moringa. Take the time to do your research as I did before you purchase an inferior brand.

WHY CANE SUGAR IN THE ZIJA® FORMULATIONS?

Health Benefits of Sugarcane

- Raw sugarcane has a left-spin to it so it is utilized by healthy cells, not diseased cells, such as cancer. Processed sugar has a right-spin to it so it is utilized by diseased cells, such as cancer. Raw sugarcane does not stimulate cancer growth.
- Sugarcane is low on the glycemic index and contains phosphorus, iron, magnesium, calcium and potassium as trace minerals.
- Sugarcane juice has been found to be very beneficial for preventing as well as treating sore throat, cold and flu.
- Since sugarcane has no simple sugar, it can be enjoyed by type 1 diabetics without any fear, however, the intake should still be limited for people suffering from type 2 diabetes.
- Cane sugar provides glucose to the body, which is stored as glycogen and burned by the muscles, whenever they require energy. Therefore, it is considered to be one of the best sources of energy.
- Increases intracellular hydration
- Cane sugar improves the urinary flow and also helps the kidney to perform its functions smoothly, and is beneficial for gonorrhea, enlarged prostate, cystitis and nephritis.

- Cane sugar consists of carbohydrates, in good quantities, and serves to refresh and energize the body. It supplies instant energy to working muscles and for this reason, it is also known to maximize performance in sports and endurance. Cane sugar is good for digestion and can effectively work as a mild laxative because of its high potassium content.

Zija® has four world class Moringa Oleifera based product lines: Weight management, Pure Nutrition, Energy and Skin Care. Within these categories there are sub-categories that allow tailor made programs for detoxification, athletic performance and dealing with the stress of everyday life.

NEVER SAY NEVER

I can remember the day when a very good doctor friend of mine called me up and said, *"Darrell, have I got something amazing to show you."* Well, let me backtrack a bit before we get into the *'amazing'.* After 26 years of being in the health business, I had created a worldwide presence that now kept me running just to maintain control. Great! My dream came true, a big successful health business, hundreds of products and a staff to help manage 100-150 calls a day.

I was starting to rethink and reevaluate the direction of my life and profession.

I can remember the day when I mentioned to a patient that I needed to reevaluate my passion, for I felt it was no longer simple and effective the way Natural healing was meant to be. As soon as I said this I could hear a quiver in her throat and to say the least, it made me think deeper. If I am doing my job effectively then I should be empowering those I consult. I then mentioned it to a few others and Bam, same type of reaction. The reaction I am talking about was one of fear. Until that time I truly thought that I had been empowering my patients to the best of my ability. This is why our focus is no longer on treatment but training because people must learn to Be The Cure they are searching for!

I decided at that point that if I could not come up with a system that totally empowered my patients to stand on their own two feet, take back their life, their health, their power, then I would no longer be able to continue along that path.

To make a long story short, 6 months later I am now living in the country of Panama, with the responsibility of going to the vegetable market, fish market and surfing with my kids. A year and a half later, after climbing the mountains of Nepal by myself, for myself, searching within to tap into my next great adventure, I then made my way back home to Kelowna. I knew at this point that I wanted to create a simple yet effective program that would put my patients back in the driver's seat. I wanted to educate people so they could take back control and Master their own health.

I had written two books previously and I never wanted to write another, but this crazy book would not leave my thoughts. No matter how hard I tried to push it away it kept pushing its way back into my thoughts, my dreams, my life.

I told him that I was writing a book and that this time I wanted to create a system that empowers people to become their own healer. This, after all, is where it all begins and ends. If we're not totally empowering our patients then we are doing a great disservice to them. I knew for sure I did not want to hear about the latest, greatest product and definitely did not want hear about a referral system or be part of some type of 'Rah Rah' hype marketing. I have been there, where the story is amazing but the product is not.

In many cases I was able to duplicate the products for a fraction of the standard cost. A year and a half later, through my own research, I realized that my doctor friend was truly onto something. This was the perfect match; the most simple and effective product that I had come across in my 30 years of practice. The most powerful health product nature has ever created is brought to the forefront with the help of a world class formulator who was able to break the code to enhance the delivery system and make the worst tasting product in the world be a delight to drink. This is a true health practitioner's dream. To deliver all the nutrition in a great tasting drink that the human body needs not only to maintain, but also to have the health you always knew you were entitled to. It is so important to me to have found a product that is foundational to everyone. A one size fits all product in regards to age, gender or any health condition. Even more important, a company that is in alignment with my journey.

When we align ourselves with like-minded people anything is possible. Invest is short for investigate, I did my research, make sure that you do yours. *Some will say if it's so good why haven't I heard of it before?* I did not hear of it until almost 2 years ago and it's been around since the Egyptians. It's the planet's most valued nutritional superfood when it comes to human existence for our children's children and us. It doesn't end here. Zija® has created an equal playing field, where everyone shares, everyone learns and everyone pays the same price for the planet's most dense phytonutrient superfood. This is what I am about, what this book is about, what life is about; creating equal opportunity for all.

In my business when you mention marketing or money it is felt to be taboo but the reality is many people have not financially built into their budget a nutritional support system that helps protect their health and way of life. Zija® is a company that thinks outside the box because when you have the world's most powerful superfood and a world where the majority of the population is malnourished and on a crash course to disease, we must create a financial bridge so all are equal on the playing field of health and wellness. Remember you're being 'marketed to' all the time. *Ask yourself, what is Dr. Wolfe trying to market to me right now and does he have my family's best interest and mine at heart?* Be an example to your loved ones, Be The Cure **U** Wish To See, Be The Light.

"TOMORROW'S BODY = WHAT YOU PUT IN IT TODAY"

When the majority of the population discovers The Whole Truth about Whole Plant Based Superfood Nutrition then our full potential will become limitless. United we stand; Nature's Way, the only way. The World Watch Institute reports that the number of people who are *"overfed but undernourished"* is at 1.2 billion, now equaling those starving from lack of food.

The Moringa tree can provide real solutions to the ever rising *"epidemics"* of diabetes, obesity, and the other degenerative diseases caused by nutritional deficiencies. In the years ahead, we will be hearing a lot more about this miracle-tree superfood. Zija® International™ is the world's largest sustainable grower of organic Moringa. It owns millions of locally maintained acres in India, where the climate is optimal to produce the most nutritionally potent crop. Become part of the Moringa Family Tree.

United we stand, No one gets left behind.

LIVE LONG CORE STRONG

"You can't exercise your way out of a bad diet. 80% of the results U will achieve are through Structured Water, Whole Plant Based Food and Super- food Nutrition."

- Dr. Darrell Wolfe, Doc of Detox

THERE'S MORE TO THE CORE THAN A SIX PACK

There are 4 foundational keys to having and keeping a functional body throughout life. Your body is a walking, talking credit card; use it wisely. Remember, if you don't make regular healthy payments, or if your payment is counterfeit, **U** will no longer be functional.

Hydration - See Water the Structure of Life Chapter
Nutrition - See Foods and Frequency Chapter
Gentle Daily Whole Body Cleansing - See Nature's Way Chapter
Exercise - Keep Reading This Chapter

The most important group of muscles in the body is the core muscles, not the back muscles like most therapies focus on. 60-70% of your immune system resides in the core. The core, literally, is what gets you up, holds you up and keeps you alive and healthy. Your core plays a major role in almost every movement of your body. Core muscles allow you the ability to complete the tasks that you need to perform every day.

It is the vital 'foundation' of all your body's movements, whether you are walking, carrying a heavy grocery bag, picking up your grandchild, making love, keeping your balance on a slippery sidewalk, playing sports and let us never forget about digestion, assimilation and elimination. Most people are becoming increasingly inactive; we spend most of our 'awake time' sitting, with our core muscles relaxed.

WHAT ARE YOUR CORE MUSCLES?

Relaxed is one thing but the average person has grown comfortable with the major part of their immune system falling down and out, this would be the large intestine along with the core muscles. This is why the Supercharge Your Life – Advanced Training Course was created. To guide anyone who wishes to Master his or her own health on a permanent basis. We must teach and deliver total health to our patients because as practitioners we must restore that which has been taken from them. Health Independence.

Many people think that their "abs" or abdominal muscles, are the only core muscles. The core muscle group includes all of the muscles that make up your torso which keeps your body stable and balanced. It takes many different muscles working in harmony to keep your body aligned during all of your many daily activities.

Your core muscles are comprised of 2 types of muscles: *stabilizers and movers*. The 'stabilizer muscles' are attached directly to the spine and support its every movement. The 'movers' are the muscles that support the stabilizer muscles and work with them to move your body with ease.

BENEFITS OF A STRONGER CORE

Your core includes your back, shoulders, chest, sides, hips, pelvis, buttock muscles and the abdominal muscles. The core forms a sturdy bridge that links your upper and lower body. Similar to the trunk of a tree, your core muscles need to be strong, but always flexible. A weak or inflexible core *(due to internal scar tissue formation)* will drain you of your energy, making you susceptible to injury.

No matter where movement begins, it ripples upward and downward through the core. That means a strong, flexible core is vital in everything you do.

Everyday Activities - Even the most basic activities of daily living, like bathing or dressing, call on your core muscles.

The Work Place - No matter the task, whether lifting, twisting or typing, a strong core makes for good posture. Good posture prevents injuries and makes you look and feel younger.

A Healthy Back - Low back pain can be prevented with core exercises such as: Yoga, Core Master Twisting, Rebounding and Core Vibration.

Sports and Other Activities - All athletic activities are powered by a strong core, even sexual activity requires core power and flexibility.

Housework and Gardening - Lifting, bending, twisting, carrying, hammering, reaching, mopping, vacuuming, and dusting all rely on a strong core.

Bathroom - Without a strong core your large intestine will sit limp within your pelvis and you will need to push to have a bowel movement. This will cause hemorrhoids and may even cause a hernia.

Balance and Stability - When you begin to lose your balance or become unstable, look to core exercises that will create a strong foundation and restore your balance as well.

Good Posture - Poor posture leads to injury, creates wear and tear on the spine and interferes with your breathing. Shallow breathing is shallow living. Good posture from a strong core projects confidence and prevents both injury and muscle pain.

When exercising, if your main focus is on your abdominal muscles, you will create an imbalance in your hips and back muscles. This can lead to injuries and reduce your athletic ability. This is where whole core exercises for strengthening, lengthening and toning are essential. Your core muscles are responsible for all your body's strength, including your arms and legs. I have seen countless people at the gym with a weak core and no matter how much they work their arms and legs they do not achieve their desired affects.

Your core is everything. It houses your digestive tract, liver, pancreas, stomach, lungs and heart, but most importantly; the Mother of All Organs, your Large Intestine. You will never reap the rewards **U** deserve in your exercises if your focus is only on the External Core and not the Internal Core, composed of your organs. When your organs lack tone and stagnate with waste, you will be kissing more then your butt goodbye. You know the roll that is hanging over your belt; well that is the Mother of All Organs, your Large Intestine in a comatose state. *How's that for down and out?* For the ins and outs on this very intoxicating topic please read *The Scoop on Your Poop* and *The Domino Effect of Acidosis.*

But, as we have seen time and time again, when we restore our core externally but not internally the aging process goes into high gear and the Poop hits the fan and causes us to lose more than just muscle mass and strength. We lose our Health. Just ask Woody. He's stiff as board (snap, crackle, pop). You now have a choice; follow the herd or lead the pack.

Your core abdominal muscles play a major role in some of your most important bodily functions, such as breathing, vomiting, coughing, urination and excretion. Do you experience two, 5-7 inch long bowel movements a day without grunting, with the feeling of complete elimination? If no, then you have entered The Domino Effect of Acidosis. How many times have you heard this one? *"I just bent over to pick up something and snap went my back..."* or *"I reached for my pills and my back went out..."* The rest of this story is: There's no more core, it has fallen on the floor.

CORE BENEFITS

Now we've established how important it is to tone and detox your Internal and External Core. Your aim here is to achieve and keep core stability.

That means you need to balance core strength exercises, with core flexibility exercises, which will strengthen, lengthen, twist, detox and tone.

A strong 'Internal' and 'External' core supports overall circulation and digestion. The major part of your immune system lives in the large intestine. *How's that working for you?*

A strong 'Internal' and 'External' core supports your lower back. This is an area that can easily develop crystallization and internal scar tissue that can lead to painful knots. A weak 'Internal Core' is one of the main causes of internal scar tissue formation in body tissues, joints and organs. A strong 'Internal' and 'External' core will help relieve cramps and PMS around the menstrual cycle. Gently Cleansing on a daily basis, strengthening, lengthening, twisting and toning core restore exercises for a pain-free healthy body.

A strong 'Internal' and ' External' core will restore your body's strength and stamina because its job is nutrient uptake and waste elimination. Go to the source, go to the Core and Be The Cure **U** Wish To See.

A strong 'Internal' and 'External' core will restore whole body balance that affects your emotional balance. A sense of calm, steadiness, and support once established in the physical will travel to your mental and emotional health because everything is connected to the Core. If you need a reason for having a strong 'Internal' and 'External' Core your body will show you all the health benefits that support it! If that's not enough, just take a look at the so-called average, normal person's core.

Stored fat in the core area, particularly in the abdominal area, will increase your risk of heart disease, Type 2 Diabetes and some cancers. Losing fat and building strength in the core can help improve your balance, stability, posture and reduce the risk of back problems. For the fastest results, combine proper exercise with a Whole Plant Based diet, Superfood Nutrition, Gentle Daily Cleansing and ample Structured Water. **Live Long Core Strong.**

RIP AND TEAR

Moderation is the keyword when it comes to endurance or strenuous exercise, as with all things in life. We have been taught unhealthy belief systems in so many areas of life, not only regarding diet and detoxification but also in physical fitness. Unhealthy exercise does not stop at athletes and the general public. You would be shocked how many fitness trainers and so- called experts are continually injuring themselves and their clients. The no pain, no gain, run faster, run harder, run longer, lift more weights, do more repetitions, *"If you don't hurt, you didn't work hard enough!"* mentality is an epidemic of abusive exercise, mentally and physically.

Anyone who runs marathons or is involved in extreme workouts would be shocked if they could see inside their body. Running and extreme workouts create internal scar tissue buildup in the muscles, tendons and ligaments and also to the heart. Repeated extreme exercise or long-distance running will create acidity that will deplete you of your essential minerals and oxygen. It will form crystallization and internal scar tissue damage in, around and on the heart. This can lead to patchy myocardial fibrosis in up to 12% of marathon runners. Long-term exercise of this nature can cause premature aging of the heart and muscles, stiffening of the heart, joints and muscles and an increase in arrhythmia and atrial fibrillation. Enlarging of the heart and thickening of the heart muscles are known as 'athlete's heart' - go figure. The heart will heal unless it is repeatedly damaged from internal scar tissue that builds up through incorrect exercise, diet, nutrition, low quality water and ineffective therapy.

This situation is only getting worse due to the way exercise has been marketed. If a person is in pain during or after exercise they will need to rid themselves of the internal scar tissue and crystallization they have caused through the no pain, no gain theory. You will eventually lose your agility, elasticity, flexibility, strength and set yourself up for a life of stiffness, pain and premature aging, unless you are taught that there is a better way, a healthier way.

Give me an injury that other therapists have been forced to give up on or just keep trying to treat without success and I will give you and show you amazing results within the first few minutes of the first treatment. At the 'Doc of Detox' we give a money-back guarantee on all treatments that we provide while training you to Be The Cure that you search for. Almost all therapies deliver superficial and temporary results at the best of times.

In the past, it was thought that internal scar tissue damage, within the body was temporary and would subside, but this has been proven to be incorrect. A published report, by Mayo Clinic stated that internal scar tissue, within the body accumulates over time. You know the spot where you keep having reoccurring pain? When you're tired or when you're stressed? That is scar tissue. Where the real problem lies is this internal scar tissue becomes a permanent fixture for people because practitioners have not been properly trained to understand it, much less deal with it or eliminate it. The older this internal scar tissue becomes, the less elasticity and flexibility it has and the more dehydrated and brittle it becomes. This is where the old saying *'stiff as a board'* comes from. This condition is caused from being highly acidic... **but wait a minute, isn't that the major cause of cancer!?**

Most exercise programs taught today along with the average lifestyle validates the need and importance of the courses we teach at the International Training Institute of Health. Our Wolfe Deep Tissue Therapists are helping thousands to bridge the gap between just living the so-called, normal life and having a life filled with joy and a pain-free body.

Most people today have been conditioned to run from pain even though they continue to live with it each and every day, learning to wear it like a badge of honor as if there are no other answers but only specialists, drugs, alcohol and marijuana: Drugged up and dumbed down. Just know that with our advanced training with internal scar tissue, we are the answer for those searching for a pain-free life, without drugs. When you invest into a Wolfe Deep Tissue Therapist - Whole Life Coach you will then be taught how to become the Master of your health and well-being and live pain-free on a permanent basis. It's training over treatment that patients need for permanent success to become The Cure they have been searching for.

As a physical therapist, I see this day in and day out, in the athletes and patients I treat. Just ask Woody, he's stiff as a board. Snap - crackle - pop! The older the internal scar tissue gets, the more brittle it becomes. Extreme sports and extreme workouts are making our International Training Institute and Wolfe Deep Tissue Restoration Therapy extremely popular in this 'take the pain' climate.

Okay, so you're halfway through your workout and suddenly you feel a twinge in your back but because you're no quitter, you push through. Moments later you hit the Wall of Pain. The pain is localized and your muscles spasm and you're now on the injured list.

The biggest mistake that trainers, athletes, or anyone performing an exercise program can make is ignoring their body's messages and continuing to push through the pain. Repetitive exercise with intensity will always show to be damaging to tissues, joints - and yes - even to the heart. Just because you lift more weights and run or cycle with a large group where everyone pushes through their pain, does not make it right or healthy. Don't be caught up in the herd *(hurt)* mentality.

The problem that most people do not realize is that the continual inflammation, caused through improper over-contracting exercise, places extreme stress at the joints and creates micro tears in muscle tissue throughout the body. This continual inflammation causes the body to continually create fibrin as a protective mechanism to wall off the pain. This will lead to severe internal scar tissue build-up, which will, in time, shorten the muscles, tendons and ligaments. This in turn will reduce the range of motion, elasticity and flexibility and will even cripple you as this internal scar tissue hardens as we see with the majority of the elderly and those who are drugged. Runners, weightlifters and extreme sport athletes need Wolfe Deep Tissue Restoration to counterbalance these over-contracting, high impact sports, if they wish to not pay the price as they age.

Inflammation and pain is the first sign of internal scar tissue formation. There is nothing worse than an injury that won't heal. It does not matter how much ice, heat, Advil, Motrin or anti-inflammatories you take or apply, they may suppress your pain but only to have you unknowingly rip and tear because they have numbed out the warning signs of re-tearing the internal scar tissue that has never been addressed properly with the correct therapy to break it down and remove it in the first place. Sometimes a chronic injury will last for months or even years with no real end in sight.

Repeated visits to the doctor for prescriptions to numb the pain, visits to physical therapists, registered massage therapists, chiropractors and acupuncturists will help reduce the problem but until the crystallization and internal scar tissue is removed and the patient is taught how to prevent it from returning, their search will go on. The major cause of injuries now and always will be the invisible bonds that bind and restrict; internal scar tissue formation that eventually turns into knots will shorten the muscles, ligaments and tendons they are attached to. This cannot be stretched out, even though most therapists and trainers teach this, for it will only rip and tear again because of the lack of circulation and elasticity due to it being fibrotic internal scar tissue. The same scar tissue that attempts to prevent damage also constricts future movement, binding tissues and organs, causing unnecessary pain and suffering when the *healing* has supposedly already completed. A transverse penetrating technique is clearly necessary if such tissues are to be restored to their healthy state. Proper guidance on diet and detoxification is essential to restore and maintain your health on a permanent basis.

In the majority of the population the internal scar tissue has hardened like cement and a change in diet alone will not be enough for true healing to take place. Tissue that was once elastic, pliable, toned and self-healing now receives hardly any blood flow due to its fibrous, crystalline structure. This tissue now lacks needed oxygen and vital essential nutrients and has the consistency of beef jerky. From a frozen shoulder to a cancer tumor you will have crystallization and internal scar tissue formation when incorrect information and ineffective treatment is given. The patient needs to be trained to be the cure they have been searching for if permanent success is their goal.

When you remove the hardened internal scar tissue, crystallization and scar tissue knots, then you will be free of pain and able to perform at your optimum once again, as a healthy active person at any age. This hardened internal scar tissue must be manually broken down and then flushed out of the system with ample quality Structured Water, Gentle Daily Cleansing, a Whole Plant Based Diet along with Superfood Nutrition and Core Exercises. This is why we believe at the International Training Institute of Health that any physical therapist without proper training in the art of deep tissue restoration and a correct foundation of nutrition and detoxification will never provide what their patients truly need – whole body healing requires a whole body approach.

The slight limp in your walk, the inability to raise your arm above your head or touch your toes or being unable to shoulder check while driving has become a normal of life for the majority. When the majority suffers from it we call it normal because we've been taught herd mentality. This is what happens when incorrect information and ineffective therapy seems to be the only choice.

These troublesome conditions are due to lack of counterbalance exercise such as stretching, foam rolling, yoga and core twisting. Other factors that increase acidity within body tissues include: an incorrect diet, incorrect or insufficient water - and excessive contractual exercise. When a muscle, tendon or ligament is damaged the body has only one repair method, internal scar tissue formation, all due to a safety mechanism called inflammation that only you can turn off.

Internal scar tissue delivers great short-term benefits by restricting movement of the injured area thus preventing further damage. But here's the downside; internal scar tissue also brings with it negative, long-term affects if not broken down and removed. The same internal scar tissue that attempts to prevent damage will also constrict movement and binding tissues and organs, causing unnecessary pain and suffering when the 'healing' has supposedly completed *(oops).* Over time this internal scar tissue will harden like cement. The decreased range of motion that this causes locks the muscles, tendons and ligaments of the body in place causing decreased circulation, thus weakening muscles and eventually draining the life force from you.

This is why the average, so-called normal person suffers from premature aging, which leads to that old saying, *"I just can't do that anymore but I wish I could."* Until you are prepared to take proper action by backing off excessive contractual exercises, by loving and respecting your body with core building, strengthening, lengthening and toning exercises, **U** will continue to suffer!

Traditional treatment techniques require months to fully resolve injuries to tissue and joints if they ever truly do. *Do these other therapies really heal or has the body just walled off the pain again with more internal scar tissue until the patient rips the so-called healed injury again a year or two later?* With Wolfe Deep Tissue Restoration Therapy along with a diet based on whole plant based foods, Structured Water and daily gentle detoxification sets the pace for life-changing instantaneous results on a permanent basis no matter the condition or the age of the patient, this I promise.

For sports related injuries and sports performance enhancement you must eliminate the internal scar tissue that binds **U**. It's vastly important to recognize and eliminate the true cause, not just ignore and cover it up, or you will have a full-blown injury that will put you on the sidelines for life.

We don't have to stop these constricting, contracting exercises we love, but we need balance through restorative exercise and therapy to keep internal scar tissue at a minimum.

If you run or workout at the gym for 30 minutes, match that with 30 minutes of stretching, yoga or core twisting. You will be pain-free, injury-free and in balance.

My personal prescription to prevent injury and to really rid the body of pain is to properly hydrate with ample Structured Water, eat a Whole Plant Based diet, Superfood Nutrition, Gentle Daily Cleansing, Core Master Twisting and Rebounding, Foam Rolling and last but not least, find a yoga studio that has maintained the true philosophy of Yoga. Set yourself free from the invisible bonds that bind **U**.

Our society is drowning in dysfunctional belief systems when it comes to effective bodywork and patient empowerment. When you experience a sports injury or any other type of injury, if you do not have the internal scar tissue broken down after the injury has supposedly completely healed, I guarantee you it will come back to haunt you when you are older.

How many times have you heard someone say, *"Yeah, this pain is back from when I..."* and *"This pain is back from when I..."* and *"This one is from when I...."* People wear their injuries like a badge of honor because they don't know any better, because their doctors and therapists do not know any better. But I know better. So when you're tired of reminiscing over the war wounds that haunt you, I'll bet you that if you have this internal scar tissue broken down and you implement the guidelines we have discussed in this book, this will be the end to your painful story. We cannot do better until we know better or should I say you cannot do better until you find a practitioner that can treat and teach you to know better.

This is why the Supercharge Your Life – Advanced Training Course, the Family Retreat Treatment & Training and the Couples Retreat Treatment & Training were created. To guide anyone who wishes to Master his or her own health on a permanent basis. We must teach and deliver total health to our patients because as practitioners we must restore that which has been taken from them. Health Independence.

YOGA

THE ART OF MASTERING THE BODY

"Yoga is a physical discipline which lengthens, strengthens, tightens and tones while performing a deep relaxing detox on the tissues and organs of the body. Yoga is about allowing and opening up on many levels with its foundations being in awareness itself. Awakening the ability to notice and feel the movement and muscles themselves. I was 8 years old when I first heard the word 'yoga'. I was at church when the Pastor said India was trying to infiltrate their religion into North America by the way of introducing an exercise known as Yoga. I forgot about this until we started this chapter. Actually, Yoga is about not controlling, or some restrictive dogma. It is the science of the body, about allowing without judgment and letting go that which does not serve U. Such as stiff joints, tight muscles and body pain. Release your invisible bonds."

- Dr. Darrell Wolfe

THE PERFECT COUNTER BALANCE FOR A CONTRACTED CULTURE

The art and science of yoga is dedicated to bringing you more in tune with your body. Its objective is to assist you in exercising the breath and body in unison for a greater awareness of your potential. This can be a perfect compliment to the drive and effort of other practices. In short, it is about creating balance and harmony with and throughout your whole body. Yoga's breathing techniques can and will improve an athlete's performance- enhancing powers along with their mental and psychological focus. Simply knowing Yoga's breath management techniques can help build resilience. The deeper effect that comes from practice is an overall sense of well-being. That sense eventually becomes the motivation to practice; a deep part of **U** seeks well-being, not accomplishment.

What does basketball superstar LeBron James, tennis champion Andy Murray and all the NFL players of the Seattle Seahawks have in common? They all used this same technique to recover from their elite workouts: Yoga.

With sports such as hockey, tennis or football, we only use 10-15% of the body, whereas with yoga every muscle, joint and organ is put to the test. Yoga works every body system: cardiovascular, skeletal, muscular and endocrine. Yoga oxygenates the blood, generating more energy when you finish the exercise as opposed to draining the body of it like many other workouts.

Athletes like Wayne Gretzky, Kareem Abdul-Jabbar and John McEnroe have heightened their performance levels through practicing yoga. By combining mental, physical and emotional strength, they became better athletes at their chosen sport. Yoga is not just an exercise; it teaches us how to calm the mind and body, enabling us to handle stressful situations more successfully.

HOCKEY & YOGA

Ryan Getzlaf practices yoga, he says, to "keep limber." But what about the spiritual side of the practice? *"I'm not really that kind of a yoga guy,"* says the Anaheim Duck's Captain. *"It's more just the stretching."*

Net-minder Tim Thomas says, *"My whole career has been about proving to people that I can play in the NHL and be successful, so Yoga is a part of that journey."*

Retired NHL forward, Georges Laraque kept his 6-foot, 243-pound frame flexible by sticking to a strict training exercise program that included Yoga.

"I'm strong, but not because I bench-press six plates," he says. *"If you do yoga, you don't need to do weights that much because it's like a weight exercise, but instead you're using your body."*

Laraque explains, *"When you work on your flexibility it makes you less prone to injuries."* He adds, *"I believe yoga is really something that will help young athletes get stronger, improve their core and become better athletes."*

In addition to the physical benefits, Laraque also enjoys the calming aspect of Yoga. *"The game can be stressful on your body and on you mentally,"* he says. *"You go there and it's just really relaxing. It's really quiet and it's hard to explain but you don't think of any problems or anything else. It's so relaxing and purifying."*

There are some top NHLers who use yoga Nidra as a relaxation practice. Yoga Nidra is a guided resting practice, a full body meditation led though audio.

Some use it to prepare on game day, after the morning practice or to completely relax (a power nap!). Some use it for post-game or next day recovery relaxation. It is a deeply restorative practice.

More and more athletes and people who just want to stay fit are realizing that with proper yoga they are able to recuperate from strenuous workouts and injury much faster, especially for those reaching middle age. Yoga also helps to prevent the typical aches and pains commonly associated with aging and an inactive lifestyle.

What Is the Counterbalance to Intense Workouts?

Professional and amateur exercisers are turning to yoga to restore their body between other sport and intense exercise programs. Even Tony Horton's best-selling "extreme" fitness DVD series, P90X, has an accompanying Yoga program, *"Yoga X"* Tony recognized this need to balance out his aging *(54 year young)* body and natural contraction from resistance training. Extreme workouts are contractual and shortening in nature. Yoga will counterbalance this with its strengthen, lengthen and detox techniques.

Athletes often carry tension in the core of the body. Specifically in the Illiopsoas, the deepest hip flexor. When that muscle is out of balance, or over tight, it can cause other muscles to react and so on. I know of an interesting experiment regarding this muscle, sometimes called an emotional muscle, as it can react to fear, etc. When a group of healthy people go to a scary movie, the psyche does not know it is just a movie, and the body reacts. When those people get up out of their seats after the movie, they feel 'old' and hunched over. That is the Illiopsoas! So, play that out in life. When there is fear, anxiety, suffering there will be a reaction in the body.

Athletes need to recognize this. One of the NHLers, who has to fight, has learned to relax through the Yoga Nidra mentioned above. From his relaxing yoga practice he can relax his deep core, the pelvis and hips, and in turn the groin. He has had no groin injuries since beginning this practice. The moral of the story is sometimes we have to release muscles (especially deep in the body), instead of work them.

Pounding The Pavement

Runners in particular need yoga to counterbalance this over-contracting high impact sport if they wish to not pay the price.

During the course of an average mile run, your foot will hit the ground 1,000 times. The force of impact on each foot is about 3-4 times your body weight. It's not surprising to hear runners complain of bad backs, knees, tight hamstrings and sore feet.

The pain most runners suffer from is not from the running itself but from the imbalances that running causes. If you bring your body back into proper alignment through the practice of Yoga, you can run long and hard for years to come. In fact, running and Yoga make a good marriage of strength and flexibility.

Strong physical activity stresses our body similar to the *'fight, flight or freeze'* response of the autonomic nervous system. Yoga has been proven to re-set the autonomic nervous system to a more parasympathetic *(relaxed)* state, which is what is needed for the body to heal and recover. In its basic philosophy, the science of Yoga, it does not have to be scary, in fact it takes the scare away from life's reactivity.

If restoration and detoxification of body tissues is the goal then an athletic yoga practice would be counterproductive. Athletes need to lean towards a yoga that calms the nervous system, rests and restores the body.

If yoga is your only form of exercise then you may want to lean towards a more fast-paced, flowing style using more intensive deep stretches.

Would an athlete become too flexible from doing Yoga? The answer is no. When Yoga is done correctly using proper breath techniques and the ego is left on the sidelines, Yoga will help prevent injury and give the athlete a competitive edge at their chosen sport. A proper Yoga practice will take you to the edge of sensation, but not push through it. Very flexible people should focus on stabilizing techniques and muscle engagement in their yoga practice, rather than expansion and flexibility. The more muscular person would want to focus on lengthening and releasing. The battle of the sexes can definitely show up in a yoga class. Women tend to be more allowing, and even have a natural flexibility, while men do not. If men do not leave the ego at the door *(and some women!)*, there will be a battle in the body. Don't let that be **U**.

Technically speaking, the more athletic a person is, the tighter they will be. Especially in the sport specific muscle groups that are affected, for example: runners-hamstrings, throwers-shoulders and one-sided sports. These individuals should use caution when starting yoga. An aggressive approach without proper guidance and body awareness will only get you into trouble.

Usually the more athletic a person is the more contracted their muscles are. Yoga is a valuable tool to restore balance in this situation, but must be respected; this is where aggressive becomes more passive.

If your exercise of choice were weightlifting, Yin Yoga would be a perfect counterbalance, as these classes focus on slow stretches with deep breathing.

Yoga is the best form of exercise in relieving stiffness from other sports or just life itself.

When muscles become fatigued, they build up with lactic acid, and yoga, with its strengthening and lengthening postures, relieves the tension and the waste is flushed away. Yoga does not deplete energy from your body like a gym workout where your body can become fatigued after the workout. Instead, it will not just increase but restore your energy, making you feel more balanced and invigorated.

If you are new at yoga you may want to participate in a class that focuses on alignment and a balance of strength and stretching. Yoga done correctly will develop strength to the same degree as it develops flexibility. A perfect blend not just for the athlete but also for all walks of life.

When it comes to Yoga, I recommend that you do an authentic style. You want to make sure that you get the emotional and psychological benefits of yoga practice rather than just a physical workout. Yoga does not care how you look or the shape you're in, it welcomes all. Yoga will test your personal boundaries by increasing your flexibility, endurance and muscle strength at a level comfortable for you.

Always remember, if you can leave your ego and expectations at the door, you will create a partnership of understanding with your body and you will begin your own yoga journey. For the first time in your life, you will pull back the curtains, release the invisible bonds and Master your mind and body and tap into your true potential.

In finishing, I would like to say that we live in a world of contraction, we need counterbalance. Somewhere we can create a new Belief System that opens our minds and our bodies. For myself, My fitness center of choice is called *'Oranj Fitness'*. Find a yoga studio that provides a wide range of levels of fitness to suite your needs with a flexible schedule to fit your lifestyle. If you would like to experience yoga and you're in my neighborhood, tell Oranj Dr. Wolfe sent you and your first session is free! *Live, Laugh, Love, Lengthen, Strengthen, Detox & Tone!*

REBOUND YOUR WAY BACK TO VITAL HEALTH

The Best Exercise To Rebound Your Immune System!

It's quoted by NASA as *"The most efficient and effective exercise yet devised by man."*

Rebounding is also known to be the most effective exercise for the prevention of cancer and for assisting the body to heal from cancer.

Who Can Rebound?

Moms, dads, children, grandparents... Rebounding is suitable for all ages and abilities! Rebounding is a rhythmic movement from one foot to the other with moderate height and a gentle pace.

Stabilizing bars can be fitted if you are unsteady, disabled or handicapped. When you incorporate weights, rebounding benefits are amazing for building and toning. Rebounding is the rhythmic movement from one foot to the other - to a moderate height - at a gentle pace.

Bouncing or jumping on a rebounder is a Cellular Exercise, your body has about 60 trillion cells. The 2-4 G forces *(gravitational pull)* involved in bouncing squeezes out the toxins. During the brief weightless period when the body is suspended in the air, the lower pressure in the cell promotes the movement of nutrients into the cells. Thus the flow of materials to and from cells is improved. It is like every cell individually exercising in your body.

When cells become weak they can rupture easily, this weakens the immune system and shows up in the form of inflammation, pain, internal scar tissue formation and eventually disease. When your cells are strong, you will have more energy and vitality. This cellular exercise results in cells being 5 times more active due to the increased G-force response.

What Is Rebounding?

Rebounding is a safe, cardiovascular muscle-building exercise with very low impact. It is a series of controlled movements performed on a mini trampoline. Running and jogging are very stressful on the feet, ankles, knees, hips, back and the spine. Rebounding decreases the shock and stress by 95% while still giving you a cardiovascular muscular workout as beneficial as running. 20 minutes of rebounding equals 1 hour of running as a cardiovascular workout. Rebounding is more effective for fitness and weight loss than cycling, running or jogging. 12 minutes of rebounding burns about 10 more calories than 12 minutes of jogging.

Cardiovascular Fitness - Exercising on the trampoline lowers the risk of cardiovascular disease in 3 ways:

1. By strengthening the legs so that they act as an auxiliary pump for the cardiovascular system. This lessens the strain on the heart.

2. The increased pulse rate strengthens the heart.
3. The strengthening of both the voluntary and involuntary muscular systems makes the entire system work more efficiently.

Rebounding = Lymphatic Detoxification of the Body

The body's lymphatic system is a network of vessels that transports nutrients and drains toxic products from tissues. This system does not contain its own pumping mechanism and relies on external pressure, including breathing and muscular contraction, to propel its contents through a system of one-way lymphatic valves.

Rebounding greatly increases lymphatic circulation more than any other exercise. Rebounding causes a pumping action that pulls waste out of cells and pushes nutrients and oxygen in. The most important fluid to immune function in the body is lymphatic fluid. Lymphatic fluid clears the system of toxins and waste products. Two-thirds of your body's white blood cells are found in the lymphatic fluid and are responsible for eliminating bacteria, viruses, parasites, fungi and cancer cells.

Rebounding is a zero-impact exercise that provides many benefits for U, all the way down to the cellular level.

The benefits of rebounding include:

- Reduces body fat and water retention *(lymph congestion)*.
- Firms legs, thighs, abdomen, arms, and hips.
- Increases agility and improves sense of balance.
- Lowers blood pressure, triglycerides and cholesterol.
- Promotes regular elimination and relieves constipation.
- Strengthens the musculoskeletal system - core building.

- Protects the joints from chronic fatigue.
- Gentle impact increases circulation of heart and lungs.
- Rehabilitates heart problems by assisting circulation through low impact exercise.
- Strengthens the heart.
- Improves resting metabolic rate as calories are burned for hours after exercise.
- Prevents chronic edema.
- Promotes tissue repair.
- Benefits the alkaline reserve of the body.
- Benefits body alignment and posture.
- Enhances digestion and elimination processes.
- Promotes deeper and easier relaxation and sleep.
- Helps to reverse aging process of muscle degeneration.

Rebounding is a year-round exercise that can be done inside or outside and is easily portable for those who travel. It's fun, it's easy, it's safe and you can do it at home to your favorite music or even while your watching TV!

Buying A Rebounder

You get what you pay for! Inexpensive models can be stiff and don't offer adequate cushioning and support. They will be hard on joints and lower back. If you cannot buy a good one, I would suggest you wait until you can. Your joints will thank you for it!

Invest In A Quality Rebounder

- A stable 6-leg design - cheaper 4 leg models are known to topple over
- Detachable legs – for easy storage

- A solid, but responsive, spring system – to ensure adequate support for your joints
- A non-slip mat – for those trickier maneuvers!
- Spending 20 minutes on a rebounder a day will help you tone and firm your body in just six weeks.
- The reason it's so effective is because your body feels an increased gravitational (G) force at the bottom of the bounce. This can be equivalent to 2 or 3 times your bodyweight with minimal stress to the joints and tissues of the body. Every cell in your body will respond to this perceived 'stress' by strengthening and toning, creating a more vibrant, resilient **U. BE THE Master OF YOUR BODY REBOUND BACK TO HEALTH.**

For the Best Quality Rebounder Made, go to: www.docofdetox. com/ultimaterebounder

TWIST YOUR WAY TO A HEALTHIER LIFE

STRENGTHEN - LENGTHEN - TWIST, DETOX AND TONE

Everybody that is not in good physical shape runs from the word 'twist'. I guarantee you that, if you're the type of person that runs from the word, twist, then you're probably not in shape. When you gently twist while you exercise, you are performing an important movement that stretches, tones and detoxifies your core. This movement helps to readjust and align your spine on a daily basis. This is one twisting action you don't want to be without.

"Age is not a factor when it comes to health and vitality," but this statement is not correct if you are the *average, normal* person that follows the herd.

Are U the type of person who is sick and tired of rip and tear exercises that tone and strengthen but accumulate toxic waste *(acidity)*? Over time, these exercises will create inflammation, pain and internal scar tissue formation.

This will cause strength, elasticity and mobility to decrease while pain and injury increase. When you continually tighten to tone, you need counterbalance to keep your body's circulation open to maintain peak performance. If circulation is not maintained, waste will build up in joints, tissues and organs. This will block nutrients and oxygen from reaching and entering tissue cells, interrupting the rest, repair, restore and tone phase at the cellular level.

Are U the type of person who would like to tone up and build muscle along with having a cardio workout that is in perfect balance from beginning to end?

Are U the type of person who would like to have a full body, muscular workout while restoring mobility back to joints and aligning your spine to creating a stronger, straighter and more flexible you?

Are U the person that wishes to rid your body of pain and premature aging? Are you the type of person that wishes to detoxify your joints, tissues and organs of that which does not serve you?

CHAPTER 26 - LIVE LONG CORE STRONG

Say goodbye to those love handles and that muffin top and say hello to a strong core, toned tummy and a smaller waist due to less waste.

The answer is a fun, easy and effective twisting exercise that detoxifies the body while giving you a great cardio workout. This exercise strengthens, lengthens, stretches, tones and detoxifies your body tissues all at the same time. Weightlifting, running, biking and other exercises like this are mainly a *contracting* movement.

They cause a build-up of acidity in the body tissues. They block and eat up your nutritional reserves and create internal scar tissue. This is why we must stretch, twist, rebound and practice Yoga to counterbalance these *contractual* exercises. Products like The Core Master facilitate a twisting action effectively removing toxic waste from the muscles and organs while increasing circulation, nutrition and oxygen into the tissue cells, similar to the twisting action you would use to wring out a wet towel.

This will probably be the smallest, but most powerful, piece of exercise equipment you will ever own. Core Master not only improves strength, flexibility and endurance of the abdominals, but also tones all of your muscles and internal core organs. The rotating platform will improve the balance and coordination of a person at any age, which in turn will restore healthy posture. Even 20 minutes a day will send you on your way toward your desired goals. There are techniques for stretching and toning and others for stretching and muscle building, but they all detox due to the twisting action on tissue, joints and organs.

Always build your workout gradually. As you become more familiar and confident with this equipment you will increase the intensity of the exercise. Do not over-twist and make your muscles sore. Love your body and start slowly to prevent injury.

In with the good and out with the bad as you become a lean, toned, health machine. Why not have the body you desire without the downside of rip and tear. Let's do the *twist*, love your body as **U** build, tone and detoxify creating a pain-free, energetic life. **Take Life On.**

To Order Your Core Twister, go to: www.docofdetox.com/coretwister

BEAUTIFUL SKIN

THE ONLY FOUNDATION YOU WILL EVER NEED

"True beauty grows from the inside out and from the outside in. Build a strong foundation. Drink Life In & Stay Young."

- Dr. Darrell Wolfe, Doc of Detox

LOVE THE SKIN YOU'RE IN

The beauty about the body's largest organ is that you can nourish it from the outside in and the inside out. We know the food chain is broken and we are not getting enough nutrients from the food we eat. To add insult to injury, the skin care industry has learned very well from its big brother; the pharmaceutical industry. Some of the ingredients in beauty products aren't that pretty. US researchers report that one in eight of the 82,000 ingredients used in personal care products are industrial chemicals, including carcinogens, pesticides, reproductive toxins, and hormone disruptors. Many products include plasticizers (chemicals that keep concrete soft), degreasers (used to get grime off auto parts), and surfactants (they reduce surface tension in water, like in paint and inks). Imagine what that does to your skin, and to the health of your loved ones. We do have choices. You can prevent premature aging and yes, even turn back the hands of time.

It's unfortunate that many doctors and skin care specialists will ignore any connection between diet, skin health and the large intestine.

Many people unknowingly miss the opportunity to make major improvements in their skin. That ends here. Simple life changing strategies for healthy skin from the inside out and the outside in.

What is the largest organ in the body?

YOUR BEAUTIFUL SKIN!

What organ is responsible for one quarter of the body's detoxification everyday?

YOUR AMAZING SKIN!

What organ eliminates two pounds of acidic waste daily?

YOUR RESILIENT SKIN!

What is one of the most important elimination organs of the body?

YOUR AWESOME SKIN!

What organ requires 33% of all the blood that is circulated in the body?

YOUR LIFE-GIVING SKIN!

When the large intestine, liver and blood become overloaded with toxic waste, what organ will display this with problems?

YOUR MIRACULOUS SKIN!

What organ is the last on the list to receive nutrition, yet the first to shows signs of malnutrition or deficiency?

THE SKIN YOUR IN!

Are U ready to learn Simple Life Changing Strategies to turn back the hands of time and truly love the skin you're in?

Your skin mirrors your inner health. The look, feel and texture are all indicators to the state of your health from the inside out and the bottom up.

The large intestine is the mother of all detoxification organs. When your skin becomes sluggish due to lack of Whole Plant Based Nutrition and Gentle Daily Cleansing and Structured Water your body will become polluted.

Guess who must pick up the slack? Your skin is a primary indicator of a toxic large intestine. As soon as your internal body becomes toxic, it will spread out, into and through your skin. This will cause your skin to become slack, irritated, itchy, wrinkled and yes, now you look and feel older than your age. Remember your skin is a mirror of your internal health. Every time you look in the mirror you will get a gentle reminder of things to come when you slack off with nutrition, hydration and detoxification.

When your internal well-being starts to crumble, skin conditions such as rosacea, acne, boils, psoriasis, rashes and premature aging will result because you lack an understanding in the art of body talk. You either pick up the slack or more than your skin will crack.

One purpose of your skin is to keep your organs, tissues, capillaries, muscles and bones in place. Your skin is known as the third lung; it inhales and exhales, allowing your body to breathe. How cool is that! It's alive!

Your skin is a respiration organ. This is why it is so important to nourish, hydrate and detoxify your body's largest organ, from the inside out and the outside in. When we use toxic substances on our skin, whether it's chlorinated water for drinking, showering, bathing or your so called skin care products, just know that you are choking the skin you're in.

This is a living and breathing **organ**, so if you can't eat it, don't **treat** it to your skin.

Eliminating waste through your skin is essential for remaining vibrantly healthy. Sweating helps to cool the body and eliminate acidic toxic waste. Your pores must remain healthy and open for business 24/7. If you decide to use deodorants, antiperspirants and toxic skin care products or bathe/ shower in chlorinated water, just know that you will be shutting down your body's largest organ and triggering unwanted symptoms.

Studies have shown a link between these toxic products and breast cancer, liver cancer, skin cancer and other forms of cancer. These products shut down the body's natural ability to open up and eliminate toxic, acidic wastes through the skin. The next time you see someone with skin problems, you now know the answer is not just an external one. It also lives deep within the bowels.

POISONING THE SKIN YOU'RE IN

Your skin and your large intestine must remain flexible to stay healthy. A healthy large intestine and healthy skin do not sag or crack. They hold their tone and shape. Minerals, amino acids, enzymes, fatty acids and vitamins are all needed for tissue integrity, but they must be able to reach the cellular level or they will have little or no effect on your body.

Just because a company tells you they have a natural product with all the nutrients to achieve the health your body deserves does not mean it is in the correct formulation that the body can recognize or assimilate on the cellular level. This is true whether it is a nutritional supplement or a skin care product. Read 'Superfood Nutrition' for a deeper understanding. Buyer beware, buyer be wise; there's knowledge and then there's **The Whole Truth.**

STRUCTURED WATER-*BEAUTIFUL SKIN*

Structured Water is not just important but critical for preventing disease, premature aging and degenerative conditions involving your skin and large intestine. Structured Water is essential for the uptake of nutrients from your food and for proper elimination of fecal waste from the large intestine. This is the same for your skin; it needs plenty of Structured Water to deliver the needed nutrients and eliminate toxic waste at the cellular level. Compare this scenario to a river that does not have an ample supply of water.

Stagnation will occur and the natural balance will be lost to mutation and dis-ease. What comes first the Mosquito or the Swamp? Terrain is everything. If you wish to get rid of the bugs then change the environment by increasing the water flow so natural balance is restored. If you had a manure pile in your living room, would you build a box around it to hide it or find a way to remove it? If stagnation occurs in your tissue cells, like the river, you will breed dis-ease. Like the riverbed without ample water, wrinkles will form in your skin due to dehydration. Structured drinking Water is the body's first and foremost healing food.

Water lubricates and keeps skin soft and supple. The best example of this is baby's skin; hydrated and healthy. When you lack Structured drinking Water your tissues will shrivel, lose tone and age prematurely; losing their ability to function properly. Your skin will lose its flexibility and elasticity due to the crystallization and internal scar tissue formation from lack of Structured drinking Water. It is a fact that people who drink ample amounts of Structured Water, live a Whole Plant Based

Lifestyle and cleanse gently on a daily basis look years younger than their age. Healthy skin reflects a healthy large intestine. You cannot have one without the other.

Read **'Water - The Structure of Life'** for a deeper understanding.

FEEDING THE SKIN YOU'RE IN

There's a saying that all answers lie within. The food chain is broken and so now is our health. When a person suffers from nutritional deficiencies, especially minerals and amino acids, they will appear to age much faster than usual. This is known as premature aging due to malnourishment and acidosis. And you thought malnourishment was a third world problem. You're witnessing a nation that is suffering from the stiffening and hardening of their fibrous connective tissue in their skin. Read *Web of Destruction* and *Scarred For Life* for a deeper understanding. Hardening body tissue is crystallization and internal scar tissue formation that can be found all the way down to the cellular level. The skin no longer snaps back into place. It has entered the wear and tear phase just like your joints going snap, crackle, pop. All disease and body pain have crystallization and internal scar tissue. *Just ask Woody.*

When you cleanse your body of toxic waste, drink and shower in life supporting water, restore the essential nutrients with Whole Plant Based Superfood Nutrition along with skin care that promotes life at the cellular level. **U** will age gracefully.

It only stands to reason that the Planet's most **dense phytonutrient plant** would contain all the ingredients, not just for a healthy vibrant body, but also for young radiant skin. **Take Life In!**

Read 'Superfood Nutrition' and 'Water: Structure of Life' for a deeper understanding on cellular nutrition.

LIFE-GIVING SKINCARE

If U Can't Eat It, Don't Put It On Your Skin. If it does not feed your skin at the cellular level then what's the point?

Beauty is more than skin deep - It's Cellular.

FACE THE FACTS

The Chinese have used face reading for thousands of years as a way to detect and diagnose diseases. This is a Chinese medical practice called, mien shiang or mien xiang (pronounced *MYEN-SHUNG*), that started in China nearly 3,000 years ago to help prevent illness. The skin on your face is able to give a glimpse of your current health and things to come. Face readings are not set in stone but they do warn of possible health issues. Your face will reflect changes in your health faster than any other part of your body.

Our faces provide clues to the path in which our health is going, by the facial lines and marks such as discolorations, spots, creases and indentations. Your face can predict the age at which certain problems may appear by the location of various marks. The bigger and darker these marks are, the more severe the problem may be. When You Face the Facts... **U** can then release the true healer from within.

DIAGNOSTIC FACE READING MAP KEY

1. Bladder/Reproductive System is the entire scalp, jawline & chin including the lower lip.
2. Small Intestines is the middle of forehead.
3. Bladder, the right side of the forehead is the right side of the bladder & the left side of the forehead represents the left side of the bladder.
4. Liver, it shows up in between eyes, outsides of eyes and as the eyeballs themselves.
5. Kidneys, the areas around, above & below each eye are the facial demonstration for both the right and left Kidneys.
6. Stomach, Esophagus & Upper Stomach on the left cheek & the Lower Stomach with the pyloric valve connecting the Stomach & Small Intestines on the right cheek.
7. Adrenal Glands, the right Adrenal Gland is on the outer corner below the eye on the right, the left Adrenal Gland is on the outer corner below the eye on the left side.
8. Heart, it shows up as the nose, upper lip area below the nose & both earlobes. Heart issues score this way, the nose 20%, the upper lip area below the nose 20% and each earlobe is worth 30%.
9. Endocrine Strip or Endocrine System (major glands), on each side of face beside the nose, from the top of the nose along the cheek, beside the mouth to the bottom of the sides of chin.
10. Lungs, the right & left lung appear in the hollows of the cheeks.

| 11. Ileocecal Valve, one each side of face, beside the nostrils we find the connection of the Small Intestine & the Ascending Colon. |
| 12. Ascending Colon, on each side of face, on the sides above the upper lip. |
| 13. Transverse Colon, on each side of face, corners of mouth. |
| 14. Descending Colon, on each side of face, below corners of mouth. |

BODY TALK

Signs & Symptoms of the Skin

It is believed that your face can tell your life story.

The ears and the top part of your face are believed to represent the earlier part of life, from preteens to early 20s. As you grow older, corresponding facial areas move downward from your eyebrows. Many prestigious Western medical journals such as *'The American Journal of Cardiology'*, have recognized a connection between a diagonal earlobe crease and coronary artery disease in people under age 70.

- **Slightly green facial hue:** Decreased liver function
- **Overly red facial hue:** Heart disease or high blood pressure
- **Yellowish facial hue:** Low function of spleen and stomach
- **Darkened facial hue:** Low kidney function
- **Whitened face:** Low lung function

EYES: Reflect the liver. A change in color can be a sign that something is wrong - especially if the color is yellow. If your eyes show yellow, contact your doctor.

- **Folding between eyebrows:** Low-functioning lymph, weakened immune system.
- **Red spots and/or pox around the eyebrows:** Increased likelihood of flu, or sign of flu in recent past.
- **Reddened eyebrows:** Overactive nervous system, lack of quality sleep.
- **Reddened eye sockets:** Inflammation in the kidneys or back pain.
- **Black eyes or black/brown spots:** Low kidney function.
- **Dark skin around eyes:** Deteriorating kidney function, likelihood of kidney 'stones'.
- **Violet swelling around eyes:** Could be ovarian, cervical, vaginal, breast complications.

NOSE: Reflects the condition of the heart. A red nose or a line through the nose can indicate heart issues. A large bulbous nose can indicate overconsumption of alcohol or enlarged heart. If the tip of the nose is swollen and has a blue hue heart circulation is poor and may indicate heart attack.

- **Reddened nose:** Bladder inflammation or back pain.
- **Swelling veins on the nose:** Deteriorating function of kidneys and bladder.
- **Black moles between nose and lips:** High levels of acid and toxins in the body.
- **Darkening of black moles between nose and lips:** Possible sign of cancer risk.

UPPER LIP: When a woman notices changes on the middle of the upper lip, she may be experiencing fertility issues, fibroids or hormonal changes.

- **Red lips:** Overactive stomach.
- **Blue lips:** Heart weakness or problem.
- **Dark lips:** Low function of spleen and kidney.
- **Pox spots or cold sores near lips:** Stomach ulcer.

CHEEKS: Reflect the condition of the lungs. A change to the hollowing of your cheeks may be a sign that you are not breathing properly.

- **Red cheeks:** Overactive liver.
- **Region between chin and ear has depressed scars, pox marks, or other anomalies:** Poorly functioning intestine. If this region becomes red, possible sign of impending diarrhea.

LARGE PORES: Indicates general toxicity.

PIMPLES OR RASHES: Indicate body toxicity, irritants, chemicals, pollutants, environmental hazards, together with deficiencies of essential fatty acids and vitamins A and C.

ACNE: Acne is a condition representing total body toxicity, poor food choices, exhaustion and nutritional deficiencies. Excessive consumption of refined salt and hormonal imbalances are also contributors. If acne is located in the chin area, it is typically due to hormonal or ovarian disturbance. It represents an excess of estrogen and a lack of progesterone. This imbalance produces deep nodular acne.

Acne that appears on the back and other areas of the face are due to excess cortex hormones from overactive adrenal glands or an under active thyroid.

Adrenal hormonal involvement has a masculinizing effect and i s often accompanied by excess facial hair in women. Bacteria present on the skin's surface live off the poisons released from the pores. Excessive pore excretion combined with these bacteria block and congest pores causing the formation of pimples and redness known as acne.

All these conditions are connected to a lack of a Whole Plant Based Superfood Nutritional Lifestyle, quality water and a lack of Gentle Daily Cleansing.

DANDRUFF OR OILY SCALP: Indicates an extreme oil deficiency.

ITCHING: Itching occurs when the skin is congested with toxins or irritants. The nerve endings react to these substances, which cause us to scratch. Itching is a warning sign that there is a decrease in the blood flow because toxins and wastes are being retained in tissue. Some itching can be a result of contact with a substance that creates a topical chemical reaction. Excess body acid can also contribute to itching, as can liver insufficiency or disease, body chemicals as in excess bile, and undigested proteins in the digestive system. Anemia, diabetes, hypothyroidism, low functioning adrenal glands, stress, worry and anxiety can cause skin discomfort. Coffee and medications have been known to increase the possibility of itching.

ECZEMA: Eczema is an inflammation of skin that is seriously depleted of essential oils. The dry crusts that form are surface cells that have died in large numbers and are flaking away as a result of this deficiency. This condition can include scaling, thickening, flaking and itching.

Eczema is often referred to as dermatitis or seborrhea and contact or photo dermatitis. These conditions are often seen in individuals with tendencies towards allergies. Dr. Philip Incao has stated that vaccines induce severe outbreaks of eczema in young patients, in addition to escalating the incidence of ear infections, asthma and bowel inflammations.

PSORIASIS: Psoriasis is a chronic condition that produces small to large varying sizes of patches of silvery scales. It is a blood-born disease where the white blood cells migrate into the uppermost layer of skin. Attention to dietary habits improves such conditions immensely and often involves fats and metabolism of fat soluble vitamins. Prolonged attention to dietary changes and daily bowel cleansing is essential to eradicate any existing evidence of psoriasis. When psoriasis presents itself, we can be sure that there is a lack of coordination and efficiency of both detoxifying and eliminating systems. This causes congested lymphatic fluids resulting in the seepage of toxins into the gastrointestinal tract. Poor carbohydrate metabolism is related to deficiencies of calcium, magnesium and zinc.

A balance of sodium and potassium is necessary for relief from psoriasis and other related skin conditions. When the nails and scalp are involved, this condition will most likely spread to other areas of the body. Conventional treatments include such things as applications of cortisone cream and coal tar, which we know addresses the external manifestation rather than the internal origin.

Until you treat the cause, you will always be chasing symptoms. Please understand that a nutrient deficiency is still a symptom. Single supplementation will never address the root cause. Whether it's a pimple, psoriasis or cancer, what we need is whole body healing. This is accomplished through Whole Plant Based Superfood Nutrition, quality water and Gentle Daily Cleansing. End of story!

SKIN CANCER: There are many different types of skin cancer. The two most common being basal cell carcinoma and squamous cell carcinoma. The good news is that both are successfully treated if caught early enough. Malignant melanoma is a more serious disease and is more rare than the other types.

Skin cancer often, but not always, originates in moles although moles are not necessarily risky. It is highly advisable to monitor any changes that occur in moles such as asymmetry, borders, red, white, blue or black moles and moles that grow beyond ¼ inch in diameter. The key is and always will be a healthy body. A healthy body does not fall prey to sickness.

READING THE SKIN YOU'RE IN

Our bodies are amazing and they speak to us, if only we would listen! The following symptoms may be clues to possible conditions within the body.

- **Bruises:** Lacking rutin, Vitamin C
- **Dry skin:** Lacking natural oils of the skin
- **Calluses:** Crusty edges of feet, lacking essential fatty acids
- **Cold puffy hands:** Hypothyroid
- **Corns:** Poor nutrition and circulation

- **Crusty skin:** On base of knuckles of fingers and/or on elbows or knees indicates lack of quality oils in diet (coconut, olive oil)
- **Dry peeling skin between toes:** General circulation, allergy to gluten, wheat, sugar, and tension
- **Elasticity loss:** Low rutin, proteins, collagen, zinc
- **Flabbiness:** Drooping of skin under jaw, tiredness, poorly functioning adrenal glands or pituitary gland.
- **Flakey:** Lack of natural oils in skin
- **Gooseflesh:** Fear, anxiety, tension, lymphatic congestion
- **Gray sallow skin:** Excess toxins, lack of oxygen, lung related disorders, asthma, serious illness
- **Hair growth excesses in abnormal locations:** Fever, anemia, emotional disorders, heart conditions
- **Moist, sweating:** Toxicity, overactive thyroid, high blood sugars, and kidney stress
- **Moist palms:** Liver problems. If palms are cold, there are adrenal and sugar problems. If warm, thyroid over-activity.
- **Moles, warts or small-localized skin growths:** Often indicate existence of toxicity of internal organ associated with this point
- **Night sweats:** High sugars, 'fever' response of body to release toxins
- **Oily skin:** Lacking oil. Oil deficiency triggers sweat glands to secrete excess sebum as an oil substitute. Can also indicate vitamin B deficiency.
- **Orange hands/palms:** Frequently seen in diabetic individuals.
- **Pale skin:** Poor blood circulation, anemia, exhaustion or burnout.

- **Pigment spots near base of thumb and forefinger:** Left hand = fatigue, low functioning spleen.
- **Pigment spotted skin:** Watch for specific acupuncture points, use as indicators.
- **Redness:** Overactive adrenal glands, lacking antihistamines, excess stress, fear, and anxieties.
- **Redness (dark):** Of face, lips = poor circulation, inefficient heart, congested liver, alcoholism, infection.
- **Red (lower arms/legs):** Circulation
- **Redness of skin of soles of feet:** Liver congestion, blockage.
- **Rough skin of nose with soreness and pimples:** Low vitamin A, liver congestion.
- **Scars, thick heavy:** Vitamin A, C, E and protein deficiencies.
- **Sensitivity to sunlight:** Lack of body oils, vitamin A, E, F.
- **Skin tenderness:** Toxins or pollutants in skin.
- **Slow healing:** Lack of proteins, vitamin A & C, zinc, silicon and calcium.
- **Small red spots:** Same as bruising, lacking digestive enzymes & vitamin C.
- **Stretch marks:** Lacking quality proteins, kidney stress, and lymphatic congestion.
- **Visible capillaries:** Spider veins on cheeks - liver problem.
- **Thin wrinkled skin:** Protein deficiency, lack of vitamins, (A, C, E and F) rutin, damage from toxins.
- **Yellow or orange skin:** Blockage of liver, gall bladder, jaundice or anemia.

As you can tell, different symptoms show different nutritional deficiencies. It may seem that there are many different causes for all these different conditions. I assure you, there is only one cause; the food chain is broken. Embrace a Whole Plant Based

Nutritional Lifestyle, Gentle Daily Cleansing and quit poisoning your skin. Let your body do what it was meant to do. Heal You!

HEALTHY SKIN TIPS

- Whole Plant Based Superfood Nutrition
- Healthy, regular bowel movements
- Dynamic Structured Water - drinking and bathing
- Fresh and raw foods, organic when possible
- Quality air & deep breathing techniques
- Steam baths, saunas
- Natural skin care
- Dry skin brushing
- Coco Salt Glow
- Core exercises
- Rest and relaxation

Nothing is written in stone. Use these tips as a gentle guide to better health. Your body will continually talk to you even if you're not listening or answering its call to action.

Let us find the strength to Face the Truth that we are the Masters of the Skin We Live In.

CASTOR OIL PACK

Healthy skin reflects a healthy large intestine. You cannot have one without the other. *What is the most important muscle group in the body?* The abdomen. This muscle group helps decide whether you will digest and eliminate effectively. If you're flabby on the outside, expect worse on the inside. A toned abdomen will give you a well-toned, healthy body.

Rubber Ball Roll

While lying down rub a tennis ball or hand ball around the abdomen from right to left in a clockwise circular motion 25 times; focusing on areas that are tender or blocked. Rubber ball roll can be done at any time or just prior to a castor oil pack.

Castor Oil Pack

The castor oil pack can be used on any body part to help reduce pain and increase range of motion and detoxification. Due to our modern so-called civilized diet, lack of exercise and the continual presence of gravity, our abdominal organs slowly but surely fall into the pelvic girdle that is located at the waistline. The main contributor to this problem is the colon. It is the last seven feet of the digestive system.

The digestive system has three main steps; these are digestion, assimilation and excretion. These three steps are performed in the abdominal region. The abdominal region is responsible for your health and vitality. Your large intestine is the body's waste disposal unit.

Through improper diet, constipation, pregnancy, or lack of exercise, this muscle, known as the colon, has not received proper nutrition or tone so it's now falling down and out, or down and in with thinner people. The majority of the population has a prolapsed *(dropped)* colon. I have yet to meet a person whose assembly line is not knotted and twisted and fallen on itself, even the best food will be left to putrefy.

This problem will not just cause blocks in the large intestine but it can lead to the following:

- Prostate Problems
- Cramps
- Internal Problems
- Intestinal Gas
- Impotence
- Low-Back Problems
- Endometriosis
- Kidney Problems
- Tipped Uterus
- Hiatus Hernia
- Swelling (Edema)
- Stomach Ulcers
- Painful Period
- Scar Tissue & Cysts
- Hemorrhoids
- Digestive Disorders
- Varicose Veins
- Pregnancy Disorders
- Constipation
- Colon Disorders
- Abdominal Distension

Reason For Use

1. Improved Digestion
2. Glandular Imbalance
3. Detoxification
4. Joint Difficulties

Materials Needed

1. Wool or cotton flannel cloth
2. Plastic covering (plastic wrap)
3. Electric heating pad
4. Towel

Instructions

Unrefined castor oil has a drawing action on the body, helping to get rid of toxins and tension build-up; also, it increases circulation to the area, speeding up the body's process of healing. The rectal implant is done after the castor oil pack routine.

Flannel or wool cloth must be used if the best results are to be achieved. The wool cloth should be three or four layers when folded. The abdominal pack should measure roughly 10 inches in width and 12 inches in length. Pour unrefined castor oil on the wool cloth covering the area. Make sure it is wet but not dripping with oil. Place it against the skin. Cover with plastic and then place the heating pad over medium and then high if the body can tolerate it. The pack should remain for at least one hour, two hours if time permits, as often as needed. After use, the cloth can be wrapped in plastic and placed in the refrigerator for re-use; this prevents the oil from evaporating. When the flannel cloth becomes discolored throw in wash. After 20 uses replace flannel.

Note: This pack can be used anywhere for tension, when tired or to alleviate pain.

Directions

- Soak flannel cloth with castor oil and place on desired body part
- Wrap with plastic around body to secure the castor oil pack
- Apply medium to high heat for at least 1-2 hours.

SKIN BRUSHING

The practice of dry skin brushing may not be new but it is a foundational anti-aging skin therapy. I thought it was important to share this amazing technique that is not only a great way to maintain healthy skin, but also helps you to maintain a healthy beautiful body. The ability of the skin to excrete toxins is of paramount importance to you. Unhealthy skin will not only make you look older but you will feel older than you truly are.

Dry brushing the skin may be one of the easiest and best ways in helping to support your body to detoxify. The skin is estimated to eliminate over a pound of waste each day through its pores and with the sloughing off of dead skin cells.

Where do you think all that dust in your house is coming from?

Dry brushing is an effective way to maximize the toxic elimination of backed up waste within the skin. Those who have inactive lifestyles or occupations, such as sitting in front of a computer screen all day, will experience stiff and sore necks and shoulders which can even affect the circulation in their arms, spine and lower back. Increased blood flow from skin brushing will help reduce stiff muscles and increase energy levels. Wherever there is stagnation there will be degeneration, which leads to crystallization and internal scar tissue formation. Increased circulation is revitalization of your life force.

Your skin, hair, fingernails and toenails are made up of a network of dead epidermal cells. All of these are a form of pulling toxins out of the body. Your sweat glands also play an active role in flushing toxins out of the body through perspiration. So again, I repeat do not clog your pores with unhealthy water, toxic skin care and antiperspirants.

As skin cells get closer and closer to the outer surface of the body, they lose their blood supply and die. This is an effective strategy of the body to eliminate wastes in these cells by sloughing off these old dead cells.

Dry brushing sloughs off old dead skin cells and the toxic debris within them, while initiating the development of new healthy skin cells. Every minute we lose over 30,000 dead skin cells, which are replaced by new healthy skin cells.

Dry skin brushing also helps renew your skin by aiding in the increased circulation and absorption of needed nutrients by eliminating clogged pores. Healthy, breathing skin is a major contributor to overall wellness.

Cellulite is produced by the body for storing toxins and acidic waste. Cellulite is comprised of toxic material that has been accumulated in your body's fat cells due to ineffective elimination. By improving lymphatic flow with skin brushing, it can help prevent the formation of unsightly cellulite. So, rather than liposuction surgery, how about using dry skin brushing, along with a Whole Plant Based Nutritional Lifestyle, Gentle Daily Cleansing, Structured Water and an enjoyable exercise routine. Together these daily routines will eliminate the toxic, acidic deposits from your body through your elimination organs, resulting in a happier, healthier **U**.

When you feel an itch what do you do? You scratch it, and in turn, the area turns red with a fresh blood supply and the natural healing process has now been turned on.

This is the same healing process that will follow a skin brushing session.

HOW TO DRY BRUSH CORRECTLY

Skin brushing sets into motion the natural healing process within your body. Dry skin brushing calms and rejuvenates the nervous system by stimulating nerve endings in the skin. Skin brushing also helps to improve circulation, firms your skin and tightens your muscles. Dry skin brushing stimulates the lymph canals to drain toxic mucoid matter into the colon; thereby, helping to purify your lymph system. This enables the lymph to perform its house- cleaning duties by keeping the blood and other tissues healthy and vital. Just another great reason to gently cleanse your colon daily so that you do not cause a back up and create a traffic jam that could lead to a break down. Increased circulation from skin brushing improves brain function and increases energy. So spoil yourself. **U deserve it.**

It is important to find a brush with natural bristles. Synthetic bristles often contain chemicals. Skin brushes are typically available at your local health food store. Purchase a brush with a long handle, so you are able to reach all areas of your body. Best-case scenario would be one that has a removable head with a strap for your hand. I enjoy a brush with firmer bristles.

Skin brushing should be performed once to twice a day. Skin brush when you wake up and before retiring. This will refresh the body in the morning and relax it before bedtime.

If you are feeling ill, please do it gently twice a day until you feel better. Skin brushing should take about 10 minutes.

Skin brushing in the morning dry and naked before your shower. Please sit if you have a problem with your balance.

It is best to begin brushing with long sweeping gentle strokes. Over time your skin will become toned and resilient, then you may wish to go deeper. The strokes should move toward the heart to improve lymphatic flow back through the venous system towards the heart.

Start at the bottom of the feet using a rotary or circular motion towards your heart. Apply very light pressure to start, avoiding broken skin, skin rashes, cuts, burns or areas where the skin is thin, such as the face or inner thighs. After you've finished both legs, move on to your arms. Brush from your fingertips, again towards your heart. Reach around and brush from your back towards your stomach or get a buddy to do it.

When dry brushing the stomach it is best to go in a clockwise motion as that works with the natural digestive flow and elimination. Brush scalp regularly to remove dead skin and to help promote hair growth. If you brush facial skin, be very gentle; better still, use a facial skin brush.

The skin should glow afterwards but should not be red or sore. A shower should always follow skin-brushing. This will remove uric acid crystals along with any dead skin that has been loosened.

Always start your shower with warm water and end with cold. When the water turns cold, let it hit your legs first. Do not let it hit your heart or head first as this can cause a slight shock to the body. Once the water is cold, do not linger.

Avoid hot showers unless a Structured Water unit is used. When showering in high temperatures, toxic chemicals are carried in the steam and into your lungs. Invest in a shower filter to prevent toxic poisoning to your body from chlorinated water. Your skin is a living breathing organ, keep it that way.

Baths can be unsanitary unless Structured Water is used. When the pores open, they allow the toxins to be reabsorbed. Also hot baths are more energy draining then relaxing. They can drain vital energy from you.

Soaps should always be used but do not soap the entire body. Areas to be soaped are the underarms, groin region and feet.

After getting out of the shower, dry off vigorously and massage your skin with pure organic coconut oil. Rub it into every part of your body and be generous. The only side effect is younger feeling and looking skin - Guaranteed.

Don't forget to clean your skin brush using soap and water once a week. After rinsing, dry your skin brush in an open, sunny spot to prevent mildew. For a thorough lymphatic cleansing, perform skin brushing daily for a minimum of three months.

Most individuals notice that they feel refreshed and energized after dry brushing. After several days of dry brushing, you may notice the gelatinous mucoid material in your stools. This is visual proof how the large intestine and skin are connected.

U GLOW

Your skin will feel silky smooth after this whole body exfoliation experience. Do not forget the icing on the cake. Lather your skin with organic coconut oil for that baby skin look and feel after every shower or bath. There is no body skin care on the market that will accomplish what you can do with organic coconut oil. Become self centered enough to focus on your health from the inside out and the outside in. **U** are worth it... Rub Life In.

When your skin needs a boost because you have that big date or you want that mini spa beauty treatment, it's time to put a Glow on. We have the icing on the cake skin treatment: The Coco Salt Glow Rub; also known as a salt scrub. If you're looking to remove old dead skin cells and to leave your skin hydrated, smooth and silky as a baby's bottom, we have the answer. This wonderful in home spa treatment is made up of epsom salts, Muscle Restore Essential Oil and organic coconut oil.

It is mixed into a paste-like substance that can be gently massaged over the body. Count on this treatment to give you that radiant glow **U** have been looking for.

The high concentration of magnesium in Epsom Salt really adds to the therapeutic value of this treatment. As discussed in *Contraction, The Chain Reaction*, magnesium is the one most neglected and under used by the majority of North Americans. This mineral is known as the relaxant, healing mineral along with being a great sleep aid. Epsom Salt also has other supportive minerals, which help in nourishing and hydrating your skin.

The National Eczema Association and the National Psoriasis Foundation recommend using the salt glow as a method to reduce the itching and inflammation caused by skin diseases. It can relieve the symptoms of certain skin disorders, such as eczema and psoriasis, but be cautious to avoid sores and inflamed areas with salt glow. Your focus is on the surrounding areas to support the body's natural healing process.

With areas of inflammation and sores, mix coconut oil with tea tree oil and apply often to encourage healing.

THE COCO SALT GLOW

BODY BOOST PROCESS

A Salt Glow helps to draw the toxins from the tissues, increases skin blood circulation thus promoting the growth of new skin cells. A Salt Glow will boost your immune system in fighting infections and illness.

- The pure essential oil Muscle Restore is used in the Coco Salt Glow. This special blend not only smells great, but also energizes and cleanses as it stimulates the senses and calms and relaxes the body.
- The Coco Salt Glow is simple but a very powerful therapy that has been used for beauty and to support the body.

- Coco Salt Glow should **not** be done after a skin brushing. These two are done on separate days. So put a Glow on.
- Take a large soup bowl, fill halfway with Epsom Salt and moisten it with quality water. The Epsom Salt should have the texture of wet sand *(granular, not soupy)*. Whatever the volume is of Epsom Salt use 10% organic coconut oil.
- Use 5 drops of Muscle Restore pure essential oil for every cup of Epsom Salt. Mix thoroughly into the moist Epsom Salt. Congratulations, you have just prepared a $100 spa treatment for $2.50.
- Step into the shower and have a warm shower to open your pores.
- Stay in the shower stall or tub. If there is nowhere to sit you may want to use a stool for comfort and safety. Make sure you are secure so you do not slip.
- With your hand, scoop about one tablespoon at a time, of the Coco Salt Glow into your palm. Start by rubbing mixture onto your right foot. Use the same routine as skin brushing.
- Rub briskly up and down in a short friction-type movement, rubbing the skin firmly enough that a red glow develops. Now friction rub the opposite foot. Repeat the procedure on both legs front and back, then the groin, hips and buttocks. Continue to the abdomen. Tighten the abdominal muscles and rub **U** Glow mixture in a clockwise motion from the right side of your abdomen to the left side. Be thorough. Moving upward, rubbing onto the chest with a light but friction type action.
- A towel can be used, which has been rubbed with some of the Coco Salt Glow to do the friction rub to the back. Continue until every area of the body has been covered.

Be very gentle on your face and neck. Do not skimp on the Coco Salt Glow.

- Now rub off the Coco Salt Glow from your body.
- Then shower with lukewarm water; going from warm to cold. When the water turns cold, let it hit your legs first. Do not let it hit your heart or head first as this can cause a slight shock to the body.
- Regular Salt Glows will help increase circulation of blood and lymph, ease constipation, swelling, skin conditions, fatigue, stiffness, headaches, tenseness, arthritis and hangover.
- If you feel like you're getting a cold or have one, then one of the best ways to stimulate circulation and your immune system is with a Coco Salt Glow. When you have finished, go to bed and rest for at least thirty minutes to enable the treatment to do it's magic. Self Indulge - You're Worth It - Rub Life In.

COO-COO FOR COCONUT OIL

1. Coconut oil is the best oil for cooking. Use it for baking, stir-frying and as a replacement for butter. Coconut oil is also great for deep-frying. It is better for high temperature cooking than vegetable oil or olive oil.
2. 2 tablespoons ingested daily will help boost metabolism, energize and alleviate pain.
3. As a replacement for cream in your coffee.
4. The best daily body lotion.
5. Can be used in making homemade lotion and deodorant bars.
6. Is a great eye makeup remover.

7. Reduces the appearance of age spots when rubbed directly on problem area.

8. Use during pregnancy to prevent stretch marks.

9. For all the nursing mothers out there. Use on sore, cracked nipples. Your little one will get the added benefit.

10. Use as a diaper rash cream on a baby's bottom.

11. Great for ridding baby of cradle cap. Massage into scalp and rinse with warm water.

12. Ingesting coconut oil supports thyroid function.

13. Excellent as a sunscreen to avoid burning.

14. Excellent for eliminating and preventing yeast and fungus infections when taken internally and applied externally to affected area.

15. The best massage oil ever. Add your favorite scent of Essential Oils for that ultimate massage.

16. For the hair, a little dab will do ya'. Excellent for split ends, anti-frizz and that healthy shine.

17. For an intensive oil treatment rub into dry hair, put a shower cap on or a plastic bag and leave on for several hours or just go into a sauna as I do.

18. A great body scrub for soft smooth skin: Mix with Epsom salts 10 to 1, rub on entire body then rub off and shower.

19. Goodbye chap stick, Hello coconut oil.

20. Heals skin injuries and infections faster when used topically.

21. Will sooth and heal perineum after birth.

22. Rub on feet to fight athlete's foot or foot fungus.

23. Helpful against psoriasis or eczema.

24. May support the body against Alzheimer's when ingested.

25. Mixed with apple cider vinegar, it is a great treatment for lice.

26. Use to make brainpower snacks for your child's lunch box such as coconut clusters.
27. Boosts energy levels and brain power when added into your smoothie.
28. Rub inside nose to help relieve allergy symptoms.
29. To increase milk supply nursing mothers can take 3-4 Tbsp a day.
30. Research has shown that coconut oil aids in digestion and the elimination of fungus, bad bacteria and parasites.
31. Has been shown to aid insulin levels.
32. To help improve the health of your gums, mix coconut oil and a drop of oregano or any other essential oil that can be ingested.
33. Helps improve cholesterol balance.
34. Mix a Tbsp into a hot lemon and honey drink to help speed recovery from a cold, flu or sore throat.
35. Use to replace vegetable oils in all of your favorite recipes.
36. Helps reduce appearance of varicose veins.
37. Speeds healing of sunburn. Use only when the heat from inflammation is gone.
38. Coconut oil is a great source of energy for the body when eaten and is not stored as fat.
39. As a personal lubricant that doesn't disturb vaginal flora.
40. Use as an antibacterial skin cream.
41. Makes for a great shaving cream.
42. Can help get rid of cellulite when used regularly on the body.
43. Keeps cast iron skillets in great condition.
44. Coconut oils anti-inflammatory properties can help reduce arthritis.

45. Can reduce itch from rashes, chicken pox, poison ivy and insect bites.
46. Can aid against acne when ingested on a regular basis.
47. Can stimulate hair growth when rubbed into scalp.
48. Aids in the absorption of calcium and magnesium.
49. The beneficial fats found in coconut oil have been shown to aid against depression and anxiety.
50. Can be used as a natural deodorant.
51. Mixed with baking soda it is a natural whitening toothpaste.
52. Excellent for pets with skin problems.
53. Has been shown to be helpful in some cases of Autism.
54. A great homemade vapor rub when mixed with the essential oil of Eucalyptus.
55. A tablespoon taken before each meal can sooth and improve digestion.
56. There is no better natural baby lotion than coconut oil.
57. A great hand moisturizer for beautiful skin.
58. Can soothe and aid healing of hemorrhoids when used topically.
59. Helps nails grow when rubbed on cuticles.
60. Helps in healing cold sores when ingested internally and applied to the area of concern.
61. **Before you or your children enter a chlorinated pool or salt water pool** rub coconut oil all over the body. This will provide protection against this very unhealthy environment. Just because everyone else swims unprotected in chlorinated water does not mean it's healthy.

OIL PULLING: NATURE'S MOUTHWASH

Oil pulling dates back to ancient times and is an Ayurvedic remedy that involves swishing a tablespoon of organic cold pressed oil in your mouth in the morning on an empty stomach for 20 minutes and then spitting it out. This procedure pulls out toxins from your body to improve not just oral health but overall health.

Reported Benefits

- Migraine headaches
- Hormone imbalances
- Tissue & joint pain & inflammation
- Gastroenteritis
- Skin Disorders
- Bronchitis
- Kidney functionality
- Sinus conditions
- Vision
- Insomnia
- Hangovers
- Allergies
- Heavy Metals
- Bleeding Gums
- Dry mouth
- Gums & throat conditions
- Whiter teeth
- Cavities and gingivitis
- Better Breath
- Stronger teeth and gums
- Jaw pain (TMJ)

HOW TO OIL PULL

Always use a high quality organic oil. Coconut oil is generally the oil of choice due to its strong antibacterial properties, but you can use any other high quality organic vegetable-based oil such as, sesame oil. Take a tablespoon of oil and swish it around in your mouth for 20 minutes.

This is a 20-minute process, so be gentle and swish slowly to prevent a stiff jaw. The oil will double in size as it pulls in saliva and body toxins.

Do not swallow, as the oil has been absorbing your body's toxins.

When you start, only go as long as you are comfortable with but your goal is to oil pull for 20 minutes. When complete, spit the oil out into the garbage because you will clog the drain. Then swish your mouth with warm water and natural organic salt. Finally, brush and floss as you normally would.

WHAT DOES OIL PULLING DO?

Oil pulling creates an environment that cleanses the mouth, as vegetable fat is an emulsifier by nature. This process has the ability to cleanse out harmful bacteria and reduce fungal overgrowth as well as reduce the toxic load on lymph nodes and other internal organs.

Coconut oil makes a great organic substitute for mouthwash as it has antibacterial and anti-fungal properties thanks to the lauric acid and monolaurin.

Coconut oil also contains easily digestible, fat-soluble vitamins such as, A, D, E and K. Vitamin A is known to be an immune booster. Vitamin E is known to have strong anti-oxidant properties, which aids skin providing protection against UV rays. Vitamin D is great for strong bones, teeth and immune system functionality. Vitamin K is good for blood-clotting and cardiovascular health. So open your mouth and pull the toxins out.

BEAUTY AND SKIN TONE

There comes a time in everyone's life when their skin begins to look and feel older. A time when they search for a way to slow down or even reverse an accelerated aging process. Aging tends to break down the polymeric bonding that gives young skin its fresh, smooth appearance. But where the fuel hits the fire, is that the food chain is broken leaving the majority of the population severely malnourished, toxic and dehydrated without realizing. On top of this we also use toxic skin care products, bathe in chlorinated water and take in other environmental pollutants, which severely escalate the aging process of the skin. As the skin area begins to exceed the face area, bags, folds and wrinkles increase due to the absence of these vital essential nutrients needed for cellular tone, elasticity and longevity. When you're hungry and toxic, you become weak and may even feel like you could fall down. How do you think your face feels?

BEAUTY IS MORE THAN SKIN DEEP

The surface of the skin is a direct reflection of the health of your large intestine and vital life giving nutrients that are made available for cellular rejuvenation of the skin. As we grow older, we deplete our cells of vital nutrients, thus, losing elasticity and tone to the facial muscles. True beauty is a reflection of the nutrition we feed the skin from the inside out and the outside in.

Just because an all natural nutritional supplement or a skin care product boasts that it contains all you need for healthy skin does not mean that it's in the proper form to be assimilated at the cellular level, where all the magic happens for youthful skin. Your outer skin is made up of several layers called epidermis. It is this outer surface that becomes rough, wrinkled and slack due to the decreased circulation caused from lack of Whole Plant Based Superfood Nutrition, a Whole Plant Based diet, skin care that reaches the cellular level, Gentle Daily Cleansing and ample Structured Water. Without these life support systems we build up lactic acid and uric acid in our cells.

This leads to crystallization and internal scar tissue build up in the deeper layers which causes decreased circulation to the skin. In turn this condition will starve your skin of its vital nutrients and oxygen also depriving it of cellular detoxification, which our skin must have on a daily basis in order to maintain its healthy look and feel. Healthy skin radiates a youthful look at any age. Read *Acidosis: What the Cell is Going On, Web of Destruction* and *Scarred for Life* to get a deeper understanding. **Love the Skin You're In and Face a New U.**

FOR A LIFETIME OF BEAUTIFUL SKIN CLICK HERE:
www.docofdetox.com/lighttherapy

LET'S GET MENTAL

"You were given this Life because you are Strong enough to Live it. Create Consciously! You are EVERYTHING!"

- *Dr. Darrell Wolfe, Doc of Detox*

MASTER YOUR EMOTIONS
OR THEY WILL MASTER YOU

The very definition of emotion can be exemplified with the first letter that constructs the word itself - The E standing for ENERGY. When E *(energy)* is combined with motion, Energy In Motion is created, with emotion being the final product. In turn, it is critical to learn to embrace emotions. Yo u can discover your emotional body by declaring that you believe that emotions can be trusted, are good, are safe, are beneficial and are there to guide you, not rule **U**. They should be seen as the beneficial pathway as opposed to being viewed as a blockage or hindrance. They are not in the way; they are the way. Anytime emotions are experienced within you, it is important to envision and experience what they are both causing and creating internally. It is a false belief of many that emotions are uncontrollable. You know the person, *"I can't control myself; this is who I am."* We can control emotion instead of allowing the emotion to control and consume us. This is achieved through neither feeling good nor bad about what is going on internally, just simply taking the time to recognize that these feelings exist. We need to live consciously. As long as emotions Master us, knee-jerk reactions will create pain and suffering for the body and for life itself. **The mind reacts, the heart creates. When you introduce the 'Healthy To 100' tools, tips and strategies, you will then become the Master of your emotions.**

A STAR IS BORN

Your life is a movie in the making. That's right, a movie where you get to be the writer, director and of course, the leading star. **You have created and orchestrated everything in your life**, for good or for bad *(law of attraction)*. You direct and create your own experiences. In turn, if you allow someone else to write your script it becomes random creating and it is no longer your movie. Although random creating allows us to potentially get what we want, it opens the possibility for us to also get what we don't want *(oops)*. You choose your experiences and life adventures. Once you realize this universal law of attraction and truly own it, you are able to empower yourself to live with passion, purpose and rise to your greatest aspirations. There is a saying: *"You are what you eat."* You must take this a step further if you desire to claim your true life's purpose. I believe a more precise statement would be, ***"You are what you eat, think and talk about."*** No matter what situation you find yourself in, it is your thoughts that got you there. Your thoughts are what shape you mentally, physically and emotionally. Intention with purpose is everything. Throw passion, love and gratitude into the mix and all desires become possible.

How do you spend your time? Where does your focus lie? Do you spend your time and energy on useless or negative thoughts and information related to past events, or do you spend your time and energy in fear, doubt and worry for your future? If your answer is yes, to any of the latter, you are unintentionally destroying the greatest gift of all, the present.

We can only experience the present, because the past has long gone, and the future is not here yet. That's why it is so important to just live for the moment and be happy now. Do not fall into playing the mind game of *"when I get this, do this, or get there, then I will be happy."* Just simply be happy now.

Yesterday is history, tomorrow is a mystery, and today is a **gift**. That's why they call it the **PRESENT**.

ASK YOURSELF

Ask yourself, *"What is this emotion doing to me and how is it serving me?"* It is possible to feel the emotion from the core of your being without letting it overpower and own you. Recognize it for what it is and where it takes you. The next critical step is to disengage from the event that brought about the emotion and continue to process it from your heart. This will reveal how you operate, who you really are and how you may be tripping yourself up. Embrace emotions and discover where you may be hiding your inner truth. When we continue to suffer we are running an emotional chaos program that will handicap us from experiencing the life that we could have. The Whole Truth is, when you are finally willing to take total responsibility for everything, especially the pain and suffering you are experiencing, instead of blaming it on others, this in itself will set you free and relieve you of your mental and physical bondage. Never be afraid to feel love for all your emotions, do not fear them. It is truly the experience of feeling, which connects you to humanity. Feeling is what ultimately keeps you alive. Life is an adventure filled with emotion. Learn to embrace it. Learn to navigate it.

HEALTH IS A STATE OF MIND

Your mind is like a sponge. Do you filter out that which does not serve your greater good: such as anything that diminishes your happiness, peace of mind and vibrant health? If it's a health-related problem you are dealing with, do you focus on the desired result of achieving vitality, or do you focus on the fear, doubt and worry of the sickness itself? Negative emotions will empower a negative state of health, whereas focusing only on the desired outcome will create a proper foundation for healing to take place. There are those who will never experience total health due to negative subconscious beliefs, which will undermine their true heart's desires, if not dealt with. Their sickness has become a part of them, like a marriage, *'for better or for worse'*, but mainly for worse. There are those who have been healed on only sugar pills. Then there are those who have died with the greatest health minds at their beck and call. No one, no where, no how, can make you do what you have not ordained. **It's always been U.**

THE GUILT TRIP
(hopefully a short one)

This situation will show up when a person has been given a strong belief of self-guilt. Something or someone, somewhere in their past has made them believe they are guilty and they have accepted this lie as the truth. When a person is made to believe this, they will judge themselves harshly. Their punishment will usually show itself in the form of some type of anxiety, pain, illness or self-abuse. This misbelief of guilt must be addressed and resolved for healing to take place on any level. An example of this is called Sinner's Syndrome; an illusionary curse that can make you sick and if not dealt with, stay with you for a lifetime. When you believe you are a sinner, a heavy burden will be yours to carry both mentally and physically until you let yourself off the hook. Trust me I have played this card for years because I judged myself harshly and allowed others to do the same. When I was young I was taught by my peers to believe that I was born a sinner.

In my mind I was doomed for life and no matter how much I suffered for these sins, I would never be good enough. Talk about *Hell on Earth*. We all know what comes along with viewing one's self as a sinner and that is judgment. Judgment, whether done by someone else or yourself is very destructive for one's mental and physical well-being. What comes after judgment but punishment. With punishment, comes affliction and the deprivation of the abundance that no one, not even ourselves, has the right to take away. We deprive ourselves of love, happiness, money and let us not forget, our emotional and physical health, all in the name of '*The Illusionary Guilt Trip*,' hopefully a short one.

YOU CHOOSE

You now get to choose how long your sentence should be. One year, two years or life. *Should I just have chronic fatigue, or should I get cancer and go out with a bang to let everyone know that I have suffered greatly for my sins?* Why play these self-abuse games, even for a short time? This will depress you emotionally as well as physically, through your immune system. The definition of sin is to miss the mark. Learn from your mistakes *(sins)*, for that's all they are. I'm going to make a bunch today, and enjoy every one of them. Learn from them and know that success is just around the next corner. Live life big! Take risks and embrace failure with forgiveness and compassion for yourself and everyone else; for this is the way to truly set yourself free. A Minister once said, "*Get off the cross, love and forgive yourself, for love heals everything and you are perfect already*." There are also those that **unknowingly play the role of the victim**. They use their sickness on a subconscious level for attention and control to get the love they feel is being kept from them. This can become a sickness in itself. If you find this situation among your family or friends, help them to find the courage inside themselves to be all they can be through exercising love and compassion. For in the end, all answers lie within. There are also those who use sickness as an excuse to not move forward in life. This occurs due to the fear of failure or feeling that one is a failure *(lie)*. It is important to understand that there cannot be significant growth without mistakes and failures. Often, those who have had the greatest successes have also had the greatest failures. What an amazing movie this will be! Let's call this one an adventure and name it, *'How I Took a Risk and Won'.*

UNCONSCIOUS DOWNLOAD

There are always those unfortunate ones who have been misinformed that their health is and will always be out of their control due to genetics, family history, the cure has not been found yet or the pity party for attention. The greatest example of all is when we are led to believe that we are helpless and hopeless in the area of our own health; that we could never have the intelligence to look after ourselves. So we always wait until something breaks and as a consequence, run with fear, doubt and worry to those wearing the white coats. Yet we need to realize that logic and self-love do not need a degree. No one will love you or take care of you on a daily basis as well as you will, when you finally learn how. For myself, I have spent thousands of hours listening, reading and practicing that which I truly want. That being physical, mental and spiritual independence from those who wish a piece of me.

It's taken work to reprogram years of church, school, government, medical and all the other force-fed information out there helping to sidetrack me from my greatness. *Can you truly say that you have dedicated yourself to releasing that amazing, awesome, one of a kind miracle from within for the ride of your life?* Without repetition on a daily basis you will never truly Master Your Life. Decide to finally take control and truly love the most precious thing in your life, that would be **U**.

DO NOT 'WEIGHT' TO CHANGE YOUR FOCUS

Let's propose you are dealing with a weight problem. *Do you allow yourself to focus on the fear of never overcoming the problem?* If you do, unfortunately you will have to learn to live with the problem, because it's you, it's always been you. Your thoughts are everything. You are what you focus on most of the time. This is because you are the most powerful creator. If you're in emotional pain then it's a lie you're telling yourself, this is self- abuse, enough already. Imagine a better way of seeing yourself, and how it will feel on an emotional level when you achieve your goal. Believe it and you will achieve it! Once you finally let go of that which does not serve you and instead come from your heart with courage, using loving intention and forgiveness, you will be able to heal yourself and lighten up. When you finally release the emotional baggage of not being good enough, the physical will melt away. I believe in you. *Do you believe in you?* **U** are Everything.

LEAD WITH YOUR HEART

Love heals EVERYTHING. Choose wisely, lead from the heart and not from the head. *'Power comes from your heart, your head will run away from you but your heart will always remain with you'*. As I have been alluding to, all emotions have a negative or positive effect, causing a physical response of either pain or pleasure. If it is a negative emotion, it will always have a negative impact on your health. The person who spoke the words, "*I hate you*" will take up these exact feelings on both a physical and emotional level. As they say, live by the sword, die by the sword. When instant gratification does not originate from the heart, it will cause pain and suffering to the person who spoke these original words of negative intent. They just took the poison pill and will feel the ill-inducing effects. They're running a dysfunctional program that has been created by a negative belief and will only continue to undermine the quality of their life on all levels.

Show these people compassion, but choose not to accept their gift of destructive behavior. Instead, choose to honor yourself and only let love in. The way that you allow others to treat you is the level of love and respect that you hold for yourself. By teaching others to love and respect you, in turn, you will be teaching them to love and respect themselves. **Life is ' for-giving' not 'for-getting.'** Remember who **U** are.

ALIGN FIRST THEN TAKE ACTION

When a person feels negative emotion, they are out of alignment. Never take action when you are in this emotional state, for when you do, you are going in headfirst and not from your heart. In the end you will only find yourself left to clean up a big mess. Just breathe! Align first, and then take action. One of the most experienced side effects from negative emotion is felt in the abdominal region. *'You make me sick to my stomach!'* We all know that one. When we do not know how to process our emotions through the heart we tend to hide them where no one, not even ourselves, can find them. Suppressed emotions equal a painful body and life. This can consist of constipation, sickness, dis-ease, unclear thoughts, bad decision-making, a depressed immune system and depression. I guess this is what they mean by 'hell on earth.'

If emotions are not dealt with properly, they will become a toxic bomb, silent but deadly - and sometimes not so silent. Learn to deal with your poop or it's going to get messy. A gentle cleansing, physically and mentally, on a daily basis will help maintain balance for one's overall health. Get out of your head, get into your heart and ground yourself. Things can get distorted when you're not in alignment with your higher purpose. Open your heart, the world awaits its greatest gift. So unwrap it, that would be **U**.

"The Mind reacts, The Heart creates."

-Unknown

FREQUENCY IS EVERYTHING

Every emotion has a frequency attached to it. Negative emotions are low vibrational frequencies that drain you of your vital energy. The cause stems from the three culprits: fear, doubt and worry. If emotions are not processed through the heart, vital life and energy will be depleted due to misdirected thought; the mind reacts, the heart creates. You will always be able to tell if your **B**elief **S**ystems are based on dysfunctional beliefs by measuring the length and intensity of the hurt you place on yourself and those around you.

I can remember being upset with my wife for days and not remembering why; this is insanity. Only you are responsible for your happiness and health. Check yourself before you wreck yourself and others. When you allow others to be in charge or when you try to take charge of other people's lives, your frequency will drop and you will be left gravely disappointed. How can someone else truly be responsible for another's happiness *(family)* or health *(doctors)*, when most can barely manage his or her own?

HAPPY OR RIGHT

Oh, how we all love to be right; but what price are you willing to pay? How much time and energy is it worth trying to prove that you're right? Are you the type of person who would go to the ends of the earth to accomplish this? If so, then you must be quite frustrated, along with everyone else around you.

Yes, there are times when we must stand up for what we believe in, but we must remember to pick our battles wisely. You will find a great sense of relief once you surrender the notion that you must be right. When you finally release yourself of this belief, you will be left feeling much happier, with a greater sense of peace. **Oh, and I know I am Right** *(LOL)*.

GO WITHIN OR DO WITHOUT

You will know how advanced you are with your self-growth by the way you handle life when things are not going your way. You can either choose to be the change you want to see, or continue to have *'hell on earth'*.

Your perception of a situation will determine the amount of pain and the amount of time you choose to suffer. Depending on individual beliefs and perceptions, one person will cause pain for themselves and others for 5 minutes, versus another person, who chooses to endure the same for 5 days. In turn, the way you choose to view an event determines everything.

We need to shrink ourselves down and sit on our shoulder. This is an important step in becoming a neutral observer in seeing where we may have dysfunctional beliefs and perceptions based on downloaded, corrupt programs. There can be two people experiencing the same event, yet one decides life is not worth living, while the other finds the courage to rise above and seize the day. Perception is everything! *Are you the victim or the hero in your movie?* Remember, you write your own story. Everyone runs a body pain program with different beliefs. Some people may have an emotional crisis 3 times a day while others will explode like an atomic bomb once every 3 days.

We all run programs that we just keep repeating. It's vital to understand that you are your programmer, so take charge and rewrite your program. For life to change externally, internally, physically and emotionally, the change must come from within. This is because you are the answer to everything. Track your programs and see if you are robotic in the way that you set yourself up for painful situations *(pain body program)*. If so, install a new chip, **live, love and laugh!**

THE POISON PILL

Remember, when you allow negative emotion to reign, you deter yourself from the path of love, health and happiness. In essence, you have just swallowed the poison pill. This only results in physical pain and needless suffering. Even if it's another person who you wish to hurt, it will be you who suffers more. Although hurtful people hurt others, they end up hurting themselves the most. Do not underestimate your power to create; this is what you were born for, but choose wisely or suffer greatly. Most people will never realize their full potential to heal themselves or create the life that they desire *(victim program)*. This is because they have been unconsciously absorbing limiting beliefs. This is not their fault, but it is their life and their responsibility to change it. The problem here lies when people make choices from fear, doubt and worry rather than from love. When we come from the position of the fear of loss, that there isn't enough to go around or that someone has more than we do, we have just chosen to swallow the poison pill and take others along for the ride *(usually family)*. An example of this is how we kidnap our love from the people closest to us and hold it for ransom until we get what we want, no matter how much we make ourselves and others suffer. This program is widely accepted as 'normal' by many families but in no way, shape or form is it Natural. If your desire is to be the most and have the most wonderful life then whenever you see a problem arise, look for the answers and changes within yourself.

U will never swallow **'The Poison Pill'.**

THE TEN-INCH LIE

There was a very interesting study done where fleas were put into a 10-inch glass jar with a glass top. After 3 hours of jumping and hitting the glass top, the fleas were set free. In reality, these fleas will never be free or even reach their full potential ever again. Instead of jumping a few feet high, they only jumped 10 inches high for the duration of their lives. This was due to the programming of limiting beliefs. Limiting beliefs will always stop you from reaching your full life potential, even without realizing it. My question to you is, *"Could it be possible that you have been unknowingly programed to jump only 10 inches high?"* You are a dynamic spirit with unlimited potential that has been educated to believe that you are much less than what you are actually meant to become. Do not believe anyone else, about anything, until you can sit in silence and go inside yourself. You are everything. You are limitless. Let me share an example of limitless belief. *Have you ever noticed that every time the Olympics happen, records are always shattered?*

When will this occurrence of record breaking end? It will never end because it is limitless, like you. What you believe, you shall achieve. If you are stuck in a certain place of your life right now, know that you have limited yourself in your beliefs. *Do you know the definition of insanity?* It is repeating the same thing over and over again and expecting a different result.

YOU ARE YOUR BELIEF SYSTEM

Change your beliefs and you change your life. Ask yourself this question, *"How do I spend my day?"* Do you believe you are *a victim of uncontrollable circumstances? If so, you are. Do you believe there is not enough to go around and that life is unfair?* If so, it is so. As sure as the sun will set tonight, **what you eat, think and talk about** will shape both who you are and who you will become. You were born to create, so do it wisely. You are everything! We all have a set of beliefs and judgments on every aspect of life. They formulate the perceptions and choices we make. The same event can happen to 10 people and they will all perceive it differently. Many of our beliefs come from what is called unconscious installation. We think we're the ones making a free choice, but in reality, we're not. You may believe you make all your choices, but this is not the case. Your peers, parents and educational systems play a significant part in your programming whether you like it or not. You may be very surprised to realize that what you are choosing is not really a product of your free choice. I have spent years taking my **B**elief **S**ystems apart piece by piece. I am 57 years old and I can tell you that my decisions and my beliefs are finally coming from within myself. I now dance to the beat of my own band, not the system's. We become drones who are governed by our government, medical system and other groups who feel that it's their duty to tell us how we must process and live our lives.

Through subtle repeated messaging we are lead to think for the best interest of others, such as various government agencies and pharmaceutical corporations. Living proof of this is demonstrated through the fact that pharmaceutical corporations own most of the advertising on TV. They have to repeat their information until it becomes second nature to you. When a **B**elief **S**ystem is being downloaded to us that goes against our nature, it must be repeated over and over again, this is known as brainwashing. Let's talk about the average person who watches TV for a few hours a day. There has been much research on this subject because it owns so much of most people's lives *(minds)*. It has been found that, on average, the more a person watches TV, the more weight they gain and the more depressed they become. By the time a child is 14 years old they have seen 1200 murders, how's that working for us? Turn your life on. Turn the channel or better still, turn it off and let your old **B**elief **S**ystems die a quick and painless death

I CHOOSE

I stopped watching TV, listening to the news and reading the newspaper many years ago. As a result, I experienced many positive side effects such as eating better, getting into shape and re-establishing a better relationship with those I love. My focus has changed on what I perceive my reality to be: Peace, Love and an Abundant Life. When we start allowing only that which serves our greater good, those who want to possess our health, wealth and freedom can no longer **man**-ipulate us.

As a result, my thoughts are no longer media driven nor orchestrated by someone who thinks he/she knows better. There is a saying that you get what you expect. Your energy always follows your thoughts. When you put your Whole person into a thought, expect it fulfilled. Be a great creator, take back your power, protect your family and **be free to make conscious decisions that serve your greater good.**

HENNY PENNY

The media will always attempt to make you feel anxious, afraid, slightly insecure and helpless. This all works by keeping you slightly off your course of health, peace and happiness, which always seems to be just beyond your reach. By creating the illusion of chaos in your life, the prevailing powers are able to distract and divert your focus towards useless worry and meaningless information. Anxious people are great consumers, made to believe they need to shop and accumulate to create temporary happiness. We can take our lives back; we are not lab rats to be continually **man-**ipulated. Once we go within ourselves, we never have to do without. All answers lie within. My thoughts are my own. Therefore, I choose. Let's say you're a person who gets their daily dose of the news from the media. Your world must be a very scary place. The media takes all the worst events from around the globe, then condenses and sensationalizes this information into 30 minutes of disaster. This draws you in and distracts you from what is truly important. This in turn creates the illusion of a fearful future. As a result, they now not only own your time, but are also Masters of your mind. *By the way, how was your sleep last night? Did the boogeyman come calling?* Oh, that's right, **he's a lie too!**

GET OUT OF YOUR MIND & INTO YOUR HEART

When you play into the media, your focus is placed on the external world entirely. Your internal world becomes neglected, yet this is the place where all true answers await you. I can assure you that for every time something bad happens in the world, a thousand wonderful things are happening simultaneously. We become spoiled rotten not only by what we eat, but also by what we participate in, think about and talk about. **Do not seek or partake in the drama.** If you do not learn to manage your own life, someone else will gladly do it for you according to their benefit and pleasure.

EMOTIONAL ATTACHMENT

Let's talk about our emotions (*let's not*). Suppressing our negative emotions without trying to figure out the **B**eliefs **S**ystems that created them can only result in emotional and physical pain. 95% of all illness has an emotional attachment to it. This is a scientific fact that has been validated by many reputable universities, including Harvard. Many medical research facilities have come out with the same findings, one being *The Mayo Clinic*. Freedom from negative emotions can only be achieved when you are at peace with yourself. Stop taking things so personally. Stop having knee-jerk reactions to situations beyond your control. Just breathe and realize that you are everything and that you are the hero in your movie. All answers lie within **yourself;** therefore, be the change you want to see. Cleanse your mind daily of negative thoughts, replacing them with your goals, dreams and desires. Become all that you were destined to be, **everything!** Cleanse your body daily of toxic waste and feed it with Nature's Bounty. You are limitless and your soul purpose is to create. So create all you truly desire! Love what you do and do what you Love. Love is not just an emotion, it is the foundation of everything in life. So one last thought; love the one you're with. **That would be U!**

HEALTHY TIPS

- Cleanse your body and mind daily
- Avoid low energy substances and people
- Eat, live and buy Whole Plant Based Superfood
- Drink plenty of pure Structured Water and breathe Structured Oxygen daily
- Never become dehydrated
- Express feelings through writing, dance, art, music, and poetry
- Life changes when you do
- Surround yourself with those who inspire and support you
- Follow your Heart and not your head
- Allow yourself to receive
- Reduce or eliminate your exposure to TV
- Stop reading the newspaper
- You can't look forward if you're looking back
- Align first then take action
- Extend acts of kindness without needing thanks
- Find ways to keep on clearing emotions
- Be grateful for what you already have (Gratitude)
- Avoid server's disease syndrome
- Avoid being too nice
- Express anger appropriately
- Allow yourself to make mistakes and forgive yourself often
- Set goals and keep a journal

Spiritual Health

- Breathing Structured Oxygen and aligning with highest vision and purpose to reverse illness
- **U** can only change the world from the inside out

- Need for quiet time & reflection by oneself
- Prayer & meditation

Mental Health

- Breathe Structured Oxygen to open your heart
- Drink Structured Water to cool down your brain
- All thoughts give or take away energy, so choose wisely
- Fixed rigid beliefs impair health & cause emotional distress
- Be fully conscious, or you will create your life by default, not design
- Your point of power is always in the present moment. Be Happy Now!

Coping with Stress

- Always take time for yourself
- Drink Structured Water daily to stay hydrated
- Don't just breathe - breathe Structured Oxygen
- Say no often
- Make smaller lists
- Avoid unnecessary housekeeping
- Get sufficient sleep
- Seek out silliness and play in your Life
- Life is not measured by time but by the breaths you take, breathe deeply & live!
- Exercise daily
- Spend time in nature

A SPECIAL NOTE

from Dr. Darrell Wolfe

We all search for good health but how would you like to have great health and experience it on a permanent basis for the rest of your life?

Just as the medical system has made health seem complicated and beyond your reach, so has the natural health industry. By the time patients' call for a Supercharge Your Life Consultation with me, they have crashed with the medical system and most have bought into the fads, ineffective therapies and this season's latest nutritional breakthrough.

Our world is based on Band-Aid therapy, the *'you break it and we'll treat you but never train you'* attitude is a rotating door. Until you become the master of your own wellbeing on a day-to-day basis, you will always be in emergency care. **You will never have great health until you have a personalized road map built specifically for you and your needs.**

This road map is designed to protect and guide you with gentle baby steps throughout your day, each and every day. Until you become the master of your own health and wellbeing, otherwise, trained - not treated, you will always be left disappointed, continually searching for the next quick fix.

Your potential for self-healing is limitless when you have a Supercharge Your Life road map built just for you! Allow

me the honor to build you that road map and to support you along your journey.

May you always be blessed,

Dr. Darrell Wolfe

AWAKENING TRANSFORMATION CONSULTATIONS

The First & Most Crucial Step For Permanent Healing

There are two sides to every story. For this story, there is the physical but we must never ever forget the emotional. You cannot heal one without the other; they must heal together as a team. Unless you are willing to look at your emotions and assess your belief systems, you will never experience long-lasting great health or your limitless potential. If you are not trained in how to change your mind, you will never change your world. When you have the tools and techniques to change your thoughts, you will change not just your health but the world around you. **Awakening Transformation Consultations take 1 hour. Combined Nutritional and Emotional Consultations take 2 hours. Whole Body Healing!**

Consultations can be done over the phone, via Skype or in person

SUPERCHARGE YOUR LIFE CONSULTATIONS

A Health Plan Tailored Just For You

The majority of the population choose to go to Medical Doctors for their day-to-day health care without questioning the fact that these practitioners have never been trained in health care, nutrition or detoxification, they were trained entirely on emergency care and prescribing drugs. Either continue to be treated or get trained to master your own body with a health plan tailored just for you! **Supercharge Your Life Consultations take 1 hour. Combined Nutritional and Emotional Consultations take 2 hours. Whole Body Healing!**

Consultations can be done over the phone,
via Skype or in person

Welcome To Your New World Where Everything Is Possible!

Call 1 855 900 4544 or 1 250 448 4544 to book your consultation

www.docofdetox.com

Advanced Courses

SUPERCHARGE YOUR LIFE ADVANCED TRAINING

Host Us In Your City

Dr. Darrell Wolfe, a worldwide recognized health coach, has condensed over 35 years of his *'in the trenches'* experience, wealth of knowledge and hidden health secrets into this unique and empowering Advanced Training Course, which is known as the *'Game Changer of Health'*. This extraordinary life-changing training will revolutionize the way you think, feel and live the rest of your life. **Supercharge Your Life Advanced Training has a General Public course and a Professional Course designed for practitioners who wish to incorporate these methods into their practice.**

This will be the most self-empowering take action course you will ever experience when it comes to erasing dysfunctional belief systems and uncovering the only true healer - that would be you. For the first time you will truly become the Master of your body and reclaim your universal right, this being individual health freedom. You will awaken to the fact that you do possess the inner wisdom to release the invisible bonds that have been unknowingly downloaded.

Uncontrollable fear, pain, inflammation, cancer and other life-threatening diseases are all symptoms of unconscious living and unconscious thought. Transform your life, just as thousands have done before you, just like you. You will leave this advanced training with a proven road map on diet, detox, nutrition, exercise and mental well-being. This advanced training is the beginning of a life most only dream of. It was designed for those who are ready to put themselves first.

Supercharge Your Life Advanced Training will strip away the illusion that commercial health has created. You will receive foundational, life-changing step-by-step strategies for cost-effective health to put you in the driver's seat of a life filled with joy. This event will be the tipping point to pulling back all the curtains and uncovering the whole truth. Unleash your body and mind and release the warrior within and become the Master of not just your health but your whole life! Be The Cure! Host Us In Your City or Come To Ours! www.itioh.com

COUPLES RETREAT & FAMILY RETREAT
TREATMENT & TRAINING
Tailored For You

Families and couples from around the globe come to be treated but most importantly trained by Dr. Darrell Wolfe and his team. With our Family & Couples Retreat Treatment and Training, each program is specifically tailored to meet your individual needs! **When you come to the Doc of Detox for our retreat trainings, you can stay in our beautiful lake view suite.**

We teach all the foundational tools, techniques and strategies in Wolfe Deep Tissue and Whole Body Nutrition and Detoxification, so that families and couples become the masters of their own health and well-being.

Wolfe Deep Tissue is the most effective form of therapy in the elimination of internal scar tissue. **From joint pain to a tumor - it's all scar tissue - which is the major cause of disease, premature aging, pain, inflammation and physical limitation.** When you learn how to remove the hardened internal scar tissue, then you will be free of pain and able to perform again as a healthy active person at any age. This internal scar tissue must be manually broken down and then flushed out of the system for elasticity, flexibility, strength and complete range of motion to return to normal. For the first time ever, you and your partner/family are able to instantly relieve each other's pain and suffering.

Most people will tell you that they have a good diet, even a great one! For over 100 years, the health manual that most use to guide their lives was written by pharmaceutical corporations, food conglomerates and petrochemical companies and has been spoon-fed to the North American population by the media and medical system. Most people follow this manual of deception and half-truths, it is no wonder that we are confused and don't understand what true health feels or looks like - that changes now, release your full potential! **You will leave this retreat with a personalized proven road map on diet, detox, nutrition, exercise and mental well-being. Live the life most only dream of!**

Master Your Health, Heal Your Body, Awaken Your Mind!

www.itioh.com

ITIOH PROFESSIONAL TRAININGS

Whole Life Coach & Wolfe Deep Tissue Certification

Advanced Courses
- **5 Days Professional Course - Whole Life Coach •**
- **7 Day Professional Course - Wolfe Deep Tissue •**

Dr. Darrell Wolfe is known worldwide for his Whole Life Coach and Wolfe Deep Tissue Professional Certification Training Courses. His Whole Life Coaching techniques and unique Deep Tissue therapy leads the way in nutritional, emotional and physical bodywork therapeutics. ITIOH Professional Courses are designed to give practitioners and those who wish to be practitioners **the most advanced, cutting-edge strategies, tools and techniques in the art of Natural Healing in the most simplistic and empowering way.** When you come to the Doc of Detox for our professional certification courses, you can stay in our beautiful lake view suite.

His philosophy has always been, 'If you can't guarantee your work then it should be for free!' Dr. Wolfe takes this one step further, his guarantee is that this Intensive Training will give you the tools, strategies and techniques for you to become the therapist that you always knew you could be. Let us train and teach you – we will surpass your expectations and will continue to do so by supporting you with weekly online webinar and teleconference trainings, so that you remain a leader in the field of health. We will teach you how to build and maintain a successful and financially lucrative practice, featuring top industry specialists to help you with marketing, media and business planning strategies. You will also be promoted on and by the Doc of Detox and ITIOH for patients to find you easily. We make success easy!

Not only will you be teaching people how to get well and stay well physically and mentally, but with our ongoing support and guidance you will build a financially sustainable, long-lasting, successful business in the field of natural health.

Whole Life Coach Certification & Wolfe Deep Tissue Certification can be taken together or separately, depending on the student or practitioners' needs.

Go to: **www.itioh.com** or call: **1 855 900 4544** for further information

WOLFE DEEP TISSUE TREATMENTS

Instantly Increases Range of Motion & Eliminates Pain

Our guarantee to you. You will experience more results in your first Wolfe Deep Tissue treatment than you have had with all other therapies or your money back! Where other therapies have failed, Wolfe Deep Tissue succeeds. You don't have to live like this.

What do you have to lose, except your pain?

Wolfe Deep Tissue Restoration was created by Dr. Darrell Wolfe Ac.PhD. 30 years ago due to the crystallization and internal scar tissue he found in all of his patients. Wolfe Deep Tissue has been shown to be the most effective form of therapy in the elimination of internal scar tissue and crystallization, which is the major cause of premature aging, pain and physical limitation whether it is an acute or chronic situation.

When you remove the hardened internal scar tissue, crystallization and scar tissue knots, then you will be free of pain and able to perform again as a healthy active person at any age. This hardened internal scar tissue must be manually broken down and then flushed out of the system for elasticity, flexibility, strength and complete range of motion to return to normal. **It's time to release all of your physical and emotional invisible bonds that bind you!**

Dr. Darrell Wolfe

- Abdominal Pain
- Ankle Problems
- Arthritis
- Back Pain
- Bursitis
- Carpal Tunnel Syndrome
- Disc Problems
- Dislocated Hip
- Dislocated Knee
- Fibromyalgia
- Foot Restructuring
- Frozen Neck/ Shoulder
- Headaches/ Migraines
- Hip Problems
- Muscle Spasm
- Neck Pain
- Nerve Pain
- Non-Surgical Breast Lift
- Non-Surgical Face Lift
- Numbness & Tingling
- Osteoarthritis
- Overuse Syndrome
- Rheumatoid Arthritis
- Sciatica
- Scoliosis
- Shin Splints
- Sinusitis/Sinus Problems
- Sports Injuries
- Sprains & Strains
- Tendinitis
- Tennis Elbow
- TMJ
- Whiplash

For more information on treatments offered, visit: www.docofdetox.com/treatments

HEALTHY TO 100 CLUB

Doc of Detox has gone global! He has put together a unique, private club to guide your health, healing, emotional well-being, nutrition and detoxification. Unlock the secrets of living *'Healthy To 100'* - learn foundational tips, strategies & techniques in diet, nutrition, detoxification, exercise, anti-aging and longevity. If you wish to live to your full potential each and every day, then look no further, welcome home to your Healthy To 100 Club!

Club Membership: $6.95/month

Full Access to Teleconferences & Webinars
Your Questions Answered Live & On-Air
(with Dr. Wolfe, the Doc of Detox)

Interviews with the Top Leaders in Natural Health

Recipes For Life & Vitality

Special Access Downloads

How-To Videos

Educational Self-Help Audios & Booklets

Weekly Deals & Monthly Draws

When you become an Elite Member for $19.95/month you will also receive:

LIVE! Webinar Trainings on Mastering Your Emotions and Taking Back Your Life

LIVE! Wolfe Deep Tissue Webinar Trainings on Treating Each and Every Muscle and Joint

Monthly Consultation Lottery: One-on-One Consultation with Dr. Wolfe
(Emotional Awakening Transformation Consultation & Supercharge Your Life Nutritional Consultation)

Register Today at: www.docofdetox.com

ABOUT
DR. DARRELL WOLFE AC.PHD.

Author . International Radio Host . Whole Life Coach

Dr. Darrell Wolfe directed The North American Institute for the Advancement of Colon Therapy for 15 years and was also the head of one of North America's leading natural cancer treatment and preventative care centers.

Dr. Wolfe's home base is Kelowna, British Columbia, where he treats, teaches and consults patients at the Doc of Detox Clinic, locally and globally.

He is the director of the prestigious *'International Training Institute of Health'*, where he teaches and certifies practitioners with his unique techniques in Wolfe Deep Tissue Restoration & Whole Life Coaching to students, health professionals and holistic schools worldwide.

One of the biggest contributions Dr. Wolfe provides are his public courses, *'Supercharge Your Life'*, *'Awakening Transformation'* *'Family & Couples Retreat Treatment and Training'*.

Dr. Wolfe has 35 years of experience and is known as the 'Doc of Detox'. He is also known for his role in the internationally acclaimed three part cancer docu-series, *The Global Quest For The Cure'* and *'The Truth About Detox'* documentary, which have been viewed by millions around the world. Dr. Wolfe also hosts his own international radio talk show *'DetoxiFridays'*.

Dr. Wolfe's best selling book *'Healthy to 100'* is the foundation from which he created his one-of-a-kind *'Healthy To 100 Club'* where he hosts his weekly *'Empower Hour'* webinars and teleconferences to awaken the world with life-changing, foundational tools, tips and strategies.

Master Your Health, Heal Your Body and Awaken Your Mind.

GLOSSARY OF HEALTH TERMS & MENTIONED AILMENTS

Acidosis - An increased acidity in the blood and other body tissue

Ammonia - A colorless gas with a very sharp odor. Ammonia is produced in the human body and is commonly found in nature. It is essential in the body as a building block for making proteins and other complex molecules. It is toxic if levels exceed that of a healthy level in the body.

Anti-Oxidants - Anti-Oxidants are substances that may protect your cells against the effects of free radicals. Free radicals are molecules produced when your body breaks down food, or by environmental exposures like tobacco smoke and radiation. Free radicals can damage cells, and may play a role in heart disease, cancer and other diseases. Anti-Oxidants are found in many foods. These include fruits and vegetables, nuts, grains, poultry, fish and in some meats.

Arterial Blood - Arterial blood is the oxygenated blood in the circulatory system found in the lungs, the left chambers of the heart, and in the arteries.

Arthritis - A form of joint disorder that involves inflammation of one or more joints. There are over 100 different forms of arthritis. The most common form, osteoarthritis (degenerative joint disease), is a result of trauma to the joint, infection of the joint, or age.

Cancer - A broad group of diseases involving unregulated cell growth. In cancer, cells divide and grow uncontrollably, forming malignant tumors, and invading nearby parts of the body. The cancer may also spread to more distant parts of the body through the lymphatic system or bloodstream. Not all tumors are cancerous; *benign tumors* do not invade neighboring tissues and do not spread throughout the body. There are over 200 different known cancers that affect humans.

Candida - A genus of yeasts and is currently the most common cause of fungal infections worldwide. Many species are harmless commensals or endosymbionts of hosts including humans; however, when mucosal barriers are disrupted or the immune system is compromised they can invade and cause disease.

Cholesterol - Cholesterol is a lipid (fat) which is produced by the liver. Cholesterol is vital for normal body function. Every cell in our body has cholesterol in its outer layer.

Chronic Fatigue - Chronic fatigue syndrome is a complicated disorder characterized by extreme fatigue that can't be explained by any underlying medical condition. The fatigue may worsen with physical or mental activity, but doesn't improve with rest.

Diabetes - A group of metabolic diseases in which a person has high blood sugar, either because the pancreas does not produce enough insulin, or because cells do not respond to the insulin that is produced. This high blood sugar produces the classical symptoms of polyuria (frequent urination), polydipsia (increased thirst) and polyphagia (increased hunger).

Pre-Diabetic Condition - Pre-diabetes means that your blood sugar level is higher than normal, but it's not yet high enough to be classified as Type 2 diabetes. Still, without intervention, pre-diabetes is likely to become Type 2 diabetes in 10 years or less. And, if you have pre-diabetes, the long-term damage of diabetes - especially to your heart and circulatory system may already be starting.

Diabetes (Type 1) - Results from the body's failure to produce insulin, and currently requires the person to inject insulin or wear an insulin pump. This form was previously referred to as 'insulin-dependent diabetes mellitus' (IDDM) or 'juvenile diabetes.'

Diabetes (Type 2) - Results from insulin resistance, a condition in which cells fail to use insulin properly, sometimes combined with an absolute insulin deficiency. This form was previously referred to as non insulin- dependent diabetes mellitus or 'adult-onset diabetes.'

Dialysis - Dialysis is a treatment: it does not cure kidney disease or make kidneys well again, and it does not fully replace your kidney function. Unless you receive a kidney transplant, you must continue to have dialysis for the rest of your life. Two types of dialysis are used to treat the later stage of chronic kidney disease: hemodialysis and peritoneal dialysis. - See more at: http://www.kidney.ca/page.aspx?pid=337#sthash.8AvLPueM.dpuf

Diverticulitis - Occurs when one or more diverticula in your digestive tract become inflamed or infected. Diverticula are small, bulging pouches that can form anywhere in your digestive system, including your esophagus, stomach and small intestine.

However, they're most commonly found in the large intestine. Diverticula are common, especially after age 40. When you have diverticula, the condition is known as diverticulosis. You may never even know you have these pouches because they seldom cause any problems, such as diverticulitis. Sometimes, however, diverticulitis occurs. This condition can cause severe abdominal pain, fever, nausea and a marked change in your bowel habits.

Emphysema - Emphysema occurs when the air sacs in your lungs are gradually destroyed, making you progressively more short of breath. Emphysema is one of several diseases known collectively as chronic obstructive pulmonary disease (COPD). Smoking is the leading cause of emphysema.

Endotoxin - A heat-stable toxin present in the intact bacterial cell but not in cell-free filtrates of cultures of intact bacteria. Endotoxins are lipopolysaccharide complexes that occur in the cell wall; they are pyrogenic and increase capillary permeability.

Q: What foods have the greatest content of Endotoxins? **A:** Based on the very small number of published papers on this subject and the small number of foods tested the foods commonly containing endotoxins were ground meat, yogurt, cheese, chocolate, ice cream, bread and precut bags of salad vegetables.

Enzymes - Are large biological molecules responsible for the thousands of metabolic processes that sustain life.

Fecalomas - A 'stone' made of feces, is a hardening of feces into lumps of varying size inside the colon, which may appear whenever chronic obstruction of transit occurs, such as in megacolon and chronic constipation.

Fibrin - An essential protein in the human body that is produced during inflammation. The body utilizes fibrin as a blood clotting protein, containing blood loss and keeping infection at bay, especially after an injury. Fibrin accumulation is one of the first steps in the body's attempt to recover.

Fibroids/Fibroid Formation - Fibroids are non-cancerous (benign) tumors that grow from the muscle layers of the uterus (womb). Fibroids are growths of smooth muscle and fibrous tissue. Fibroids can vary in size, from that of a bean to as large as a melon.

Fibromyalgia - Fibromyalgia is a disorder characterized by widespread musculoskeletal pain accompanied by fatigue, sleep, memory and mood issues. Researchers believe that fibromyalgia amplifies painful sensations by affecting the way your brain processes pain signals.

Symptoms sometimes begin after a physical trauma, surgery, infection or significant psychological stress. In other cases, symptoms gradually accumulate over time with no single triggering event. Women are much more likely to develop fibromyalgia than are men. Many people who have fibromyalgia also have tension headaches, Temporomandibular Joint (TMJ) disorders, irritable bowel syndrome, anxiety and depression. While there is no cure for fibromyalgia, a variety of medications can help control symptoms. Exercise, relaxation and stress-reduction measures also may help.

GMO - Genetically Modified Organisms refer to the plants or animals created through the gene splicing techniques of biotechnology. GMOs and genetically engineered (GE) foods refer to the same thing. They are foods created by merging DNA from different species. The safety of GMO foods is unproven and a growing body of research connects these foods with health concerns and environmental damage. For this reason, most developed nations have policies requiring mandatory labeling of GMO foods at the very least, and some have issued bans on GMO food production and imports. In Canada we do not.

Hemorrhoids - Hemorrhoids (HEM-uh-roids), also called piles, are swollen and inflamed veins in your anus and lower rectum. Hemorrhoids may result from straining during bowel movements or from the increased pressure on these veins during pregnancy, among other causes. Hemorrhoids may be located inside the rectum (internal hemorrhoids), or they may develop under the skin around the anus (external hemorrhoids). Hemorrhoids are common ailments. By age 50, about half of adults have had to deal with the itching, discomfort and bleeding that can signal the presence of hemorrhoids. Fortunately, many effective options are available to treat hemorrhoids. Most people can get relief from symptoms by using home treatments and making lifestyle changes.

Ileocecal Valve - Valve between the ileum of the small intestine and the cecum of the large intestine; prevents material from flowing back from the large to the small intestine.

Inflammation - Inflammation is the body's attempt at self-protection; the aim being to remove harmful stimuli, including damaged cells, irritants, or pathogens and begin the healing process.

Insomnia - Insomnia is a disorder that can make it hard to fall asleep, hard to stay asleep, or both. With insomnia, you usually awaken feeling unrefreshed, which takes a toll on your ability to function during the day. Insomnia can sap not only your energy level and mood but also your health, work performance and quality of life.

How much sleep is enough varies from person to person. Most adults need seven to eight hours a night. Many adults experience insomnia at some point, but some people have long-term (chronic) insomnia.

LDL's - An LDL particle is a microscopic blob consisting of an outer rim of lipoprotein surrounding a cholesterol center. LDL is called low-density lipoprotein because LDL particles tend to be less dense than other kinds of cholesterol particles. LDL is a "bad cholesterol" that collects in the walls of blood vessels, causing the blockages of atherosclerosis. Higher LDL levels put you at greater risk for a heart attack from a sudden blood clot in an artery narrowed by atherosclerosis.

Leptin/hormone Leptin - A protein hormone that plays a key role in regulating energy intake and energy expenditure, including appetite and metabolism. It is one of the most important adipose derived hormones.

Lesion - Any abnormality in the tissue of an organism (in layman's terms, "damage"), usually caused by disease or trauma.

Low Libido - Sex drive is determined by biological, psychological, and social factors. Biologically, levels of hormones such as testosterone are believed to affect sex drive; social factors, such as work and family, also have an impact; as do internal psychological factors, like personality and stress. Medical conditions, medications, lifestyle and relationship issues may affect sex drive. A low libido is the low desire for sexual intimacy often in relation to physiological traits, stress and related to low levels of testosterone in women or men.

Lymph - The fluid that circulates throughout the lymphatic system. The lymph is formed when the interstitial fluid (the fluid which lies in the interstices of all body tissues)[1] is collected through lymph capillaries. It is then transported through lymph vessels to lymph nodes before emptying ultimately into the right or the left subclavian vein, where it mixes back with blood.

Lymph Nodes - Your lymph nodes, also called lymph glands, play a vital role in your body's ability to fight off viruses, bacteria and other causes of illnesses. Common areas where you might notice swollen lymph nodes include your neck, under your chin, in your armpits and in your groin.

Metabolized - To change (food) into a form that can be used by your body: to process and use (substances brought into your body) (Merriam-Webster Dictionary)

Microbes - Microbes are single-cell organisms so tiny that millions can fit into the eye of a needle. They are the oldest form of life on earth. Without microbes, we couldn't eat or breathe.

Mitochondria - Mitochondria are known as the powerhouses of the cell. They are organelles that act like a digestive system that takes in nutrients, breaks them down, and creates energy for the cell. The process of creating cell energy is known as cellular respiration. Most of the chemical reactions involved in cellular respiration happen in the mitochondria. A mitochondrion is shaped perfectly to maximize its efforts.

Mitochondria are very small organelles. You might find cells with several thousand mitochondria. The number depends on what the cell needs to do. If the purpose of the cell is to transmit nerve impulses, there will be fewer mitochondria than in a muscle cell that needs loads of energy. If the cell feels it is not getting enough energy to survive, more mitochondria can be created. Sometimes they can even grow, move, and combine with other mitochondria, depending on the cell's needs.

Nutrients - A nutrient is a chemical that an organism needs to live and grow or a substance used in an organism's metabolism which must be taken in from its environment. They are used to build and repair t issues, regulate body processes and are converted to and used as energy.

Osteoarthritis - Osteoarthritis is the most common form of arthritis, affecting millions of people around the world. Often called wear-and-tear arthritis, osteoarthritis occurs when the protective cartilage on the ends of your bones wears down over time. While osteoarthritis can damage any joint in your body, the disorder most commonly affects joints in your hands, neck, lower back, knees and hips. Osteoarthritis gradually worsens with time, and no cure exists. But osteoarthritis treatments can slow the progression of the disease, relieve pain and improve joint function.

Osteoporosis - Causes bones to become weak and brittle - so brittle that a fall or even mild stresses like bending over or coughing can cause a fracture. Osteoporosis related fractures most commonly occur in the hip, wrist or spine.

Bone is living tissue, which is constantly being absorbed and replaced. Osteoporosis occurs when the creation of new bone doesn't keep up with the removal of old bone.

Palpation - Palpation is used by various therapists to assess the texture of a patient's tissue (such as swelling or muscle tone), to locate the spatial coordinates of particular anatomical landmarks (e.g., to assess range and quality of joint motion), and assess tenderness through tissue deformation (e.g., provoking pain with pressure or stretching). In summary, palpation might be used either to determine painful areas and to qualify pain felt by patients, or to locate three-dimensional coordinates of anatomical landmarks to quantify some aspects of the palpated subject.

Parasites - A parasite is an organism that lives on or in a host and gets its food from or at the expense of it's host. Parasites can cause disease in humans. Some parasitic diseases are easily treated and some are not.

PCBs - Were widely used as dielectric and coolant fluids, for example in transformers, capacitors, and electric motors. Due to PCBs environmental toxicity and classification as a persistent organic pollutant, PCB production was banned by the United States Congress in 1979 and by the Stockholm Convention on Persistent Organic Pollutants in 2001. According to the US Environmental Protection Agency (EPA), PCBs have been shown to cause cancer in animals, and there is also evidence that they can cause cancer in humans.

PMS (Premenstrual Syndrome) - Premenstrual syndrome (PMS) has a wide variety of symptoms, including mood swings, tender breasts, food cravings, fatigue, irritability and depression. An estimated 3 of every 4 menstruating women experience some form of premenstrual syndrome. These problems tend to peak during your late 20s and early 30s. Symptoms tend to recur in a predictable pattern. Yet the physical and emotional changes you experience with premenstrual syndrome may be particularly intense in some months and only slightly noticeable in others. Still, you don't have to let these problems control your life. Treatments and lifestyle adjustments can help you reduce or manage the signs and symptoms of premenstrual syndrome.

Processed Foods - The definition of what constitutes a processed food can vary slightly, but it usually refers to foods that are packaged in boxes, cans or bags. These foods need to be processed extensively to be edible and are not found as is in nature. In addition to going through many complex processing steps such as over heating (killing most if not all nutrition if ever there was any nutrition to begin with), processed foods often contain additives, artificial flavorings and other chemical ingredients.

Avoid processed foods and base your diet on whole food to get the most nutrition and maximize your health.

Putrefaction - is one of seven stages in the decomposition of the body of a dead animal. It can be viewed, in broad terms, as the decomposition of proteins in a process that results in the eventual breakdown of cohesion between tissues and the liquefaction of most organs.

Scar Tissue - is fibrous, connective tissue made primarily of **fibrin** --which the body uses to replace previously healthy tissue that has been destroyed by injury or disease. Under normal conditions, internal scar tissue should be the final result during typical inflammatory response. However, when inflammation has become prolonged – fibrin, along with other proteins such as collagen, can begin to transform original soft tissue into a tough fibrous matrix. Differentiated and sequestered apart from healthy tissue, this fibrous matrix still maintains the biological markers of inflammation, such as swelling, redness and pain.

Serotonin - Serotonin is a chemical your body produces that's needed for your nerve cells and brain to function.

Sleep Apnea - Sleep apnea is a potentially serious sleep disorder in which breathing repeatedly stops and starts. You may have sleep apnea if you snore loudly and you feel tired even after a full night's sleep. There are two main types of sleep apnea: Obstructive sleep apnea, the more common form that occurs when throat muscles relax; Central sleep apnea, which occurs when your brain doesn't send proper signals to the muscles that control breathing. If you think you might have sleep apnea, see your doctor. Treatment is necessary to avoid heart problems and other complications.

Toxemia (dirty blood) - A condition in which the blood contains toxins produced by body cells at a local source of infection or derived from the growth of microorganisms. Also called blood poisoning.

Toxic Dilation aka "Megacolon" - is an acute form of colonic distention. It is characterized by a very dilated colon (megacolon), accompanied by abdominal distention (bloating), and sometimes fever, abdominal pain, or shock.

Toxic megacolon is usually a complication of inflammatory bowel disease, such as ulcerative colitis and, more rarely,

Crohn's Disease, and of some infections of the colon, including Clostridium difficile infections, which have led to pseudomembranous colitis.

Toxicity - Toxicity is the degree to which a substance can damage an organism. Toxicity can refer to the effect on a whole organism, such as an animal, bacterium, or plant, as well as the effect on a substructure of the organism, such as a cell (cytotoxicity) or an organ such as the liver (hepatotoxicity).

Ulcerative Colitis - Is an inflammatory bowel disease (IBD) that causes long-lasting inflammation in part of your digestive tract. Like Crohn's Disease, another common IBD, ulcerative colitis can be debilitating and sometimes can lead to life-threatening complications. Because ulcerative colitis is a chronic condition, symptoms usually develop over time, rather than suddenly.

Ulcerative colitis usually affects only the innermost lining of your large intestine (colon) and rectum. It occurs only through continuous stretches of your colon, unlike Crohn's Disease, which occurs anywhere in the digestive tract and often spreads deeply into the affected tissues.

HEALTHY TO 100: FUN TERMS KEY

Throughout this book, as you read you may have noticed some terms that stood out!

For your benefit we have listed these words complete with their intended meanings... Enjoy!

(**Zombie**) or (**Zombie Nation**) : An individual, or a large body of people, void of all feeling and emotion, populating a zombie nation and living in a sleep-like state of unconsciousness. Because they all share the same unconsciousness, Unconscious of The Whole Truth, they accept it as...'*normal*'.

Hell-th: An evil plot designed to lead you to believe that you're on a path to health, but when The Whole Truth is digested it becomes clear this is a one way ticket - Destination?...Hell.

(evil plot): An enslaving method contrived for your body, mind and spirit, in the name of greed and profit benefiting only the almighty few.

man-ipulation: The process of charging more, promising more and delivering less. Processed and GMO foods are prime examples.

U: Everything that's beautiful; the '*REAL YOU*'.

Pooh-Tea time: A cleansing tea break for toddlers.

Structured Water: A water molecule free of toxins, chlorine, chemicals and fluoride. Structured Water supports life as it was designed to; through hydrating and fueling a physically

Structured body to its fullest capacity providing optimal performance for the human body to thrive.

Dis-ease: To live in a state of fear or discomfort; focused on negative feelings, emotions or thoughts that may contribute to illness and impaired **'normal'** functions of the mind, body and spirit.

Frequency: Universal Law states that everything in the Universe moves and vibrates. Everything is vibrating at one speed or another. Nothing rests. Everything you see around you is vibrating at one frequency or another and so are you. Every healthy living cell of every organ/tissue in your body has its own vibrational frequency. Unhealthy cells, e.g., cancer, vibrate at lower frequencies. In a similar manner, fresh, unprocessed foods vibrate at a higher frequency than those which have become processed or stale. Frequency is Everything.

Unconscious living: is to lead a **'normal'** life ultimately downloaded since birth, day in day out practicing a lifestyle burdened with habits, carrot dangling and false hopes which leads you to believe you are free and as powerful as you wish to be. In reality this unconscious lifestyle which so many embrace has been designed and perfected by the almighty few to empower and benefit the almighty few.

Take Life In: To embrace Nature, To embrace a Whole Lifestyle. To take in The Whole Truth you have always known deep down inside.

Whole Plant Based Superfood Nutrition: The most complete highly absorbable nutrition, the world's most Phytodense

Nutrient Superfood on the planet known as none other than Moringa Oleifera.

XM Plus: A Moringa Oleifera energy mix produced by Zija® International LTD. The all-natural powder blend of XM+ is a convenient way to consume cell-ready nutrients, anti-oxidants, minerals, omega oils and proteins that provide the energy you need to fuel your entire body throughout the day. Please go to: www.docofdetox.myzija.com for more product information and details about Moringa Oleifera.

Wasteline: The area of the human body where fat is most easily stored; commonly referred to as the *'gut'*. Year after year, toxins, fecal matter and toxic waste build-up, compact and putrefy in and around the waistline. For many today, the outcome of unconscious choices regarding nutrition is - THE WASTELINE.

Lighten the Load: Through awareness of The Whole Truth, the tools you now possess, you are enabled to release the Thin Within. It's time to

Cleanse, Restore and Zija® Build. Take Life In, upgrade and become THE REAL U. Lighten the load!

Stinkin' Thinkin': Occurs when your focus is out of the now, shadowed with worry, fear and doubt. It is the process of negative, repetitive, empty energy trapped on the mental merry-go-round of your mind!

Gentle Daily Cleansing: The act of daily maintenance on your body, the most vital tool **U** possess. It is said that; *'your body is your temple'* and for very good reasons. Treat it as such and gently cleanse daily with *'Doc of Detox'* Daily Cleansing Tea for optimal performance.

It's Tea Time: A cleansing tea break designed to release the real **U!**

Invisible Bonds: A fibrous matter defined by internal scar tissue, crystallization and emotions cemented, invisibly to the naked eye, beneath your tissues. These bonds can birth through both physical and emotional trauma and can weave a wicked web inside us. Over time they cripple us physically, mentally, emotionally and ever so unnecessarily. Go Deep and Release your Invisible Bonds!

Hunger Trigger: A trigger that can be enabled through emotion, trauma and unconscious habits. Commonly found in a Zombie Nation lifestyle fueled by little to no nutritional value. Pull the trigger on hunger and embrace a Whole Plant Based Superfood Nutritious Lifestyle to Release the Thin Within.

HEALTHY TO 100: REFERENCES & LINKS TO

Dr. Drucker *(ref on: p.43)*

Dr. Carolyn Dean MD, ND *(ref on p.58)*

Ty Bollinger *(ref on: p.67,)*

Marcia Angell MD *(ref on: p.69)*

Dr. Mark Hyman *(ref on p.94, 269)*

Dr. Robert Lustig *(ref on: p.95)*

Dr. Theodore A. Baroody *(ref on: p.157)*

Dr. Otto Warburg *(ref on: p.79, 157)*

Dr. Charles Northern *(ref on: p.158)*

Dr. Patch Adams *(ref on: p.178)*

Dr. Blaser *(ref on: p.220)*

Dr. Oz *(ref on: p.230, 445)*

Dr. Robert Becker MD *(ref on: p.268)*

Albert Szent-Györgyi *(ref on: p.268, 272, 402)*

Alexander Viardot *(ref on: p.233, 272)*

Pascal Imbealt *(ref on: p.232)*

Albert Einstein *(ref on: p.268)*

Dr. Kikuo Chishima *(ref on: p.268)*

Dr. Gallard *(ref on: p.269)*

Heinrich Hertz *(ref on: p.269)*

Bruce Tainio *(ref on: p.270)*

Dr. Royal Rife *(ref on: p.271)*

Nikola Tesla *(ref on: p.272, 385)*

Sandor Katz *(ref on: p.297)*

Ann Lotwin *(ref on: p.301)*

Janice Skoreyko *(ref on: p.301)*

Dr. Gerald Pollack *(ref on: p. 340)*

Dr. Carey A. Reams *(ref on: p.347)*

Dr. Konstantin Korotkov *(ref on: p. 369)*

Dr. Royal Lee *(ref on: p.370)*

Magda Havas *(ref on: p.382, 405)*

Marcel Wolfe *(ref on: p.383-390)*

Dr. Fritz-Albert Popp *(ref on: p.405-407)*

Dr. Finsen *(ref on: p.409)*

Professor SA Muyibi *(ref on: p.447)*

Dr. Russ Bianchi *(ref on: p.449)*

Dr. Howard Fisher *(ref on: p.455)*

Dr. Duke *(ref on: p.455)*

Dr. Philip Incao *(ref on: p.510)*

The Mayo Clinic *(ref on: p.551)*

itioh.com

docofdetox.com

docofdetox.myzija.com

NOTES

NOTES

NOTES

Master Your Health, Heal Your Body and Awaken Your Mind!

www.docofdetox.com